TO END
— A —
PLAGUE

TO END
—A—
PLAGUE

AMERICA'S FIGHT
TO DEFEAT AIDS
IN AFRICA

EMILY BASS

PUBLICAFFAIRS
New York

PublicAffairs

Hachette Book Group

1290 Avenue of the Americas, New York, NY 10104

www.publicaffairsbooks.com

@Public_Affairs

Printed in the United States of America

First Edition: June 2021

Published by PublicAffairs, an imprint of Perseus Books, LLC, a subsidiary of Hachette Book Group, Inc. The PublicAffairs name and logo is a trademark of the Hachette Book Group.

The Hachette Speakers Bureau provides a wide range of authors for speaking events. To find out more, go to www.hachettespeakersbureau.com or call (866) 376-6591.

The publisher is not responsible for websites (or their content) that are not owned by the publisher.

Print book interior design by Six Red Marbles, Inc.

Names and identifying details of some individuals in this book have been changed to preserve privacy.

Library of Congress Cataloging-in-Publication Data

Names: Bass, Emily, author.

Title: To end a plague : America's fight to defeat AIDS in Africa / Emily Bass.

Description: First edition. | New York : PublicAffairs, 2021. | Includes
    bibliographical references and index.

Identifiers: LCCN 2020054321 | ISBN 9781541762435 (hardcover) |
    ISBN 9781541762459 (ebook)

Subjects: LCSH: AIDS (Disease)—Prevention—Government policy—
    United States. | AIDS (Disease)—Prevention—International cooperation. |
    AIDS (Disease)—Africa. | Medical assistance, American—Africa.

Classification: LCC RA643.83 .B37 2021 | DDC 362.19697/920096—dc23

LC record available at https://lccn.loc.gov/2020054321

ISBNs: 978-1-5417-6243-5 (hardcover), 978-1-5417-6245-9 (ebook)

LSC-C

Printing 1, 2021

For Cissy, Lillian, Milly, and Yvette,
our daughters and sons,
and all of the next generation

CONTENTS

PROLOGUE

O N JANUARY 28, 2003, the night that President George W. Bush launched America's war on AIDS in Africa, he brought the whirlwind with him. In fact, it had seldom left his side. In his 2001 inaugural address, the president twice quoted a letter to Thomas Jefferson from his friend and fellow slave-owning politician John Page. "We know the Race is not to the swift nor the Battle to the strong. Do you not think an Angel rides in the Whirlwind and directs this Storm?"[1] Page penned those words after congratulating Jefferson on the Declaration of Independence, conjoining American governance and divine Providence. Some of Bush's supporters did much the same, seeing divine intervention in an election settled by a Supreme Court decision. At first, the president's whirlwind seemed merely metaphorical. But 235 days after his inauguration, twin columns of air roiled at the bottom of Manhattan Island. Ever since, even on clear days, America had dwelt within a storm.

"In a whirlwind of change and hope and peril, our faith is sure; our resolve is firm; and our Union is strong," the president said on that January 28, in his 2003 State of the Union address.[2] If he did not name the angel this time, perhaps it was because he intended to assume its earthly, avenging form. Like many viewers of the speech who hadn't voted for Bush, I tuned in dreading a declaration of war on Iraq. Two months prior, Congress had authorized use of force; millions of people around the world had taken to the streets to protest, but the White House's zeal for war had not slackened. I'd turned on the speech because I understood witness as an act of resistance. He would not catch those who vehemently opposed violence and vengeance by surprise.

In the opening minutes of the speech, Bush hardly projected holy clarity. His eyes darted, and his mouth seemed a separate living thing, wriggling, flattening, and bunching up with helminthic volition. But after his promise of hydrogen-powered cars, his voice softened, grew hoarse with sincerity. My sense of watching a badly dubbed soap opera disappeared. He began to talk about something that interested him: getting drunk. He'd met a Louisiana addict in recovery. "God does miracles in people's lives," that man had said to the president. "You never think it could be you."

The putty of Bush's face softened with an inwardly directed tenderness when he spoke these words. He could not make himself the subject, of course. But he had been frank about his own alcoholism and recovery. Against my will, I warmed toward him just then. We knew each other, drunks and recovering drunks. On that January night I was twenty-nine years old, sitting in my apartment in downtown Brooklyn, wrapped in the duvet I had brought to college my senior year. I was, if asked, an AIDS activist and journalist. That was what I did; but I was not always sure who I was, and so I loved nothing more than when, after a third or fourth glass of wine, I could at last hear my voice at a distance.

Bush finished the story about recovery in Louisiana with a plea for people to embrace God's "wonder-working power," then hopscotched from a condemnation of partial-birth abortion to a call for a law against human cloning, staking the state's claim to control corporeality in all its forms, from womb to cell. Divine might manifested as governmental jurisdiction over bodies. His voice was firm and his sentences flowed. Something was coming.

Just after 9:30 p.m., Eastern Daylight Time, he looked at the camera again. "Today, on the continent of Africa, nearly thirty million people have the AIDS virus, including three million children under the age of fifteen," he said. I recognized the facts that were a catechism for me and many others working on "global AIDS"—an American neologism for the epidemic beyond US borders. "There are whole countries where more than one-third of the adult population carries the infection. More than four million require immediate drug treatment. Yet across that continent, only 50,000 AIDS victims—only 50,000," he repeated himself, as we activists did in our own speeches, marveling at the inhumanity, "are receiving the medicine they need." Bush continued,

> A doctor in rural South Africa describes his frustration. He says, "We have no medicines, many hospitals tell people, 'You've got AIDS. We can't help you. Go home and die.'" In the age of miraculous medicines, no person should have to hear those words.... [T]onight I propose the Emergency Plan for AIDS Relief, a work of mercy beyond all current international efforts to help the people of Africa. This comprehensive plan will prevent 7 million new AIDS infections, treat at least 2 million people with life-extending drugs and provide humane care for millions of people suffering from AIDS and for children orphaned by AIDS. I ask the Congress to commit $15 billion over the next five years, including nearly $10 billion in new money, to turn the tide against AIDS in the most afflicted nations of Africa and the Caribbean.

His words ended years of American negligence. With a scant handful of sentences, Bush launched the largest disease-specific foreign aid effort in the history of the country and the world. He also brought to an end an era of shameful American heel-dragging over whether people in Africa living with HIV and dying of AIDS deserved access to the medications that had changed HIV from a death sentence to a chronic disease in people who could afford them. In the years to come, members of Congress would call the president's plan the most effective American foreign aid since the Marshall Plan—the legendary post–World War II effort to rebuild Europe and head off Soviet alliances. The program that would be known as the President's Emergency Plan for AIDS Relief (PEPFAR) would meet the goals Bush set in the State of the Union ahead of schedule and go on hitting or surpassing them across three presidential administrations and eight Congresses.

That night Bush laid out his vision for one war that would maim and another one that would heal. One lethal and ill-fated, the other surprisingly adept at saving lives. Americans would become all too familiar with the death and destruction caused by the war on terror; the plague war would receive far less notice. Ten years after its launch, Nobel laureate Harold Varmus declared with surprise that "few Americans...understand how successful the [PEPFAR] has been and how it was conceived and carried out."[3] In subsequent years, assessments of Bush's presidency would cite the AIDS war as his primary positive achievement, sometimes with gotcha headlines like "George W. Bush Was a Much Better President Than Liberals Like to Admit."[4] Such stories suggested that the program's most salient feature was its surprising progenitor and obscured the extent to which Bush's work of mercy was also a feat of engineering—of policies, attitudes, activist strategies, and public health programs. The COVID-19 pandemic that began in 2020 made it clear that the country could ill afford this mischaracterization. Even with compromises that put cracks in its foundation, PEPFAR is America's most sustained and effective fight against a pandemic of the twenty-first century. An unprecedented achievement in promoting public health instead of public death, it offers lessons in how the US government can organize and implement a long-term plague war.

We who worked on AIDS knew none of this that night. But we did know that while a virus can cause illness, it is human actions that allow the virus first to spread until it inhabits enough bodies that an "outbreak" has occurred and then to continue to spread until its presence has reached "epidemic" or "pandemic" proportions. We knew that the actions that fueled the epidemic were not condom-less sex acts or shared syringes but the laws passed and stigma dispensed by members of society who despised homosexuals, denigrated women, and deplored drug use. HIV lived in blood and body fluids; each act of transmission occurred as a result of two people drawing close. But we knew that the propagation of pathogens to epidemic levels is not inexorable except in the context of human negligence.

The president and the advisors who'd mapped out the plan to wage war on what was then the worst plague of the twenty-first century knew this too. The global pandemic had reached an astonishing daily death toll after effective medications were licensed and made available in the wealthiest nations in the world. To wage war on the virus was, then, to wage war on the human-derived scourge of inequity: a lofty idea, and one for which President Bush might have earned praise even if he'd simply written a giant check. But while the other war he'd launch that night would prove to be based on faulty intelligence and half-truths, the President's Emergency Plan for AIDS Relief was rigorously researched and scientifically sound. It was indeed a plan. In an effort to save the lives of predominantly Black and brown people whose health was imperiled by a sexually transmitted infection, he'd commissioned and endorsed a marriage of meticulous research and audacious assumptions, then endorsed the plan and the funding level—unprecedented in US disease-fighting history—that it required. It would be seventeen years before the United States took another global epidemic as seriously as AIDS, and by then the most astonishing thing about the program would be not how it started but that it had endured, with its lineaments more or less intact. The original plan had been sufficiently well devised to preserve the program's bipartisan support. The mere fact of PEPFAR's persistence defied the flea-like American attention span for public health emergencies, which wandered once the adrenalin wore off and the outbreaks had been quelled among the most privileged members of society.

Those who watched the speech that night in 2003 also knew the toll taken by years of inaction by this man's predecessors and his global peers. As he paused for applause, his mouth wriggling into a line of suppressed satisfaction, I began to sob, feeling gratitude and then—an instant later—shame. I had allowed hope to be kindled by a man who occasioned little but despair. As my mood shifted from optimism to self-castigation, I knew with a rare and sudden clarity that my life had changed too. I wanted to know what the president's announcement meant and whether hope was warranted at all. I knew that this was not a simple question and that the search for an answer would define my life for years to come.

I was not alone in the force of my reaction. The vast majority of people living with HIV, as well as scientists, activists, doctors, nurses, and politicians who had been fighting for access to AIDS drugs for all, had not seen it coming. In hotel rooms and homes, groping for our phones, exclaiming, sweating in the hot flush of committing sodomy, as one friend did ritually with his husband on the occasion of Bush's State of the Union address, we felt the words in our blood. Or perhaps we felt our blood in the president's words. We heard him say things we had said for years prior: the same statistics and figures, the same insistence that the medications that saved some lives should save all lives. He'd claimed the plan as his—the president's—but we knew whom else it belonged to. Because we worked on HIV, we knew that symptoms of the virus can take years to appear. The moment the virus arrives in the body is not the moment it announces itself. Often, the first symptoms come after years of unseen attempts at self-protection by the body and its brilliant immune system. Such is the subterfuge of infection and historic change: that which is visible is not the beginning but the result of a struggle that has been going on for some time.

CHAPTER 1

THE INSIDE-OUTSIDE GAME

"ALL ENZYMES ARE PROTEINS," I muttered to Anne-christine d'Adesky in 1996, then looked down at my hands. D'Adesky, *Out* magazine's HIV reporter, cut a dramatic figure in the SoHo office. She had ragged, black-dyed hair and pearl-white skin. She wore leather pants, thrift-store cowboy shirts with shiny, pearlized snaps, and bodega musk oil that, on her, smelled rich and intoxicating.

I thought d'Adesky was magnificent. I was also gripped with depression both merciless and mundane and on many days could hardly look anyone in the eye. That day, I tried. As *Out*'s fact-checking temp, I spent hours on the spellings of couturiers and colognes. Each fashion spread carried credits for the scent you would have smelled if you'd been there. I majored in biology in college because I thought that it was as good a language as any for a writer to know. I'd devoured the atlas of the body and the vocabulary of the actual, only to find myself phoning Issey Miyake's press contact to confirm a scent in pages that smelled of nothing but ink and shine. I needed to get d'Adesky's attention so that she'd ask for me to work on her pieces and maybe give me a chance to write something of my own.

"'Enzyme protein' is redundant." I choked out. I put a line through the word "protein." "You don't need to say both."

A descendant of what she described as a "convoluted family tree of Belgian and Haitian colonizers and colonized," d'Adesky had produced Pulitzer Prize–nominated coverage of political upheaval and everyday life in Haiti throughout the early 1990s before returning to New York, where she ate fire with the Lesbian Avengers and joined the direct-action powerhouse activist group ACT UP. At the same time, d'Adesky gravitated toward the journalistic work of digging into the science of the opportunistic infections that were killing her friends.[1] She liked wreckage, remedies, potential, intuition. That day in 1996, she looked at me as though noticing me for the first time. A few months later, when she persuaded *Out* to launch an HIV-focused quarterly called *HIV Plus*, she hired a performance artist as the managing editor because she was a Virgo, enlisted her ex-girlfriend and current roommate Cindra Feuer as one member of the editorial team, and brought me on as the other.

To write my articles, I tried to mimic d'Adesky's lucid sentences and loose-limbed metaphors. To research them, I read the daily fax blasts from Housing Works, the New York organization spawned by ACT UP that focused on addressing the housing, mental health, and substance abuse needs of people living with HIV. I flipped through the slippery pages of the *Lancet* and the *New England Journal of Medicine* that arrived in hard copy every month. Mostly, though, I picked up the phone. D'Adesky had a single-spaced list of phone numbers for HIV-positive activists, scientists, doctors, and social workers who had been fighting AIDS for years even as the city, state, and country looked the other way. She gave me a copy of her list to pin above my desk. Call Spencer, call Mark, call Michael, call Gregg, she'd say after assigning me a piece. Spencer Cox, Mark Harrington, Michael Marco, and Gregg Gonsalves—these were some of the beautiful, science-savvy survivors of the first wave of American AIDS who had, like other activists focused on housing and mental health, impelled the National Institutes of Health, the US Food and Drug Administration (FDA), drug companies, and the US government to accelerate research on drugs to treat HIV and the opportunistic infections that afflicted the weakened immune system. Their ceaseless demands to move faster and work more closely with people living with HIV had resulted in the antiretroviral (ARV) medications that, when used in combination, stopped the virus from making copies of itself. When viral activity halted, so did the assault on the immune system. Combination antiretroviral therapy (ART) changed HIV from a death sentence into a chronic, manageable disease.[2]

I began working with d'Adesky within weeks of FDA approval of the first protease inhibitor—a new category of ARVs that was highly effective when used together with other ARVs. When I joined her team, she was still laughing about having won a queer dance contest with JD Davids at the 1996 International AIDS Conference in Vancouver. The pair triumphed, drenching themselves with water that made Davids's green hair dye run until he looked like a topless, gyrating Medusa. They had been irresistible and triumphant, though the next day, when a researcher d'Adesky was about to interview offered her wry congratulations on her victory, she blanched.

AIDS activists had never stopped dancing or making art, even during the killing years, and in Vancouver there had indeed been cause for celebration. The meeting featured the first full presentation of data on the effects of the antiretroviral "cocktail" of medications that included the new protease drugs along with compounds like AZT and ddI, which had been available for some years. People who'd canceled their insurance policies and were waiting to die found themselves facing the rest of their lives. One of the participants at the meeting was a slim, handsome Californian named Chris Collins who'd made a film about AIDS, then set aside cineaste ambitions and turned to wrangling legislation to fund virus-fighting efforts in the office of Nancy Pelosi. He found a friend in tears. "Tony Fauci just told me I'm not going to die," the friend exclaimed, referring to the tough, diminutive scientist who'd headed the National Institute of Allergy and Infectious Diseases since 1984.[3] Fauci had been the target of activist ire and a close collaborator, hosting dinner meetings with the same people who took over the campus of the National Institutes of Health, working to develop a shared scientific agenda.

The meeting's scientific news was welcome, but it did not expunge the sense of grief for all the comrades who had not lived long enough to hear Fauci tell them that their lives were saved. People who have survived a war mark victory not with light hearts but with mourning. Nor did it eliminate a sense of dread. The pandemic was global; the drugs, priced at more than $10,000 a year, were a luxury for the vast majority of people living with HIV. "Are you listening yet? The headlines that PWAs [people living with AIDS] want you to write from this conference would read: 'Human Rights Violations and Genocide Continue to Kill Millions of Impoverished People with AIDS.' That is the truth about AIDS in 1996," Eric Sawyer exhorted participants during the opening session.[4] A tall former football star from a working-class family in upstate New York, Sawyer was an ACT UP member who'd acquired HIV in 1979, before it even had a name. A decade later, he and other ACT UP members, including Charles King, Keith Cylar, and Virginia Shubert, ruffled feathers when they demanded time in the weekly Monday evening meeting to advance an activist agenda on Medicaid, housing, and social services. Sawyer and his allies ignored the critiques that they were "diluting the energy ... taking up too much time on social justice issues" and went on to found Housing Works.[5]

At the Vancouver meeting in 1998, Sawyer was a grimly passionate Cassandra. He himself was white; still, he knew that Black people, poor people, and people who used drugs had been and would continue to be left behind. "Greed equals death," he shouted, bringing the crowd along in the chant, updating the "Silence equals death" slogan that had been created by a small artists' collective and become synonymous with ACT UP.

I began working for d'Adesky a few months after the Vancouver meeting and quickly understood that while I had arrived at a moment of change in the AIDS epidemic, there were different ideas about what had changed and for whom. The year 1996 was a sharp dividing line between two eras: "before" and "after" effective combination AIDS treatment; it also marked the beginning of the gap between those who had access to the medications and those who did not.

While d'Adesky put former junkies, homeless people, and Black and brown women and their children on the cover of *HIV Plus*, the ads inside were thick with pictures of mostly white muscled men in chaste yet suggestive "brother's keeper" hugs, one muscled arm across another man's chest, or else rock climbing or biking, showing acres of unblemished skin. But American AIDS didn't look the way it looked in the drug company advertisements. Between 1988 and 1990, the number of Black Americans diagnosed with HIV surpassed the number of diagnoses in white Americans for the first time, in spite of the fact that Black Americans account for just 14 percent of the US population.[6]

Racial disparities in rates of HIV diagnoses were widening at the precise moment that the antiretroviral cocktail became available. In 1996, when AIDS ceased to be the leading cause of death for all Americans, it remained the number one killer of Black Americans.[7] In 1997, rates of new HIV diagnoses in gay men and other men who have sex with men who identified as Black, indigenous, Latinx, or of Asian and Pacific Island descent surpassed those in white gay men— and would remain higher every year thereafter. In that same year, the first full year in which the potent antiretroviral "cocktail" was available, AIDS deaths dropped by 47 percent overall, the largest single-year decline in a disease-related death rate ever recorded; but the odds of survival were not equal.[8] As one paper on people with HIV receiving Medicaid noted, "Black patients have approximately ten times and Hispanic patients four times the mortality rate from HIV/AIDS compared with white patients." The same paper noted that white people with HIV were more likely to receive antiretroviral medications than were Black or Latinx people and that men with HIV were more likely to receive the medications than women. All of these gaps, present at the moment that the American plague ended, would persist for years to come.[9]

Communities of color impacted by HIV weren't the audience for the slick drug company advertisements for ART. At home in West Philadelphia, JD Davids looked around and realized that many members of the local ACT UP chapter—unique among national chapters for its robust membership of people of color, former veterans, and incarcerated people—didn't know much about the medications at all. "There was such a gap between who was getting this information and who wasn't," Davids said.[10] He cofounded Project TEACH (Treatment Education Activists Combatting HIV) and started explaining the science to former drug users, people who'd been incarcerated, people who were not affluent and white. He understood that drugs that treated the virus in the blood did not remediate what public health experts called the "structural determinants" that drove the epidemic, including lack of access to high-quality, clear information and health services.

A pathogen moves from one person to another on its own. To move through vast swathes of a population, it is aided and abetted by the negligence and violence of the state. The ordeal of AIDS as a whole was not over; nor was the epidemic. I had arrived at the moment when the search for treatment ended and the work of ending the plague had just begun.

— —

AT *HIV PLUS*, I spent the next two years mastering the science of the drugs and their specific actions within immune cells. Untreated, HIV can make up to one billion copies of itself every day. I saw the viral mechanics as a vast and clanking printing press; the drugs were a set of saboteurs. Nucleoside reverse transcriptase inhibitors prevented the virus from translating its genome into the language of the cell. I watched them slip the wrench into the works. The protease inhibitors that stopped the virus from launching new particles in the cell were the squad that slashed the tires on the factory trucks. One or two drugs alone had not been sufficient to stop the virus. With three drugs, three different teams of saboteurs, the mad work of copying shut down. I came to know each squad and each agent editing the table of meds that ran in every issue of *HIV Plus*.

Each drug had a brand name and a generic one. Merck's Crixivan, one of the earliest protease inhibitors, was known in generic form as indinavir. Generic name, brand name: the crux of the gap in access to the drugs lay in that chemical taxonomy. A pharmaceutical company like Glaxo Wellcome, Pfizer, Boehringer Ingelheim, or Merck made the most money when a drug for which it held the patent was only available in its branded form. As long as a patent held, the company named the compound and, far more importantly, set the price. But most pharmaceutical products and commodities come in branded and generic forms. Not all plastic bandages are "Band-Aids," and Advil is just one company's name for ibuprofen. Like other products, pharmaceutical compounds could be recreated, and when the drugs came off patent, they were. So-called generic manufacturing led to competition; the prices dropped.

I learned about drug pricing and patents through the listservs that were, in the mid-1990s, emerging as new spaces for sharing information and ideas. The staff of *HIV Plus* shared a single dial-up internet connection; our AOL password was based on d'Adesky's astrological sign. In those listservs, I left the molecular realm and began to learn about the global policies and practices that kept drug prices high. I relied on John James, a Brooklyn-born gay rights activist who'd edited one of the first newsletters for people with HIV and their allies that helped break down the complex science. Many people, including myself, read *AIDS Treatment News* for scrupulously researched updates and clear explanations. James often wrote about drugs and the cells in the body, but by 1998, he had expanded to the geopolitical, offering a pellucid explanation of the General Agreement on Tariffs and Trade (GATT), which bound rich and poor nations into compacts, enforced by the World Trade Organization (WTO), over imports, exports, intellectual property, and more. "Perhaps the worst single feature of GATT was the decision to include pharmaceutical patents—effectively locking in a system which cuts off most of the world's population from almost all access to new medicines, until 20 years later when the patents expire," James wrote.[11]

Many of the places that needed AIDS drugs the most were not markets for the companies that had their headquarters in the Western world. A cheaper AIDS pill on the shelves in Gaborone or Lusaka would not displace a more expensive one. Companies did not make their money in Botswana or Zambia. But in a globalized world, the principle of patent protection mattered. A cheaper version of a drug anywhere—even in a country that wasn't a market for the full-priced medication—was a threat to profit everywhere. James had lived through and documented the years in which there hadn't been any pills at all. He knew how to envision change. "It seems impossible to change the GATT treaty itself, because so many countries willingly or unwillingly signed on. But it would still be surprisingly feasible for an activist movement to save lives," he wrote.

By the time I encountered James, I'd learned that AIDS activists had a sense of the movement as a body. The muscle was activists in the street. The heart was service delivery organizations and support groups that cooked meals, washed sheets, and fought for housing and comprehensive services for people with addictions and mental health issues. The brain was the science geeks—a group of laypeople who'd learned immunology, virology, drug development, and the mechanics of clinical trials in order to teach one another and to formulate potent demands. I first heard the heart, brain, muscle analogy from Carlton Hogan, a midwestern AIDS activist whose "how to be a problem patient" columns laid out in delicious, furious detail the ways that people with HIV could navigate the jargon encountered in their doctors' offices.[12] I modeled my work on that of people like Hogan, who explained statistical trial design to me whenever I needed help, and JD Davids, who cowrote "An Assay Is a Test" as a guide for regular people trying to understand scientific presentations.[13] I learned that plainspoken, precise, and irreverent language that emerged from and explained the body was valuable.

If I was seldom happy, as long as I was working, I was at peace. I liked to be useful, and I was good at what I did. When I left the office and stepped out onto Greene Street, though, I struggled to find my bearings. I did not know what I wanted to do or where I wanted to go. On some evenings, I followed d'Adesky and Feuer to activist meetings. I was too uncertain and unhappy to accept their invitation to zine launches, loft parties, potluck holidays. Conversation was a challenge; contributing facts and drafts of press sheets came far easier.

One evening in October 1998, I followed them to the old red-brick building holding the Lesbian and Gay Community Center and climbed a narrow staircase to a room filled with queers who were outraged and heartbroken over the recent brutal murder of Matthew Shepard, a young gay college student in Wyoming. The room held authority and experience. Many people were all too familiar with the alchemy of grief, anger, and purpose that begets activism. Ideas appeared, morphed, elided. A political funeral, in the ACT UP tradition? Yes. Seeking a permit from the city? Maybe. A pale-skinned, freckled woman with dark hair pinched her first three fingers against her thumb and made small circles in the air as she spoke. I guessed that if she could, she'd be smoking. "That makes no sense whatso-fucking ever," Sharonann Lynch said in a surprisingly sweet-toned drawl, then laid out a counterplan.

On Monday, October 19, the evening that the Shepard political funeral began, I followed Lynch off the curb of the sidewalk in front of the Plaza Hotel. "You're under arrest, you're under arrest, you're under arrest," a cop jerked his thumb at her, then me, then the person next to me. She stepped forward, sat down, and waited to be hauled off. I stepped back, tightened the pink ribbon around my forearm that designated me as a marshal—an activist who would help organize the protest as it moved—and spent the next several hours racing down the center of Fifth Avenue hand in hand with others, marked by ribbons, seeking to avoid the police and to guide the crowd so large it seized Fifth Avenue. The crowd flowed down the East Side artery, and we raced alongside it, seeking to steer it this way, then that, to avoid the infuriated police who menaced with horses and billy clubs. The city was a body; we were the bloodstream, the throng as large as our grief and anger. I had seldom felt so alive.[14]

After that, I would go to any meeting Lynch called in her Alphabet City apartment, smoke-filled sessions discussing AIDS in prison or the feasibility of chaining oneself to the Rockefeller Center Christmas tree. The activists I met there were, like Lynch, largely unsmiling, unphased by getting arrested during civil disobedience. Most were white, queer, and enthralling. They made wheat paste to slap up signs for upcoming protests; when the cops busted them, they jumped turnstiles. Later, they laughed. They seldom mentioned where they'd gone to college, if they'd gone at all, or what they wanted to be, as though they only wanted to be themselves. If I was careful to remain taciturn and tactical, I could get dates—but only if I could stay awake. When the meetings ended, the work began: painting banners, making signs. It seemed these activists never slept and seldom ate, save for trips across Avenue A to Teresa's, a Polish restaurant with old red booths, springs pressing hard against packing-tape-patched Naugahyde gashes, for plate-sized latkes, medicinal Jack, and cokes.

Unlike most of the activists, I was from New York City. If I wanted a home-cooked meal, I could always go uptown to my parents' apartment, book filled and warm. I could find my childhood friends, go to diners that didn't double as bars, eat french fries under twenty-four-hour golden light, watch *The X-Files*. Uptown, all I did was rest and eat. I wanted to stay there forever; I could not wait to leave.

I was accustomed to ambivalence. I grew up on the Upper West Side of Manhattan, the daughter of two Antioch college graduates, one a Jew from the Bronx and the other a transplanted southerner raised in Leonia, New Jersey. They sent me to a secular Yiddish school where my Stalinist teacher made sure we learned "Nkosi Sikelel' iAfrika," the African National Congress antiapartheid anthem, along with "Zog Nit Keynmol," the hymn of the Jewish resistance in World War II. As a child, in the Baptist and Episcopalian churches of my North Carolina family, I was transfixed by the women in the congregation, whose clothes matched their bags, whose hair didn't move, and whose foundation-heavy skin was as flat and smooth as that of a mannequin.

At twenty-two, I spiked the world around me with binaries, then told myself to choose: the church or the shul; Snow White or her queer sister; the state or the revolution; the vague, benign warmth of the natal home or the endless night of activist urgency. I myself dressed in a wardrobe filled with effort and contradiction: Laura Ashley jumpsuits; high, red Doc Martens lace-up boots; voluminous floral dresses topped with men's button-down shirts. A tendon in my neck strained when I arranged my face in what I hoped appeared to be a smile. My curly hair crackled with a testosterone frizz. I dyed it blonde, shaved it off, wore it long, but I never recognized myself in the mirror.

New York City itself rebuked me. I could come back, but I could not go home. Elected in 1993, New York's mayor Rudy Giuliani created a Gotham peopled by Black menaces and pervy queers, then enacted a raft of policies to protect a mythic populous from all that was frightening and unclean. In the name of public health, he undertook cuts to public education, encouraged privatization of public hospitals, and attempted a dismantling of the Department of AIDS. No panhandling, no squeegee men, no sex shops, no X-rated movies. Disney displaced sex shops in Times Square; public spaces bore private names.[15]

Many nights to calm my mind, I walked south toward the Twin Towers through a city that seemed to be undergoing a rapid glaciation, plate glass and silver-blue commercial lighting overtaking blocks where delis, diners, and hardware stores had once offered cluttered windows, local names. In the stores I passed, the number of objects in the window stood in inverse proportion to their prices: a pair of shoes, a dress, a single bag. In this landscape hospitable only to the enormously rich, the cost of cleanliness came clear. It was not money but other people's lives. I could leave d'Adesky's assignments on my desk at the end of the day, but I still saw the world marked by AIDS and the patterns it, like all plagues, revealed in society. All of my Jewish education had been preparation, not commemoration. Crisis was the norm. By the time I realized how frightened I was of what would happen when I accepted this, I already had.

IN JANUARY 1999, I met JD Davids for the first time at the Conference on Retroviruses and Opportunistic Infections. To stretch the *HIV Plus* budget, d'Adesky and I shared a room; to stretch his even more minimal budget, Davids bunked with us, bringing a pile of plaid shirts, black jeans, and protest T's that were hardly adequate against Chicago's frigid cold.

The hottest talk at the conference came from a German American virologist named Beatrice Hahn, who announced she'd identified a close relative of human immunodeficiency virus, or HIV. It had come from the frozen cadaver of a Cameroonian chimpanzee named Marilyn who'd been captured and held at Holloman Air Force Base in New Mexico for years. Simian immunodeficiency virus does not cause disease in monkeys, but at some point the virus leaped from chimps to humans and acquired its virulent form. Showing spiky family trees of genetic relatedness, Hahn declared that Marilyn had carried, in her blood, something close to the origin of AIDS.[16]

One afternoon, a shaggy-haired man in a rumpled suit came flying toward Davids and me in the conference center hallway. He was from the Rainforest Action Network (RAN), he said. Hahn was going to receive an award for her research, and he wanted to use the opportunity to call attention to the rapacious forces that threatened Marilyn's descendants' habitats. Over breakfast with Davids, he explained the risks posed by the trade-liberalizing legislation known as the African Growth and Opportunity Act and by a World Bank–funded Chad–Cameroon oil pipeline that posed risks to people, nonhuman primates, and the land.[17] As Davids recalled, the RAN organizer explained "why AIDS activists should care about trade policy."[18] It was the first such conversation that Davids would have, and for him it tied the inequities of West Philadelphia back to the West African region from whence so many Black Americans' ancestors had come against their will.

All of the HIV in the world could be traced to three separate instances of "zoonotic" transmission in which a chimp and a human drew close. Perhaps a hunter had been wounded while trapping one of Marilyn's ancestral relatives, and their blood had mingled, passing on the simian virus that mutated and acquired virulence in its new human host. That human-adapted virus also mutated and changed as the years passed. Some of those mutations serve as blazes on the trail back through time to viral origins. A British team that sequenced a range of HIV samples followed that trail back to 1920s Kinshasa in what is now the Democratic Republic of Congo. The virus had likely circulated for some time prior, but Kinshasa, with its congestion of underpaid male laborers, female sex workers, and, eventually, a railway line, allowed the virus to spread within and then beyond the city.[19] As Canadian infectious disease specialist Dr. Jacques Pepin laid out in his book *The Origins of AIDS*, white human behavior caused the epidemic via colonial engineering that forced African men into congested quarters and, in lieu of allowing families to join them, permitted handfuls of women to sell sex instead.[20]

The long-term consequences included AIDS and environmental devastation—as well as resistance and activism both within sub-Saharan Africa and in the Western nations that had been built on those ill-gotten gains. The ACT UP Philadelphia chapter was filled with people whose bodies and lives reflected this legacy of extraction, including the uneven distribution of quality health care that its members called America's medical apartheid. In the late 1990s, its legion of members included John Bell, a straight, Black veteran living with HIV; Kiyoshi Kuromiya, who'd been born in a Japanese internment camp and had gone on to become an antiwar civil rights activist and cofounder of the Philadelphia chapter of the Gay Liberation Front;[21] and Joyce Hamilton, a Black woman living with HIV who'd joined the group after seeing one of its protests against an impending statewide plan to move Medicaid recipients into cost- and corner-cutting HMOs that would not provide quality care to people living with HIV.[22] Asia Russell, a white activist from Silver Spring, Maryland, who had gravitated toward ACT UP Philadelphia as a teenager, paid close attention to the teachings from these and many other members. "In ACT UP Philadelphia, we were always trained to think about the hidden spaces," she said. The group fought for the rights of prisoners with HIV, concealed behind bars. Another campaign involved fighting back against Bill Clinton–era cuts to social welfare systems. "Connecting the end of food stamps as we knew them to a life with dignity for people living with HIV—that's what drew me to AIDS activism—that electrifying connection."[23]

Like Davids, Russell was interested in the connections between trade policy, aid, and AIDS in Africa. She'd picked up on the issues raised by John James and others and, in January 1999, took the train up to the SoHo offices of the AIDS Treatment Data Network to learn more.

The network offices sat just off the northwest corner of Broadway and Houston, beside a David Barton gym. A visitor disembarking on the sixth floor that night would have seen Russell—a dark-eyed, short-haired figure with coiled intensity—among a group seated in chairs drawn close together on a blonde wood floor, all watching as a man with a mop of brown curls held up Matchbox-car-sized boxes that held pill bottles. "This drug was made in India by a generic company called Cipla, and a year's supply of this drug will cost $80," said Jamie Love, a lawyer who worked with consumer-protection advocate Ralph Nader. He held the box aloft. The drug in question was AZT; in America, a year's supply cost $3,500.[24]

A bearded man, somewhat older than many of the participants, had helped organize the gathering. Dr. Alan Berkman was a self-described revolutionary who had gone underground after providing medical care to one of the participants in a 1981 botched and bloody attempt to rob a Brink's armored truck—and subsequently spent seven years in prison for his political activism. Berkman's understanding of the limitations of medical care in a white supremacist state were bone deep. Before his arrest, Berkman had treated survivors of the Attica prison riots, Native American protesters at Wounded Knee, and Puerto Rican revolutionaries. Diagnosed with cancer while in prison, he'd nearly died of sepsis, saving his own life by pinching an IV line to set off an alarm that forced a negligent nurse to his bedside.

In 1994, two years after his release from prison, Berkman became the staff physician at the Highbridge Woodycrest Center, a residential HIV/AIDS program in Harlem.[25] His partner, Barbara Zeller, also a physician, had been working on the front lines of New York's AIDS epidemic for years, serving as the director of a residential health facility for people dealing with drug addiction and HIV who had "been through the war of the streets...their medical and psychosocial problems...vast and sometimes overwhelming."[26]

Both Zeller and Berkman understood that an epidemic like AIDS required radical social justice as well as medication. In 1998, when they traveled to the International AIDS Conference in Geneva, they came face to face with the extent to which this was true within America and beyond its borders. Held two years after the Vancouver meeting, the Geneva meeting had the slogan "Bridging the Gap." But for many speakers, the gap yawned, without a bridge in sight. In Geneva, Jonathan Mann, the first director of the special program on AIDS at the World Health Organization (WHO), declared the chasm in access to antiretrovirals an emergency that required action, not out of charity but because of shared humanity and "solidarity."[27]

Mann had been urging global solidarity and massive action for more than a decade. In 1987, he called on the United Nations General Assembly to consider the emergency in terms of "three epidemics"—one of the virus, the next of the diseases that ravaged the body in the absence of treatment, and the third of reactions to both HIV and AIDS. In 1987, he'd said, "These three epidemics—of [the] AIDS virus, of AIDS itself, and of social reaction and response—together constitute what the World Health Assembly recently called a 'worldwide emergency.' "[28] By 1998—also the year in which he and his wife, Mary Lou Clements-Mann, perished in the crash of Swissair Flight 111—Mann had allies in Geneva, including Peter Piot, the bespectacled, impassioned head of UNAIDS, the agency charged with coordinating all UN work on AIDS. As a patient, physician, and former prisoner, Berkman was, like Piot and Mann, horrified by the "inertia manifested by people who were supposed to be providing leadership around global AIDS." In Geneva, his horror and "social rage" had swelled. The low-cost drugs were "a matter of right and justice."[29]

When he returned to New York City from Geneva, Berkman reached out to Bob Lederer, a fellow traveler in the anti-imperialist May 19th group,[30] who in turn reached out to Eric Sawyer, who'd warned of the coming access gap at the Vancouver AIDS Conference in 1996.[31]

Berkman, Lederer, Lederer's partner and fellow activist John Riley, and Sawyer met for dinner a few times before calling the meeting at the AIDS Treatment Data Network. Berkman would talk about the drug combinations selling "like hotcakes" and the "pornographic" profligacy of pharmaceutical company dinners held to educate prescribers and, sometimes, potential consumers about their new drugs. The luxury boutiques and big-box stores pocking the avenue below and the box in Love's hand lay on the same continuum in a world that prioritized profits over people's lives.

In the weeks after the meeting on lower Broadway, the group tried to figure out what they wanted to win. For Russell, the initial grappling with access gaps within and outside America felt like working from the middle of "a Russian nesting doll," where the most proximate layer was "the US and key debates about racism," with detention of and discrimination against Haitians—an issue Eric Sawyer had worked on at ACT UP—lying just beyond. From the initial meeting, she and others began the work of bringing gaps in more distant geographies into focus too.

In New York, other people joined the group that had met at that January meeting, including Jennifer Flynn, a queer AIDS and housing activist who hailed from New Jersey, and Sharonann Lynch, who'd helped organized the Matthew Shepard rally a few months prior. Lynch was an erstwhile Southern studies major who'd founded ACT UP Memphis then moved north. Flynn, Lynch, and a handful of other young activists had founded Fed Up Queers (FUQ)—whose acronym made Lynch chuckle—a scrappy, direct-action group that fought back against Mayor Giuliani's assault on New York. In the protests against the police shooting of Amadou Diallo, an unarmed Black man, FUQ members were the first to be arrested for civil disobedience.

One night, Lynch arrived in a basement where Lederer, Riley, and Sawyer were debating whether the group's mission statement ought to encompass "micronutrients."[32] She'd mastered ACT UP's organizing discipline. "You knock down every barrier. Behind every barrier, there's a person who can give you what you want."[33] In the weeks that followed, as winter turned into spring in New York City and

Philadelphia, the group tried to apply this discipline to the chasm in access to AIDS medications. They started with what they knew: drugs cost whatever the patent holder decided to charge—at least in the United States, where generic manufacture of a compound at a cheaper price was prohibited until the patent had expired. They quickly learned that not all countries were willing to play by American rules. Brazil recognized patents on the process by which a molecule was made but not the molecule itself. A Brazilian laboratory that could reverse-engineer a molecule could make it, even if that meant breaking the patent. Thailand, too, had both the capacity and a national framework for manufacturing cheap generic medications—resources that both the US government and PhRMA, the US pharmaceutical lobby, regularly pressured it not to use.[34]

Similarly, postapartheid South Africa had a law called the Medicines Act that enshrined the nation's right to make or import generic medications in the context of health emergencies. One of the provisions involved in exercising this right was known as compulsory licensing, a term that referred to government-sanctioned production of a patented product or process without the consent of the patent holder. Another key provision was parallel importing, in which a country obtained a noncounterfeit version of a product made without permission of the patent holder, such as a drug made under compulsory license.[35]

As the group gathered information, asked questions, and emailed experts, they also came to understand how the US government intervened to protect drug companies' patents. Starting in 1997, the US government had, at the behest of the pharmaceutical lobby, pressured South Africa to back away from the use of either compulsory licensing or parallel importing. The Clinton administration placed South Africa on the "watch list" of the Office of the US Trade Representative (USTR) and subsequently refused to request tariff reductions until South Africa made "progress" on its intellectual property provisions. Both US Trade Representative Charlene Barshefsky and Vice President Al Gore specifically raised concerns about the provisions in private meetings with the country's elected leaders, including President Thabo Mbeki.

When the activists figured out that the White House was stumping for drug companies and not the lives of newly liberated South Africans, they knew they had a media-ready story. They also knew the power of pointing the finger at a single person. Clinton occupied the Oval Office, but it was his vice president, Al Gore, whose public image was most vulnerable. Clinton was set to leave the White House; Gore was about to launch his own presidential campaign.

I'd ended up on Sharonann Lynch's "B-list" of activists—meaning I could not be relied upon to risk arrest in civil disobedience. Still, she knew she needed bodies in the streets, which was why in June 1999 I got a call for a weekend meeting in an apartment on East 11th Street. Gore was going to declare his presidential candidacy in Carthage, Tennessee, in a few days' time. At the meeting, Lynch sat with a steno notebook flipped open in her lap. What if the activists drove down to Carthage and disrupted the announcement of his candidacy? Could people do that?

There is nothing remarkable at all about the moment that a decision gets made that will change everything. People checked their work schedules; they considered who would rent a car. They talked about how long it would take to drive down. The proposition hung as a bubble in midair, and then there was an astringent certainty. People would drive overnight and confront the candidate when he declared. What would they chant? "AIDS Drugs for Africa, Gore's Greed Kills." I helped with the order of the words. Lynch grinned with one side of her mouth and produced, as if out of thin air, a sticker for me: a gold star, as though she knew that I was best suited for watching, then finding the words.

—— ——

ON JUNE 15, 1999, Lynch did hours-long stints behind the wheel of a rental car, relying on fellow Fed Up Queers member Emily Winklestein's renditions of Lucinda Williams songs to keep her awake.[36] They met up with a group that arrived in a rented van packed with freshly made shirts that read "Columbia Students for Gore." They'd donned these shirts and shoved flier-sized signs reading "AIDS Drugs for Africa" beneath them. They'd hoped they wouldn't need tickets to get into the main crowd. When it turned out they did, they'd sweet-talked a granny working the cordon into allowing them in anyway.

Mark Milano, a blazing-eyed stalwart of ACT UP, held the whistle that was the signal to start shouting. As he'd later write, "Al started talking: about women's rights (couldn't disrupt there); about voting rights for blacks (no, not there); about immigrant rights (not yet); and then about 'stronger families.' Okay, close enough to 'family values' for me—I got up on a fence, ripped off my t-shirt to reveal one that said 'GORE'S GREED KILLS' and blew my whistle. All hell broke loose. We began chanting, 'Gore is killing Africans—AIDS drugs now!' One of the women we had been chatting with for hours turned to us with tears in her eyes: 'I can't believe you're a part of this!' "[37]

The next day, the *New York Times* coverage of the June 16 kickoff event mentioned the protest and its focus on "AIDS drugs for Africa," the first time that the phrase had appeared in mainstream American media.[38] By the time the story ran, another set of activists was barreling north to Manchester, New Hampshire, for Gore's next scheduled appearance. The group detoured to fetch Rachel Maddow from her yardwork and PhD writing in Northampton, Massachusetts. This time, the fresh-faced crew got placed behind the candidate, a prime location for unfurling a banner reading, "Gore's Greed Kills."

Gore's campaign manager, Donna Brazile, followed another ACT UP Philadelphia member, Paul Davis, as he left the Manchester demonstration. "What do you people want?" she'd asked. Davis, who favored black jeans and plaid shirts wrapped around his pixie waist, had been waiting for the question. He wore a pile of proto-dreads on top of his head. But as much as he looked like an angry anarcho-punk, Davis could—and did—talk to anyone, more honey than vinegar, in a rapid-fire secret code that he never stopped to explain because he figured if you were worth talking to, then sooner or later you'd catch on to his lingo. People he believed in were "weirdos" and "chickens," new activists were "peaches," and hard workers were "good eggs." People who worked for members of Congress were "Congress critters."

He was, above all, a master of the "inside-outside game"—the activist jab-cross that applies threats, pressure, and shame in the streets and negotiates behind the scenes. He'd learned the game in Seattle, working alongside tenant organizers taking over unclaimed houses, land-trusting them, and turning them over to self-managed homeless communities. It was a staple of the American AIDS activist movement too. ACT UP cofounder Larry Kramer would excoriate Dr. Anthony Fauci in public, then call him up as if they were the best of friends.

The whole point of following Gore from place to place was to get someone like Brazile to ask someone like Davis, "What do you want?" Like all good activists, Davis had a specific, actionable answer ready. Davis wanted Brazile to help her former boss, Representative Eleanor Holmes Norton, get a letter from the Congressional Black Caucus (CBC) to the Gore campaign asking about its positions related to essential medications, compulsory licensing, and parallel importing as needed.

Brazile agreed to Davis's demand, but the vice president's office also went on the offensive, seeking to discredit the activists as willfully misunderstanding the causes of the raging African AIDS epidemic. The Gore team compiled a list of quotes in the vice president's defense from politicians and mainstream groups like the AIDS Action Council (AAC). (When AAC's Daniel Zingale told *Newsweek* that blaming Gore for AIDS in Africa was like blaming Franklin Roosevelt for World War II, Maddow fired off a blistering condemnation.)[39] While Gore's team played defense in public, they scrambled to come up with a solution. "The only way we are going to start to get out from under the current situation, which will get worse before it gets better and now includes the CBC and others, is to announce the plan that you all have been working on with Sandy," wrote Richard Socarides, the openly gay White House advisor on LGBT issues, referring to Sandra Thurman, the head of the Office of National AIDS Policy. "We need to do this in the next two weeks.

Help!" Socarides sent his email to "Sandy" and several members of Gore's staff.[40]

The "plan" in question was a $100 million investment in HIV testing and treatment for the prevention of vertical HIV transmission, also called prevention of mother-to-child transmission of HIV.[41] Known as the LIFE initiative, the project emerged out of Thurman's tireless work to garner White House funding for global AIDS. To build political will, she'd brought diverse delegations of members of Congress and their influencers on heart-strings-tugging trips to hold AIDS orphans in Africa. The LIFE initiative was a major achievement, and Thurman was "fit to be tied" when she learned that Gore, not Clinton, would announce the new funding—especially since the image burnishing did nothing to appease the activists, who'd "zap" Gore eight times in the next seven weeks, always giving the media advance notice.[42]

Gore's ambiguous response to the letter dispatched by Representative James Clyburn, chair of the Congressional Black Caucus, only fueled frustrations. "I want you to know from the start that I support South Africa's efforts to enhance health care for its people—including efforts to engage in compulsory licensing and parallel importing of pharmaceuticals—so long as they are done in a way consistent with international agreements," Gore wrote, without explaining how he proposed squaring the World Trade Organization's patent protections with South Africa's right to obtain medications.[43] On August 23, activists took over Gore's office in the Old Executive Office Building. Immediately afterward, they began publicizing a "showdown with Gore" for October 6 with a flier that spoofed the campaign logo, reading "Greed 2000," a shooting star encircling the phrase.[44] Before that action could happen, however, the government and its drug company allies changed their positions.

On September 9, 1999, the Pharmaceutical Manufacturers' Association announced that it would drop its lawsuit against the government of South Africa over the provisions allowing parallel importing and compulsory licensing in the Medicines Act.[45] On September 17, the US Trade Representative's Office announced that the United

States had "come to an understanding" with the country given the severity of its AIDS epidemic. The USTR removed South Africa from the "301 Watch List" cataloguing countries that have run afoul of America's self-interested economic agenda.[46] In under three months, a globally focused American AIDS activist coalition brought a technical trade issue into the public eye and forced the US government to take a position that ran counter to the desires of major campaign contributors in the pharmaceutical industry.

— —

SHIFTING BARRIERS TO OBTAINING cheap drugs was one part of the battle; getting funding to buy the drugs—at any price—was another. Here, the activists made less headway in 1999 and 2000 with a White House still swayed by the view, prevalent among the experts who guided the US approach to foreign aid and development, that investing in AIDS drugs for Africa meant making promises that, however moral they might seem, the government would not want to keep. The magnitude of the pandemic was such that anything but a massive, ambitious investment would be inadequate. Some officials fretted that a piecemeal response would only prompt unending demands. In the face of the greatest plague of the twenty-first century, leading development experts argued that the best way to manage America's potentially enormous obligation was to do nothing at all.

A three-part *Washington Post* series by Barton Gellman published in late 2000 laid bare the specific aversion of the US Agency for International Development (USAID) to the lifesaving medications. Gellman reported that USAID's AIDS advisor, Duff Gillespie, had written an internal memo arguing against antiretrovirals just at the time that the new medications began to change the course of disease in America. "Transplantation of Northern interventions to the South" was a bad idea, he reportedly wrote. Gillespie thought those drugs—the "Northern intervention"—would "siphon off resources" with "limited or no impact on the course of the epidemic."[47]

USAID's hesitation on the greatest humanitarian issue of the century came at a time when its reputation was already in something of a shambles. When the Cold War ended, American politicians no longer had a rationale for foreign aid. Without hearts and minds to win in the fight against communism, the case for spending overseas was harder to make, with fiscal conservatives especially hard to convince. The agency's checkered track record didn't help. Founded by John F. Kennedy in 1961, USAID had been hamstrung from the start. Congressional earmarks that dictated what the agency should spend its money on limited the ability of field missions to act on local priorities, while a "Buy American" provision drove up costs.[48]

Boondoggles abounded—even in the early years when money was flush and the Cold War logic clear. When Irvin Coker, a career foreign service officer, arrived in Senegal in 1967, as part of a West African survey trip for USAID's accounting division, he found a rice-production project with about sixteen contractors from the US Department of Agriculture sitting around doing nothing. "We had selected a site which is flooded out every year, when it rains," he recalled. "I asked: 'Did you know this in advance?' The man I was talking to said: 'No.' I said: 'Well, why didn't you know it in advance?' He said: 'Well, we didn't use any of the Senegalese experts for this project.' I found that was a waste of money."[49]

USAID did notch successes, including championing immunization campaigns, contraceptive provision, and shifts in agricultural approaches that helped double crop yields as part of the "Green Revolution." But it failed to secure staunch, bipartisan support from government officials who could never quite agree on why America dispensed aid. Was it in order to advance its own interests, via spending on uplift of political allies, or was it apolitical humanitarianism? USAID itself avowed the latter, even though the vast sums that flowed to countries where America was at war, from Cambodia to Afghanistan, belied the claims of neutrality.

After the end of the Cold War, one development expert would write, "The U.S. foreign assistance program has groped to find its bearings. No recent administration has articulated a compelling vision: what its purpose should be, how it relates to broader U.S. foreign policy and national security interests, and how aid programs should be executed."⁵⁰ Murkiness in worth and mandate took a toll. Between 1995 and 2000, the agency's staff size shrank by nearly 30 percent. President Clinton designated it a "laboratory" for innovation but also oversaw the closure of twenty-six of the agency's overseas missions—the first reduction in US development partners since the Marshall Plan. The Republican-controlled Congress teamed up with the State Department in a failed attempt to dismantle the agency and move its functions into the State Department in Foggy Bottom.⁵¹

By 2000, USAID had little political clout, power, or backing because its focal issues were not perceived as threats to national security. Winning hearts and minds in the midst of a war, whether hot or cold, was part of military strategy. Poverty, hunger, and childhood disease were terrible things—but they were not widely viewed as posing direct, material threats to domestic American life. This view prevailed even as experts warned that infectious-disease outbreaks didn't respect borders and that the history of pandemics past foretold a future in which a novel influenza virus could spark a pandemic that would bring the world to its knees.

If Bill Clinton deprioritized USAID, he did apprehend the security threat associated with HIV. His administration created the first health-focused position on the National Security Council (NSC) and staffed it with Dr. Kenneth Bernard, a passionate and loquacious physician who realized that security experts liked "point-in-time" events—wars, invasions, missile strikes—and had a far more difficult time comprehending the slow-motion security risk of an epidemic like AIDS. Arguing that anything that destabilized economies and societies was a security threat, Bernard tried to get the powerful NSC to take on AIDS as a critical issue.

Bernard had help with this argument. In May 2000, the United States declared AIDS a threat to American security—a first for an infectious disease. The virus itself wasn't the problem—it was still raging in many segments of America's population. But if an entire generation of adults were wiped out, "revolutionary wars, ethnic wars, genocides and disruptive regime transitions" might ensue.⁵² The orphans would grow up and be recruited into lawless militias, wreaking havoc at the behest of their adult commandants.

Bernard got the green light for developing a strategy and proposal for action, only to see Sandy Thurman's LIFE initiative—developed independently and, Bernard said, in secrecy—carry the day. Years later, Bernard bemoaned bipartisan American waffling over whether public health and infectious disease were indeed worthy of consideration as security issues that warranted action to protect the nation's own interests.[53] It was, in many respects, a replication of the ambivalence over foreign aid. The American government couldn't figure out whether it provided development aid to help other countries or to boost its own political interests; nor could it decide whether it fought epidemics beyond its borders in order to save foreign lives, or to protect those of Americans.[54]

At about the same time that HIV morphed into an American security threat, the *Advocate* acquired *Out* magazine and, with it, *HIV Plus*, moving the office out to Los Angeles and—when we declined to follow—relieving us of our jobs. ACT UP Philly came up to New York in force for our closing party, and a lanky artist and West Coast transplant named Kate Sorensen was among them. We'd met on a snowy night in late 1999 at a party at d'Adesky's house—I'd finally begun venturing out to gatherings that weren't meetings. Leaning in the kitchen door, Sorensen told me she had a crush on my writing. A few months later in SoHo, I implored her to buy me the vodka gimlets that went down tart and easy and loosened my tongue. I leaned on the bar and tried to get her to be Bogart to my laid-off Bacall. She didn't buy silver screen stereotypes though, and so I bought my own and tried to pretend that I knew what I would do, or who I was, now that I'd lost my job.

Once again d'Adesky offered me an answer. The International AIDS Conference would be held in July in Durban, South Africa, the first time the meeting had taken place in sub-Saharan Africa. Before we were laid off, d'Adesky was already working on a conference for HIV-positive women and their allies that she'd organized in collaboration with groups of South African women living with HIV.

While we still had a budget from *HIV Plus*, she'd bought plane tickets from a Russian bucket shop that would not refund them. We kept the tickets, and I picked up a freelance writing contract with the American Foundation for AIDS Research. I sublet my apartment for three months and left for a place I'd never been and about which I knew little save for AIDS statistics and the words to what was now the national anthem.

We took off from JFK in the swelter of July humidity and landed in Johannesburg, where the Southern Hemisphere's winter was underway, the trees autumn hued, the air smoke scented and chilled. I'd packed my camping backpack, an octopus of Fastex clips, with a mosquito net, a first aid kit, and performance fabrics. I was cold, underdressed, and on edge due to warnings about the country's high rates of violent crime. Walking to the convenience store by the hostel for eggs, butter, and a Cadbury chocolate bar, I encountered a woman in the street. "Help me, my sister," she said, or at least that was what I heard. As I backed away, I heard myself say, "Not yet. Not yet."

D'Adesky rented a tiny car to drive from Johannesburg to Durban; I claimed one of the seats because I was not ready to ride public transportation or, for that matter, to leave her side. We drove out of Johannesburg and into the dusk of low, dry, golden fields, the rolling veld. On arrival, we checked into the Holiday Inn South Beach in Durban, where the air smelled of salt and grilling meat from the never-ending *braais* of the beachfront bars. I kept following d'Adesky, first to registration in the giant conference center with the swooping glass facade of an airline terminal and then to the Durban Playhouse, where the meeting, "*Ubumbano IoMama*," roughly translated as "Woman United," was scheduled to take place.

The Playhouse was a Tudor-style building stretching much of a city block. During apartheid, those allowed into the cinema had been treated to a star-spangled trompe l'oeil sky. Decades later, the grand entryway smelled of wood polish and sawdust and—when the women organizers crowded into a basement room—of sweat, cakes of laundry soap, sweet-scented body oils, and the iron tang of blood. When the meeting started, we'd use the upstairs rooms with their wide windowsills and creaking wooden floors. That afternoon we crowded close, chair legs locking, climbing on tables, a room of Black women, a handful of whites.

One by one, people rose, gave their names, and said how long they had been living with HIV. Evan Ruderman, a petite, white American feminist who'd dropped out of high school to become an electrician, stood up. When she said she'd been living with HIV for twelve years, the room gasped. The Black women did not expect to live that long. Roughly 20 percent of the country's adult population had HIV; without treatment, the vast majority would die. In spite of the recent victory that had seen the United States remove trade-related barriers to South African purchase or production of antiretrovirals, a government-supported treatment program was nowhere in sight.[55]

Thabo Mbeki, the South African president, stated that the drugs that had prolonged Ruderman's life needed to be used with an abundance of caution, and an eye to the true motives of the profit-hungry pharmaceutical industry. He expressed public doubts about whether HIV was the causative agent of the constellation of diseases collectively defined as AIDS and used these doubts about HIV and the pills that treated it as an excuse for investigating the issues rather than launching a national AIDS response. The country was grappling with massive income inequality and poverty; it also had one of the largest economies and most robust health systems in sub-Saharan Africa. Moreover, as the newly formed activist group the Treatment Action Campaign (TAC) pointed out, the postapartheid constitution stipulated citizens' right to health. TAC had started in 1998, building on the powerful legacy of antiapartheid resistance with local chapters that identified issues in their health clinics and local governments, then turned out crowds to demand action. TAC brought passionate, meticulously-researched counterarguments and legal challenges to the AIDS denialism peddled by President Mbeki and his health minister, Manto Tshabalala-Msimang.[56]

Around the world, concerned allies made common cause. Before Durban, Alan Berkman had helped to write a "Global Manifesto" that laid out demands for governments, pharma, and the "bureaucracies" of UNAIDS and the WHO, asserting, "We demand ACTION and not statistics and press releases!"[57] More than 5,000 scientists, researchers, activists, and public health professionals signed on to the "Durban Declaration," released days before the meeting's start, which took aim at Mbeki's denialism, affirming that HIV caused AIDS and the benefits of the drugs were real.[58]

"Call me Chief," a broad-shouldered Black South African woman said to me in the basement of the Durban Playhouse. She had a gap between her teeth and a fedora on her head. "You will be *Nkosazana*," she said. It meant princess. I blushed. I had not thought aloud about what I expected from this conference of women or even what it meant to be an ally. If pressed, I would have admitted that I had not anticipated so much life.

That evening, d'Adesky, Cindra Feuer, and I left the Playhouse and walked down Joe Slovo Avenue to find a doorway in a dead-end street at the end of a dingy shopping arcade. We ducked below a metal grate pulled halfway down and rode an ancient elevator up to the unused office space rented as the activist headquarters for the week. TAC had hired out the space along with Health GAP—the group formed out of those early meetings convened by Alan Berkman that now had Paul Davis, Sharonann Lynch, and Asia Russell on its staff.

TAC and Health GAP, along with the Thai Drug Users Network, Brazil's Grupo Pela Vida, and the Indian Lawyer's Collective, were the core of a global cadre of groups that advanced national and community-based components of a common agenda focused on securing universal access to affordable AIDS medications. On the listservs, I'd come to know by name some of the Indians, Thais, and Brazilians whose countries were willing to produce and/or export cheap medications. When I emerged from the elevator into a warren of rooms filled with the black carapaces of rolling chairs and fauxwood desks with chipped veneers, it seemed like every one of the people I'd encountered in the virtual space was there.

ACT UP Philadelphia had turned out in force. The members who'd traveled to Durban included Melvin White, a Black gay man living with HIV; along with Paul Davis; Asia Russell; JD Davids; and Kate Sorensen, who'd left me with thrumming curiosity that night in SoHo. She had dyed her short hair rainbow colors with food coloring and sat on the floor beside a printer she had brought, zipped up in a plastic protective case, all the way from America. There, too, were the leaders of ACT UP Paris—Gaelle Krikorian and Khalil Elouardighi—whom I'd met when they came through New York and who now stood, unsmiling, in form-fitting black T-shirts that read, "Africa Is Burning." I recognized Brazilian activists, proud of their country's patent-breaking policies and universal AIDS drug program, and the Indians whose companies manufactured the active pharmaceutical ingredients that Brazil imported to make its medications. Rachel Cohen, Kris Torgeson, and Daniel Berman were all there from Médecins Sans Frontières (MSF) New York. The South African activists commanded the attention of everyone in the room, even when they were not trying to. Zackie Achmat, Mark Heywood, Vuyiseka Dubula, others whose names I did not know.

When the activists called their meeting to order, no one made up new names for each other. During introductions, everyone who had one gave their title. "I am the executive secretary of the Treatment Action Campaign," or "I am the vice president of ACT UP Paris." With the dingy furniture and lighting, the slept-in clothing, and the vague currents of sexual tension, it was like a meeting of a student council or yearbook staff. The group approached the issue of if, and how, to protest President Mbeki at the opening ceremony the next day. His AIDS denialism was immoral, an affront to anyone who cared about AIDS; he was also the president of a proud, liberated Black nation. If American activists did not, then, know that printers could be had in sub-Saharan Africa, we—like the other non-Africans—understood that this was not our government to blame and shame. Nor did all of the South African activists have access to the seats on the floor of the stadium where Mbeki would speak. Only people with conference registrations could get close; locals were relegated to the bleachers. The discussion proceeded with extreme care, as though we were all traversing a great height, a precipitous drop on either side.

35

The room took on the saturated hues and crisp edges of a space filled with concentration. The South African activists seated in the bleacher seats would start a chant during their president's speech. People who'd come from beyond the country's borders would follow their lead.

It was a night to tell the truth. "Will you take me home?" I asked Kate Sorensen when the meeting ended. We navigated by the board-walk building's rooftop lights, but we were never in danger of being lost. Exhausted, jet-lagged, dirty, and disoriented, each person in that room had understood where we were: on the knife-edge of history.

At the march the next day, I tried to copy the South African activists in their *toyi toyi*, the hybrid of marching and dancing originated by antiapartheid freedom fighters. I stumbled in the stomping and jumping, which surged forward then leapt back, and sang nonsense syllables to the apartheid-era songs that now had lyrics condemning the CEOs of Pfizer and GlaxoSmithKline. I had been warned of the enormous rates of crime and violence in South Africa, and so I had been scared each time I stepped into the street. Within that sinuous, swarming crowd, I could finally look around, taking in storefronts, bank buildings, electronics shops. Amid the clamor, I slipped into the place itself, a city that, with its wide streets and congested shopping districts, could have been many places in the world. Then, in an instant, it was only one place: Durban. As we marched, the sun dropped swiftly, and a chill crept into the air. I felt as though my skin had loosened from my body, as though I might shuck it off. Travel and mass protest both afford escape, however illusory, from the isolated self. Momentarily unencumbered, I felt very far from home and, at the same time, that I had arrived.

For many of the Westerners at the march that day, the focus on Africa, and on specific countries within the region, was a relatively new development. One could argue for equitable drug access without traveling to or knowing much, if anything, about the places where the drugs were lacking. For all the work that Eric Sawyer and his globally focused ACT UP comrades undertook, African AIDS—including AIDS affecting Africans in the diaspora—hadn't dominated the group's agenda.

In New York City, Kim Nichols, a white woman with a gentle voice and a wide-planed, open face, had joined the African Services Committee, which had been founded in 1981 to meet the needs of African emigrants newly arrived in the United States. By 1991, the immigrants arriving at the organization for housing or jobs were "coming with full-blown AIDS, tuberculosis in particular." When she thought back on that time in later years, she'd recall "the loneliness of working on African AIDS." Diagnosed herself in 1992, Nichols, a onetime acupuncturist, was embedded in both the city AIDS response and the New York–based activist community. "I felt I had to keep reminding people that . . . there was an immigrant presence in New York City that was very deeply affected by the AIDS epidemic. More than that, to try to connect with others who had the means, the intention, the knowledge to work in Africa or at least begin to explore some sort of a more localized response in Africa."[59]

When Amanda Lugg, a British Ugandan chef and queer activist moved to New York City in 1993, she marked the way that local AIDS activism and community support structures often replicated racial divides. ACT UP New York was not wholly white, but it also was not the sole or even the chief node of organizing for the Black, Indigenous, and people of color (BIPOC) living with HIV in the city. "I am in awe at the amount of work that ACT UP did . . . I didn't go because of my perception that the white gay intelligentsia was at the helm of the movement," Black gay filmmaker Chas. Bennett Brack later said.[60]

In New York, as in every community hit by AIDS, BIPOC organized their own support networks and services, drawing on history, tradition, and diasporic identity. In Harlem, Gay Men of African Descent offered HIV education and services intermingled with stories of gay resistance and resilience during the Harlem Renaissance.[61] Marlon Riggs, the brilliant filmmaker and writer whose life was cut short by AIDS, documented the experiences of his compatriots—gay men of color with diasporic identifications with Africa and Haiti—and dropped a pink triangle into the center of the African continent in his dizzying, delicious 1991 film *Anthem*, in which the poet Essex Hemphill, who would also die of AIDS, declaimed his poetry. "Every time we kiss, we feel the new world coming." This new world often meant BIPOC-led responses and resistance that received less attention than the media-savvy ACT UP protests. Bennett Brack worked at Gay Men's Health Crisis but "chose to put [his] efforts into [projects] targeted for black folk, in the sacred community of Lavender Light Gospel Choir and Unity Fellowship Church."[62]

There was a gap between white and BIPOC-led responses in the United States; there was a gulf between the epidemic in America and in Africa.[63] In the mid-1990s Lugg was working for God's Love We Deliver, a meal service for homebound people with AIDS. Lugg kept a map of Africa and its AIDS statistics pinned to the bulletin board above her desk. One day a colleague asked her why. "I said, 'Well, look at Africa, this is what's happening in the [global] south.' And she said to me, 'Oh, you don't want to get involved with that. It's too much. It's overwhelming. It's like we can't even think about it.'"[64] Lugg ignored her colleague and instead joined Kim Nichols on the staff of African Services Committee, where, in the late 1990s, the pair worked to pull together a scant handful of like-minded organizations interested in Africa. After Durban, Lugg and Nichols hosted a meeting between members of that group and the Health GAP team, a convening that ended the relative isolation of Africa-focused activists working in New York. Lugg would become a Health GAP board member and dynamic speaker at many of its rallies, but she also wouldn't forget the years when the epidemic in Africa and its impact on the New York–based diaspora had seemed a world apart.

— —

IN JULY 2000, YVETTE Raphael, a twenty-five-year-old Black feminist from the South African province of Limpopo, had a job counting guns. As a monitoring and evaluation officer for a government office, she collected munitions from citizens of all races who'd armed themselves under apartheid. She logged the weapons that marked the armistice, of sorts, in one war. When she realized she carried the virus in her blood, she started talking about her status right away. "If you fire me, I'll sue," she told her employers.[65]

Raphael also started treatment right away, a decision that put her in the distinct minority of her comrades living with HIV. She had the money to pay for the medications when others did not. She wasn't deterred by the government's denialism, even though Mbeki's questions left her anxious each time she swallowed the pills. She also had women friends who couldn't afford drugs and asked her to take care of their children when they died. "My power around it was if I can survive and look after my friends' kids, I should do it, and that was a decision of a group of women who were in my circle," she said.

She watched as prominent male movement leaders, including Zackie Achmat and Lucky Mazibuko, went on "treatment strikes," stating that, even though they had the resources to pay for the pills, they wouldn't take the new combination antiretroviral therapy until it was available to all South Africans who needed it. These bold stances seized international media attention and put the men's health in peril.[66] But to Raphael, the decision looked like one that only men could make. She couldn't say, " 'Yhoo, I am a strong man, if you don't give it to everyone I would rather die.' . . . For women it meant something different."

One of the women in Raphael's circle was Prudence Mabele, among the first South African women to declare her HIV status openly. An activist firebrand and *sangoma*—or traditional healer—she cofounded both the Treatment Action Campaign and the Positive Women's Network (PWN). TAC was savvy, visible, and powerful. To Raphael, it seemed as though the group often had male leaders in speaking roles at press conferences, while the women who'd done the door knocking to turn out the massive protest crowds didn't always make it into the front-page news. With PWN, Mabele emphasized psychosocial support and issues of trauma and gender-based violence.

Raphael met Mabele soon after her diagnosis, when Raphael, a "damn hard worker," was surfing internet chat rooms to learn about the virus while executing her job. Via the internet, she found AIDS activists in America and Europe like Charles King, a cofounder of Housing Works. King said that "housing was health care," and

Raphael—the granddaughter of a land activist—knew exactly what he meant.

Twenty years later, when I asked Raphael if she'd been in Durban in 2000 at the AIDS conference, she said she had. She told me that "Pru" had a hotel room at the Marine Parade paid for by one of the international groups looking to support South African activists. She'd piled four of her friends in, including Raphael, and then brought them along to the high-profile meetings she'd been invited to.

Raphael has a mobile, expressive face that slips from playful, pursed-lip pout to square-jawed defiance with liquid ease. At that conference she remembered using her body to make her point throughout the entire week of the meeting, forcing herself into the streets over and over. "When you were in the conference and people told you, 'So and so is dying,' you had to literally pick yourself up and start another *toyi toyi* and make sure there is another protest—enough for the world to hear. Because now here's the world in your country."

One day, Mabele swept Raphael into a meeting with Thabo Mbeki and Manto Tshabalala-Msimang. She'd gotten sick and tired of the president and health minister saying that the ARVs were poison. "Yvette Raphael," she'd called out. "Please stand up." She told everyone that her friend Yvette was taking antiretrovirals and was doing so well, looking so nice and fat. Raphael told me that when she went back to their shared hotel room and fell asleep, Thabo Mbeki and Manto Tshabalala-Msimang came for her. In her dream, they kidnapped her off the beach she'd just been sitting on, forcing her away with them to the Union Buildings, the official seat of South African government, many kilometers away in Pretoria.

To Raphael, the dream came from "the trauma of having to use my body" and from the drugs in her blood—one side effect of some of the medications was nearly hallucinatory dreams. She would take on the children, take the medications, pull herself into the street to *toyi toyi* in a fallen comrade's name. Her feminist principles, handed down by her grandmother and reinforced by her tribe of women friends, moved her body as much as her muscles. But when she was at rest, the fear crept in. She'd be responsible for eight children before she was twenty-five; her life, and theirs, depended on the president being wrong about the medications. Survival was an act of rebellion.[67]

Years later, Raphael told me there was video of Prudence Mabele asking her to stand up before the president. "I need to see that event," I said to her, then started combing the Durban conference program. I saw events I remembered vividly—like the historic speech by Justice Edwin Cameron, a white South African jurist with HIV who denounced the immorality of the treatment gap. I saw, too, the debate-style sessions between eminent scientists over whether it was possible to use AIDS drugs in Africa. I'd gone to one debate where Dr. Paul Farmer showed before and after pictures of Haitians brought back from the brink of death by antiretrovirals and quoted American poet Wendell Berry: "Rats and roaches live by competition under the laws of supply and demand; it is the privilege of human beings to live under the laws of justice and mercy." I recalled that Mead Over, a health economist and Farmer's debate opponent, declared that prevention of new infections was of the utmost importance and that an effective AIDS response simply had to deal with sex workers who were "epidemiological pumps"—acquiring HIV then churning it out into their clients' bodies.

But I could not find a session with Prudence Mabele and President Mbeki anywhere. I wanted to put us in the same place at the same time, to make the point that I treated the *toyi toyi* like a dance, while Raphael pounded the pavement to commemorate another death, performing because people like me were watching. "I'm obsessed," I messaged her. "I can't find it."

"Sorry, sis," she wrote back. It wasn't that conference; it was another one, in 2001. She'd received her diagnosis in December 2000; in July, when I'd been in Durban, she'd been enjoying the last HIV-free months of her life. The meetings had all seemed so big to her back then, she said. It always seemed like the world was watching.

"Sorry, sis." Raphael's apology jolted me. I realized how much I wanted her to have been in Durban in July 2000. I'd been at the opening ceremony of the conference where a young boy named Nkosi Johnson stood, nearly swallowed by his suit, his eyes giant in a skeletal head, and explained that he had HIV and wished to live. Great red balls bounced among the audience, making slow arcs from one set of patting hands to another. After Johnson left the stage, President Thabo Mbeki spoke at length, suggesting that poverty, malnutrition, and underdevelopment all caused AIDS. During his speech, the South African AIDS activists' voices had come drifting down from seats high above the stadium floor. From where I sat, they sounded faint and light, an echo of the roar that had filled the streets just hours earlier. Johnson died eleven months later in June 2001. The effect that evening was as horrifying as if we'd witnessed his execution, which—in a way—we had.

I met Raphael nearly a decade after the Durban meeting, when she was a fellow at the AIDS advocacy organization where I worked. With her swagger and playful sense that she had my number, Raphael reminded me of Chief, whom she'd also known. By the time Raphael and I met, Chief had been dead for three years. Our mutual friends thought she'd stopped taking antiretrovirals; they knew only that she'd stopped picking up her phone. I myself had been an inconstant friend, sending email replies months after she wrote, uncertain what I could offer from afar.

I was hungry for Raphael's account of her time in Durban because I could not ask Chief to tell me what had really happened, and I did not like my own Durban story, with its traveler's curiosity and naivete. The impulse to decenter myself and other white American activists was appropriate. But when I messaged Raphael that I was "obsessed" with finding the video, I realized I wanted to disappear altogether, to write her story and leave mine out entirely. That would not have been noble; it would have been a lie.

The 2000 International AIDS Conference in Durban was the beginning of the transnational AIDS activist movement's collective memory, the first time so many people who cared about the same thing were in the same place, with the eyes of the world watching. It began a shared experience. Raphael remembered Nkosi Johnson like she'd seen him speak because the movement's memories were hers to claim.

Collective memory can obscure as often as it illuminates, reinforcing a single version and offering it up as fact. The versions matter. Raphael had not been there, but she'd felt it in her body as if she had. I had been there, one of thousands of white Western people whose prior experience in other geographies afforded a sense of understanding of the situation far from home. My own body had been strung with desire for Kate, a desire heightened by the proximity of death, so near and sure it seemed to darken the shadows on the pavement beneath the marchers' stomping feet. The events that followed for years to come would be shaped by Black and white, African and American, Northern and Southern desires, beliefs, convictions. Black bodies would be offered as proof that the drugs worked; white ones would recede, even as they exercised power. All the bodies needed to be included in the telling.

The truth was in all of it: the loquacious, evasive president, the boy who had no time to waste, the march, the swiftly falling dusk, the beach, the *braais*, the certainty that sex, which the billboards said could kill, was the only possible salvation. To tell the truth, I had to include how Evan Ruderman lived just two more years, how I recoiled from Chief's intensity, how easy solidarity seems in a crowd. There was failure, disappointment, misunderstanding, and misremembering amid the certainty, glory, and bravery.

By the conclusion of the Durban AIDS conference—perhaps by the conclusion of the march on the opening night—the question of AIDS drugs for Africa changed from "if" to "how." It seemed as inevitable as that perfect orb of searing orange sun that rose each day out the beachside windows. Yet there were many answers to the questions, many nightmares, many dreams. Once the medications began to arrive, the kaleidoscopic nature of these visions became abundantly clear.

—— ——

I LEFT DURBAN WITH a combination of writer's block, heartache over parting with Kate, and a dense sense of dread. Chief, like almost all the other Black South African women at the conference, did not have treatment, and she told me that she did not know if she wanted to take it. Having joined the AIDS activist movement at the moment that antiretrovirals arrived, I'd never had friends who might die as the result of state-sanctioned violence before I saw them again.

As a parting gift, d'Adesky passed on an assignment she'd been offered by the International AIDS Vaccine Initiative to write about AIDS vaccine research in a country I knew almost nothing about. In August 2000—after reporting in Lesotho and South Africa for several weeks—I boarded a plane in Johannesburg and flew five hours north. I landed at night and rode down Entebbe Road after the owners of the small three-sided shops called *dukas* had lit their lamps. It was a drive through flickering shrines, missing sidewalks, dirt paths, and overloaded bicycles. The malls and motorways of modern South Africa appeared a shining scrim before the townships and their poverty. Uganda was, it seemed, not hiding anything. The government, under the leadership of President Yoweri Kaguta Museveni, forthrightly accepted HIV as a problem; Museveni decreed that all sectors of the government needed to respond. He'd approved of the establishment of the Joint Clinical Research Center (JCRC) as a parastatal organization that would do HIV research and, for paying clients, provide treatment.[68]

The clinic's director was Dr. Peter Mugyenyi. In 1977, Mugyenyi had hunkered down in the backseat of a friend's Volkswagen to flee the country then ruled by Idi Amin, whose vicious anti-intellectualism put educated elites like Mugyenyi in peril. On his return in 1989, after Museveni assumed power, Mugyenyi found that the fear of political violence had subsided, but a new "bad omen hovered in the air."[69] He saw coffin makers' stands crowding the roadsides and understood that a new, lethal force stalked the nation: the virus that caused AIDS.

By the time I met him, Mugyenyi had emerged as a vocal, seemingly fearless treatment activist. Disgusted by Western pronouncements that Africans could not take AIDS medications, he'd begun offering antiretrovirals to people who could pay for them—chiefs, politicians, and wealthy businesspeople. He provided them with discretion and a lifeline; they in turn offered the proof he needed. He closed most of his PowerPoint presentations with a slide stating, "Yes! It Is Possible to Treat AIDS in Africa." He'd tell the audience, and anyone else who asked, that the cost of drugs was the only limiting factor. To make his point, he imported generic antiretrovirals from Indian manufacturers, turning a sanction from the National Drug Authority into a media moment that highlighted the absurdity of a world in which it was illegal to procure the medications that saved people's lives.

In public, Mugyenyi exuded confidence and professionalism. He could not afford to let the public see his fear and exhaustion, though he felt these too. Instead he welcomed visitors, giving interviews in his office in the elegant green-roofed, white-walled JCRC building that was itself a rebuke to the notion that his country's health system was too primitive to provide antiretroviral medications.[70]

Before I was ushered into Mugyenyi's office in the JCRC complex on Rubaga hill, I'd seen the physician on *60 Minutes* and in countless media stories produced around the time of the Durban AIDS Conference just two months before. I had no new questions. No reason, really, to ask for his time. But the doctor was willing to speak to any journalist or visitor who listened. He sat behind a heavy wooden desk, brocade curtains in the window, and shuffled papers while he repeated his message. It was possible for Africans to take AIDS drugs. Cost was the only obstacle.

While I dropped a sugar cube into my tea and tried to think of something else to ask him, a knock sounded at the door. A woman entered, dressed in a matching ensemble from headpiece to skirt, striking in sapphire blue and white. She and Mugyenyi spoke for a while and laughed. She had bangles on her wrist that clanked and rang when she reached out to shake the doctor's hand. She was, he said to me, a patient from West Africa. She flew in every month from her home country. He had many other wealthy clients—politicians, tribal chiefs, and businesspeople—who did the same. He saw whoever came and was able to pay. As he did so, he thought of those who couldn't pay, people like the woman who came to his clinic every day, bringing her daughter and a bottle of carefully boiled water. "Why are you here?" he'd ask her. "Just in case you find something," she'd explain. She hoped that the doctor might produce an affordable remedy that could save her life. One day, though, she hadn't appeared anymore.[71]

Mugyenyi hadn't been able to bring himself to ask what happened to the woman or her daughter, and he knew that there were thousands of men, women, and children who were also waiting for something, anything that might stave off death. Until he had an answer, he would invite every visitor into his office and onto the wards to show them the proof—that it was indeed possible for Africans with HIV to take antiretrovirals. When an American member of Congress asked him to leave antiretrovirals out of his prepared remarks before a House of Representatives hearing, he refused. He would not change his story or turn away a witness.[72] People with the power to change things needed to see what was possible—and what was happening in the meantime.

CHAPTER 2

THE HARD THINGS

To lure people to move to Philadelphia, Paul Davis and his fellow anarchists offered a range of enticements, including a bike, a room in a squat house, six dates, five bucks and—sometimes—a spot in whatever band JD Davids was currently playing in. Davis himself was ensconced in (K)not Squat, a Baltimore Avenue row house with a deep porch whose black, whorled pillars were, for a time, striped with police-tape yellow. A bundle of twigs stood in for a banister; the ground-floor air was heavy with the smell of cumin and legumes from Mariposa Cooperative up the street. To keep up the steady drumbeat of media outreach, the Squat had landlines aplenty—all ready to jack into computers for late-night faxing. In early 2001, as Davis and other Health GAP members continued sending faxes and press releases about drug pricing and profiteering, he realized the movement had to start working on its next demand. "Holy shit," he thought, "we need another thing."[1]

In the months after the July 2000 Durban AIDS Conference, the prices of antiretroviral medications had come tumbling down. The media-savvy activist movement had persuaded the press and the public that price gouging on essential medications was morally unconscionable and that access to AIDS medications was a human right. In late 2000, the Indian drug manufacturer Cipla sought "compulsory licenses" for six antiretroviral drugs held under patent by major pharmaceutical companies. Those companies responded that they needed more time.[2] When Cipla began to export its versions of the antiretrovirals lamivudine and zidovudine to Uganda, Glaxo Wellcome dispatched a letter telling the company to cease and desist, writing, "Intellectual property protection is essential to sustain the investment needed for discovery and development of new treatments for HIV/AIDS and other diseases affecting the developing world."[3]

Cipla did not stop. Instead, in February 2001 the company pushed further—announcing that it could make and sell antiretrovirals for less than a dollar per person per day.[4] That was when Davis—and others—realized that the world needed a "thing" that would buy and distribute the cheap medications. "Sitting around in Philly, we did some cursory AltaVista searches and realized no one [was set up to] pay for [the AIDS drugs]," Davis recalled, naming the search engine popular at the time.[5] The activists thought that the US government was a poor choice. Its pro-patent stance, along with the Agency for International Development's "Buy American" stipulation, would make procurement of generics difficult, as would USAID's opposition to antiretroviral treatment. Nor was USAID or any single country's development agency the right entity to serve as the purchaser and distributor of pills to treat a global pandemic. If any single funder took charge, decisions about what to buy would be left in the hands of donor nations, not the recipient countries themselves. The World Bank seemed like a possibility, but when Davis asked around, he realized it was part of what his peers in the antiglobalization movement considered a neoliberal axis of evil.

Ever since the 1950s, the World Bank and the International Monetary Fund (IMF), collectively known as the Bretton Woods Institutions, had driven approaches to loan-based development aid to low-income countries. Many of these conditions, including salary caps, hiring freezes, and the requirement of user fees for health services, hampered provision of equitable, quality health and education. Countries ended up saddled with debt, servicing their repayments instead of their citizens, even as the cash infusions and the policy

requirements that came with them failed to transform their economies. As the twentieth century drew to a close, a coalition of church
groups, anticapitalist activists concerned about a range of issues, from
environmental degradation to reproductive justice, joined up with the
Irish rock legend Bono to demand cancellation of low-income countries' debt by 2000. The "Jubilee 2000" campaign took its name from
the prescription in the book of Leviticus that every fiftieth year see
property and land returned to their original owners, including those
who'd lost them due to debt.[6] Health GAP swiftly made common
cause with the Jubilee 2000 crew, and its smart, focused messaging had
made AIDS drugs for Africa a central demand alongside debt relief.

So no, Davis thought, the Bretton Woods groups wouldn't do.
Whatever the "thing" was, the entity had to be willing and able to buy
generic drugs in large quantities and equipped to distribute them to
the countries that needed them. Large orders from "pooled procurement" of drugs offered big money and guaranteed demand; generic
and branded manufacturers would drop their prices to compete for
giant contracts. Small and inconstant orders kept prices high. Doctors Without Borders/Médecins Sans Frontières (MSF), Health GAP,
and European counterparts at ACT UP Paris began knocking ideas
around. Davis and others made phone calls to Jim Kim, the future
head of the World Bank, who was then at Harvard and working with
Partners in Health (the organization run by Paul Farmer and made
famous by Tracy Kidder's book *Mountains Beyond Mountains*).

The assemblage of groups thinking through "bulk-procurement"
mechanisms were international, linked by the internet, and sufficiently small that Davis, Asia Russell, and other activists quickly
emerged as experts in an uncharted field. In January 2001, the director of health-sector coordination for the South African Development
Community emailed Davis asking for resources and ideas, saying, "If
you are aware of any work that has been done in the area, or experts,
we would still be interested to hear about them, in case there is not
enough material from the UN system."[7]

Over the first months of 2001, Davis led the Health GAP team's
process of working their ideas into a characteristically brainy, brazen

three-page briefing paper that paired technical analysis with audacious demands. Davis liked to say that if an ask didn't seem impossible, then it wasn't sufficiently ambitious. "The program must purchase drugs at the best world prices, regardless of patent status," the final version of the paper ran. America had to contribute funds "without strings." "Governance shall not be limited to donors. People with AIDS from participating countries must be represented."[8] Davis and Russell brought the briefing paper to the United Nations and walked through its core demands with R. P. Eddy, a former Clinton staffer assisting Secretary-General Kofi Annan with UN work on AIDS.[9]

Davis, who "bottom-lined" the group's Washington, DC–based work, also made sure that key staffers on Capitol Hill had the analysis. As the discussions about what such a mechanism might look like ricocheted from the United Nations to Congress and the halls of academia, staffers came back to Davis to find out where Health GAP stood on various proposals, including a "trust fund" for AIDS drugs that would be housed at the World Bank. This approach appealed to US lawmakers, including Representatives Barbara Lee, Nancy Pelosi, Henry Hyde, and Tom Lantos—all of whom had led on a range of AIDS-related legislation, including a 2000 law that called for the US Treasury to negotiate with the Bank to create a "World Bank AIDS Trust Fund."[10]

"Paul, is your org. [sic] going to come out in support of funding of the World Bank AIDS Trust Fund?" wrote Michael Riggs, a stalwart AIDS activist ally in Congresswoman Barbara Lee's office. Lee and Riggs had led calls for action on AIDS in Africa for years—and they took Health GAP's analysis seriously. "Also, we are working on your recommendations for the TF [Trust Fund]," Riggs wrote.[11]

Nor were the activists alone in their thinking. At the 2000 International AIDS Conference in Durban, economist Jeffrey Sachs, then at Harvard University, publicly estimated that the world needed to spend $10 billion to $20 billion a year to address the stark divide between rich and poor when it came to global health.[12] He, too, advanced a call for a "global fund" to fight not only AIDS but tuberculosis and malaria—intertwined diseases of poverty.[13] These monies could not go for prevention alone. Antiretroviral treatment was critical, Sachs argued. More than one hundred of his Harvard colleagues agreed and in early April 2001 published "Consensus Statement on Antiretroviral Treatment for AIDS in Poor Countries."[14]

By the time the Harvard faculty endorsed AIDS drugs for Africa, discussions about where such a fund would sit and who might run it were well advanced. Carol Bellamy, head of UNICEF, wrote a *New York Times* editorial proposing that her agency provide the support.[15] When Davis forwarded Bellamy's proposal on to a treatment-focused listserv in April 2001, he referenced Health GAP's inside-outside game: "We are on Capitol Hill working quietly to build support."

US support was important, but it was also essential to keep the government's hands off the steering wheel. At the top of his list of core concerns, Davis wrote, "The program must be multilateral. A US based or directed program will meet with failure in the international community of nations and funders and would be poorly designed." He signed off his email with the admonishment, "We do NOT want this program designed by the Bush Admin or the U.S. Congress."[16]

Exactly a week later, on April 26, 2001, United Nations Secretary-General Kofi Annan took the stage at a Lagos, Nigeria, summit on HIV/AIDS and other infectious diseases. He addressed the African leaders in the audience, but his remarks were meant for the world. It was time, he said, to create a "war chest" to fight AIDS, tuberculosis, and malaria. "I propose the creation of a Global Fund, dedicated to the battle against HIV/AIDS and other infectious diseases," he said, promising to pursue plans in the coming weeks so that the fund could be fully fleshed out—with contributions in place—by an unprecedented UN General Assembly special session on AIDS to be held that coming June.[17]

Months of behind-the-scenes work had paid off with a proposal that embraced generic medications and that would, as the details got fleshed out, specify that decision-making power had to sit with low-income countries and people living with and most impacted by HIV, tuberculosis, and malaria.

The Fund was precisely what was needed to get AIDS drugs to Africa. It was also a manifestation of a longed-for foreign aid model that put decision-making power in the hands of the poor. In 2001, Matthew Kavanagh had threaded his arms through PVC pipes and "locked down" with other activists to block an intersection at a Bretton Woods conference, getting arrested for the second time in his life. As a gay, not-yet-out high school student in upstate New York in the 1990s, Kavanagh, a redhead with a flashing grin, was drawn to HIV work because it was "a thing you could do that was about being queer." By 2001, he'd come out, spent a year abroad in Namibia, and thrown himself into antiglobalization work. Kavanagh, who'd go on to become a Health GAP staff member and galvanizing force in Africa-focused AIDS activism, was, at the time, thrilled by what the Fund meant for the bigger fight for a justice-based global economy. It was "a post-neoliberal dream of an entity that is multilateral and governed at the grass roots," he said.[18]

For the dream to come true, though, the activists wanted the US government to ante up without seeking to shape the agenda. But the George W. Bush administration—just ninety-six days in power—was not inclined to rubber-stamp proposals for foreign aid on AIDS or any other issue. The West Wing staff was taking careful note and developing its own vision.

—— ——

EVEN BEFORE HE'D BEEN inaugurated, George W. Bush laid out a West Wing organogram that all but ensured proposals like the Global Fund would receive close and careful scrutiny. During a hike on his ranch days before the inauguration, the president-elect told a *New York Times* reporter that he'd planned a West Wing that integrated economic and foreign policy. He wanted to ensure close coordination between his national security advisor, Condoleezza Rice, and his chief economic advisor, Lawrence Lindsey.[19] Lindsey would also run the National Economic Council (NEC), a body that Bill Clinton had established as a counterpart to the National Security Council (NSC) in recognition of market-based risks in the new world order taking shape after the collapse of the Soviet Union.[20] Its first chairman, Robert E. Rubin, had helped build its profile, but it had lost strength and clout when Rubin left to become Treasury secretary in 1995. The Clinton White House hadn't had a single staffer responsible to the heads of the NEC and the NSC; Bush's White House would. Bush told the *Times* that Rice and Lindsey would "share a desk."[21]

On January 21, 2020, almost exactly twenty years after Bush's first-term inauguration, I met the man who'd filled the position—or positions, to be exact. One individual had served as deputy national security advisor and deputy national economics advisor. "I became the desk," Gary Edson said to me and grinned.

It had taken me two years to get Edson to agree to talk to me. I'd first reached out to him because Dr. Anthony Fauci, the immunologist and AIDS activist interlocutor who'd led the National Institute of Allergy and Infectious Diseases since 1984, told me to. "Gary Edson is key," he told me in January 2018, explaining that during the time that Fauci had worked to draw up the blueprint for the President's Emergency Plan for AIDS Relief (PEPFAR), Edson was the person he'd been on the phone with "two or three times a week." Fauci added that he was often left out of the story. "Gary Edson is the name that somehow or other doesn't get discussed when you talk about the history of PEPFAR," he said.

I knew what he meant. Edson appeared, but was not quoted, in three quasi-official accounts of Bush's AIDS initiative—authored by Nobel laureate Harold Varmus;[22] Jay Lefkowitz, a lawyer who held several roles in the Bush administration, including domestic policy advisor;[23] and John Donnelly, a veteran science journalist.[24] I valued the accounts but was also vexed by how each started with the president's desire to take action and ended with the 2003 State of the Union. In these narratives of secret meetings and carefully guarded plans, the activism that forced the drug prices down hardly figured at all. Without that price reduction from over $10,000 to less than $400 a year, large-scale AIDS treatment programs would not have been feasible in low- and lower-middle-income countries. Neither George W. Bush nor his predecessor, Bill Clinton, had sought to drop the costs or overhaul patent-favoring trade policies. Clinton would, post-presidency, tackle both these issues. The monumental scale of Bush's magnanimity crowded those details to the margins. As long as there was money to buy the medications for all who needed them, the issue of who set the prices and what happened to countries and companies that sought to create competition seemed less compelling. It sometimes seemed to me as though Bush had, through his largesse, purchased the story rights to America's fight against global AIDS.

Stories about PEPFAR didn't just crowd out activist work; they also paid glancing attention to the other, major foreign aid innovations that took place at the same time. Under Bush, the volume of foreign aid rose at rates comparable only to the post–World War II period in which the Marshall Plan sent funds sluicing into Europe, and the level of aid was, in 2005, higher than at any point in US history.[25] In Bush's first term, the government created the first new foreign-aid-dispensing entity in forty years, and the White House attempted an overhaul of the entire architecture of foreign aid. While Bush was still in office, one aid scholar wrote, "No time since the administration of President John F. Kennedy has seen more changes in the volumes of aid, in aid's purposes and policies, in its organization, and in its overall status in foreign policy."[26]

Like the activist work that also got pushed to the margins, the effort to reform American aid had great relevance to the AIDS response. Antiretrovirals controlled the virus in the blood, but they were not a remedy for the social woes that drove the epidemic. One could not talk about AIDS without talking about poverty, debt, corruption, misogyny, white supremacy, homophobia, and capitalism. But one could not dismantle these issues by dealing with AIDS alone. The assault on drug prices had been a battle in a larger war against capitalism and its cruel, greed-based globalization. The establishment's rejoinder was to offer money without tearing down the system. Until the revolution came, foreign aid aimed at alleviating poverty was part of any pandemic response, even if it was not labeled as such.

The longer a pandemic lasted, the more the content in the margins mattered. AIDS might yet be vanquished by the current approaches, but long-term control of future pandemics depended on both activism and the architecture of foreign aid. I did not expect Edson to add much to the former topic, but I badgered him for an interview for nearly two years because of his role in the latter. Edson was widely credited with creating the Millennium Challenge Corporation, the wholly-new foreign aid entity launched in 2002. Edson, who had a law degree and an MBA, kept a low public profile. He'd been an entrepreneur and special advisor in Reagan's State Department and, in one of the few interviews I found, described his career as "a Jackson Pollack painting." People who worked with him, like Fauci, didn't forget his drive. "He keeps folders on all of the world's problems," one collaborator told me. When we spoke on the phone, I wanted to understand the broader set of ideas and imperatives from which PEPFAR had emerged. He agreed, noting that he'd never met someone worse at taking "no" for an answer than he was. We'd need a half a day, he said, and we needed to meet in person.

Edson booked a conference room in a marble-floored DC law firm with hallways wide as runways and with abstract, monochrome canvases in the common areas. When I walked in, he was standing by a white board that he'd filled with an organogram of the White House, the National Security Council, and the National Economic Council circa 2001. With his brush cut and black sweatshirt, he looked more Silicon Valley than West Wing. Security sat on the left of Edson's chart, economics on the right. He thumped the board with a marker. He'd sat smack in the middle.

The structure was a response to an interconnected, globalized world order in which markets and foreign economies posed threats equal to, if not greater than, military incursions and armaments. In a world where currency-related crises in Thailand, South Korea, Indonesia, Russia, and Mexico had recently threatened to destabilize countries, regions, and American investment, international economic policy and national security policy were inseparable. The structure he'd sketched was one way to achieve integration. A Kissingerian architecture that kept foreign policy focus on "hard-power" military matters, and not on the "soft-power" issues of economic growth and foreign aid, wasn't adequate for a world in which foreign policy could trigger not just wars but financial meltdowns that could—in the jargon of the day—grow contagious.

An economic collapse could trigger a security issue, as could a global pandemic like AIDS. Edson's diagram captured another shift from the Clinton administration structure. On Bush's taking office, the White House dispensed with the public health–focused position on the National Security Council that Clinton had created and that had been held by Dr. Kenneth Bernard, who created the first-ever Biodefense and Health Security Office at the White House. The incoming Bush team dispensed with that office too. (Bernard told me he hadn't even been able to present his transition memo, which detailed, among other issues, the security risk posed by AIDS and the need for a more robust US response.)[27]

Instead, Edson created a director of development on his staff, the first such position on the National Security Council; eventually, the work expanded into a directorate—an office—on development issues. Global health sat within the development arena, and so this structure did technically maintain a health focus on the NSC, albeit one that sat at a distance from matters of national self-interest. A country wracked by disease might collapse, with shock waves that had security implications. A development-oriented health focus could address that. But if a disease threat emerged in or arrived on American soil, nesting global health within development made less sense. Indeed, in the aftermath of the September 11 attacks, when letters containing anthrax arrived in congressional and media offices, Bernard was hired back as special assistant to the president for biodefense on the Homeland Security Council.

Nevertheless, the Bush White House architecture did advance an integrated economic and foreign policy closer to the NSC agenda. Edson was able to get economic advisors installed in each of the National Security Council's geographic "directorates," which mirror the

State Department's bureaus for Africa, Asia, the Middle East, and so on. He soon had a staff of eleven or twelve and, with Rice's ear, a way to bring economic and development issues from around the globe to the table at the National Security Council. "This may seem like geeky management stuff," he said.

It didn't seem geeky to me at all. In Washington, DC, all structure is political, all bureaucracy plumbing for power. For years, development, including global health, had been at the end of a dripping faucet, with little standing or relevance in geopolitics. Because of historical American ambivalence over the purpose of its development aid, USAID did not sit on the National Security Council; there was no cabinet-level position for development. The agency had nominal independence but needed its budget approved by the State Department, which, in turn, often had to turn to USAID or other agencies when it wanted funds for projects that might be classified as development. Edson's was the first West Wing role to link development, economic policy, and national security. A third component of his job was being the president's chief negotiator for laying the groundwork for the summit of the Group of 7 (G7) nations. In the United States, the holder of this role is anachronistically known as the "Sherpa." The G7 is comprised of Canada, France, Germany, Italy, Japan, the United Kingdom, and the United States. Russia was invited to join for deliberations on specific issues—a configuration dubbed the G8.

Edson drew the organizational chart on one part of the white board. On the other side, he sketched a time line. "You need to cast your mind all the way back to January of 2001 and what the world looked like," he said. "People forget, we forget so quickly." I looked over his shoulder at a pair of large canvases, black geometries on a white background.

I remembered.

It poured on Election Day in January 2001. I woke Kate Sorensen from a deep sleep to ask her if she thought I should go to Washington for the inauguration. I wasn't supposed to be there in her bedroom on the top floor of the Philadelphia anarchist house known as "Fancy House." She'd asked me to remain in New York City. For the past three months, ever since my return from South Africa in late 2000, we'd been ferrying back and forth between our two cities and, it often felt, between two different worlds.

Kate was eleven years older than me. She was also, at the time our relationship unfolded, trying to stay out of jail. The week after she'd left Durban, she'd served as a marshal for a march and protest against the "criminal injustice system" in Philadelphia, a demonstration timed to coincide with the Republican National Convention, at which George W. Bush would receive the party's presidential nomination. Kate was arrested and charged with twenty felonies, her bail set at $1 million. As criminal proceedings against Kate and other activists unfolded, they exposed the extent of the city, state, and federal surveillance and infiltration of the activist community involved in the "R2K" protests and the broader antiglobalization movement. The state took preemptive steps to disrupt the planned protests by raiding and seizing the contents of activist spaces, where puppets, signs, and banners were being made, and beginning arrests before the largely peaceful protests had even begun. The approach itself emerged in tandem with the movement, aggression matched to activist power, which exploded in disruptive protests at a World Trade Organization meeting in Seattle in 1999, then moved on to Jubilee 2000—and showed no signs of stopping.[28]

Bush was effectively trying to put Kate in prison; his father had, through his homophobic heel-dragging over a comprehensive American AIDS response, killed many of her friends. She didn't want to cuddle, at least not with someone who lacked existential dread. I was upset that Bush Junior had been elected, but I did not feel personally endangered. I thought my body was safe. When she'd asked me to stay in New York, I'd gone to Philadelphia anyway. When I pestered her about whether I should now go down to DC, she grew angry. I could take her rainsuit. I needed to leave her alone.

The rain pelting the suit's rugged plastic had added to the percussion of the day. The protesters banged frantic tattoos on their drums. I met friends from New York City at DC's Union Station, and we walked for a time beneath a giant puppet with clouds of white fabric billowing beneath its arms like wings. It seemed to me like no one in the crowd thronging the streets along the motorcade cheered for the new commander in chief, who had received fewer popular votes than his opponent, Al Gore, and been installed by virtue of a narrowly decided Supreme Court decision. People beat drums, blew airhorns, and held signs that said, "Hail to the Thief," "Supreme Injustice," "Let the People Pick the President," "End the Racist Death Penalty."

In the car on the way home, we listened to a rebroadcast of the inaugural address on NPR. When Bush invoked the angel in the whirlwind, one of my traveling companions gasped. "The angel of history," she said. Walter Benjamin had first named this being, attaching its likeness to Paul Klee's painting *Angelus Novus*. The angel that desired, and was unable to, "make whole what has been smashed," presided over modern life, including the most recent plague.[29] For a moment it was as though the apparition that descended from a crack in the sky in Tony Kushner's AIDS-focused trilogy *Angels in America*, now hovered before the window of the car.

I remembered.

"So, in January 2001, you had three million deaths from HIV per year, only 50,000 people in all of Africa on antiretroviral treatment," Edson continued. "In terms of international development, the Millennium Development Goals [MDGs] had been adopted only in 2000," he said, referring to the United Nations Millennium Declaration issued by the General Assembly in September 2000. The declaration laid out hopes for a peaceful, pluralistic twenty-first century and detailed core aspirations, including halving global poverty and hunger, ensuring universal primary education, promoting gender equality and empowering women, addressing the plight of slum dwellers, and halting the spread of HIV/AIDS.[30]

The declaration laid the groundwork for the goals, which were fleshed out in more detail in 2001. The collaborative planning reflected the fact that billions of dollars of aid had not ended global inequity. There were plenty of contributing factors, including crippling debt owed by many countries, the structural-adjustment conditions imposed on them by the World Bank and the International Monetary Fund, the failure of multinational corporations to pay taxes in the countries from which they extracted resources, and corruption among leaders in every part of the world. The MDGs did not tackle these issues head on, but they did take aim at another core problem: a lack of coordination and common agenda among major sources of aid. All too often, countries acted alone, dispensing aid that fit their singular agendas and priorities. Wealthy nations sent money and "missions" to low-resource settings without talking among themselves or even coordinating between agencies from the same country. The so-called beneficiaries were saddled with a jostling array of reporting and monitoring requirements, time lines, and targets.

In advancing a finite set of priorities, the eight Millennium Development Goals were a monumental step toward global agreement on critical aims. Endorsing them implied endorsing the substantial costs of achieving such lofty, necessary aims. The declaration didn't explicitly state the expected contributions of high- or low-income nations, but many of the United Nations member states had, since 1970, endorsed the target of wealthy nations contributing 0.7 percent of gross national income (GNI) to foreign aid. Under Bill Clinton, the United States endorsed the declaration but not the target—which the United States had opposed for thirty years on the grounds that America "did not subscribe to specific targets or timetables."[31] In fact, Clinton's FY2001 budget, in effect when Bush entered the Oval Office, allocated the equivalent of 0.11 percent of US GNI to foreign aid, a historic low.[32]

But Bush would write that he sought "a stark departure from the G8's tradition of measuring generosity by the percentage of GDP a nation spent on foreign aid." Asking wealthy nations to tithe a specific portion of their resources was, to Bush, a "handout," offered by European nations that "felt guilty about what nations like France had done in the colonial era."[33] He thought this model involved writing a check without asking how it would be spent—a form of conscience-salving paternalism. As long as the focus was on inputs—the amount of money spent—and not on outcomes, meaning the results to be achieved, the size of the check didn't matter. Bush was convinced that aid had to be tied to performance on the part of both the high-income countries providing the resources and the low- and lower-middle income countries where the money would be spent. Recipient countries needed to perform; donors needed to provide the funding. Edson said that Bush called this "shared responsibility for results."

In this conceptualization, funders need to be transparent about the criteria they used to select the countries that received aid and the criteria that would be used to judge whether the aid had impact. Setting eligibility criteria for aid could encourage countries to meet them in order to qualify; in theory it also meant that donor countries would have a harder time funneling funds into states with poor track records on human rights or use of aid—whether for strategic reasons or out of postcolonial shame.

"America did not colonize African nations. America did not create corruption," Bush snapped at Jacques Chirac during one G8 meeting.[34] Edson repeated something similar to me during our conversation. "Bush the African," as Condoleezza Rice dubbed him, wrote vividly about visiting slave forts in Ghana and the horror of the trade in human lives, but stopped well short of naming these slaves as the source of America's wealth or the country as a cruel and bloody exemplar of settler colonialism.[35] The Bush White House did not think that America had to atone for its past or account for its present role in extractive capitalism. Instead, Edson—who Bush had said, on the campaign trail, was running "to do the hard things, not the easy things"—set out to realize an ambition he shared with President Bush. The two men wanted to reshape "the entire development assistance paradigm" in the name of outcomes not inputs and shared accountability for results.[36]

The men in the West were not alone in seeking dramatic change to foreign aid. At roughly the same time, the Bush White House, the United Nations–convened global community, AIDS activists, and the broader antiglobalization movement all assessed historic approaches to foreign aid, declared them lacking, and then proposed dramatic new solutions: debt relief; an end to the Bretton Woods

Institutions; realization of the Millennium Development Goals; and the launch and full funding of the Global Fund to Fight AIDS, Tuberculosis, and Malaria.

All parties involved understood that money alone did not wipe out history or change the future. The differences emerged in the proposed solutions. To left wing, antiglobalization activists, transformation depended on redistributing power so that people from the countries receiving the aid made decisions without conditions imposed by donors and lenders and in the absence of trade-related provisions that protected the interests of wealthy nations and giant corporations.

Of all of the new initiatives, the Global Fund was among the first to attempt to put many of the principles into practice on a global scale. The Fund's success rested on the degree to which the country-driven processes would yield truly ambitious proposals. Even with a pluralistic approach to developing proposals that put people living with and affected by HIV, tuberculosis, and malaria at the table, this still meant that success depended on national governments designing and implementing ambitious treatment programs. If the governments of countries receiving grants from the Fund offered modest proposals, not only would people die but donors would not be impelled to make large contributions. By the same token, if donors did not fully fund the new mechanism, risk-averse countries might submit smaller proposals. Supply and demand for funding had to be consistent with the overwhelming need. This closely resembled the shared responsibility that Bush believed was critical. But it appeared to take the sharing too far. When Bush heard of the Fund, he was "concerned that a fund composed of contributions from different countries with different interests would not spend taxpayer money in a focused or effective way."[37]

Skeptical, Bush still decided to make a contribution. On May 11, 2001, he announced a $200 million American donation. The first governmental contribution in the world was a sum far less than estimated need. Jeffrey Sachs had estimated that the US fair-share contribution was $1 billion to $2 billion. At a Rose Garden ceremony with Kofi Annan, President Bush used much of the speech to lay out American expectations for what the Global Fund needed to do and prove, using the terms that he and Edson valued. "We must know that the money is well spent, victims are well cared for, and local populations are well served," he said. "All proposals must be reviewed for effectiveness by medical and public health experts. Addressing a plague of this magnitude requires scientific accountability to ensure results."[38] Bush also said that the new fund "must respect intellectual property rights, as an incentive for vital research and development," a stipulation that seemed to take direct aim at activists' ongoing efforts to secure access to generic medications, regardless of patent status.

Davis, Sachs, and a vast array of other activists, academics, and public health workers who'd argued for the new procurement mechanism were aghast. The United States was the wealthiest nation in the world, and other prospective donors were watching. The pledge, a fraction of the estimated need, seemed like a vote of no confidence and a signal to other donors that they too could be stingy without facing blame.

I heard about the nascent fund from Davis when Kate and I ran into him on Baltimore Avenue by the co-op, the bike shop, the Thai restaurant that served meals under a blue tarp. Davis stood close while he talked, smiling a wicked grin. I was, in that time, preoccupied with the state's case against Kate for her activities at the Republican convention the previous summer. We went to "R2K" legal defense fund-raisers where punk bands and spoken-word poetry artists performed and Kate was greeted as a celebrity. At her home, the boiler often quit—we'd touch the radiator so often it was warmed by our hands. Even when the heat came on, there was still a chill. Kate was scared, even terrified, of spending time behind bars.

In March 2001, the jury returned its decision, acquitting Kate of all charges save for a single misdemeanor. She'd been vindicated in court, but the state's commitment to policing nonviolent protest also took its toll. Now that she wasn't facing jail time, she could look for a new job, look at activist work beyond convention-related legal defense. As the immediate threat receded, so did the fear and urgency that had bound us in Durban and in Philadelphia. I imagined we would spend just as much time together as we had during the cold months of her court case. I'd seen my devotion as activist work. While the movement took on new fights and protests, I'd tried to take care of Kate. She didn't need that now. Instead, she had to find a new job, return to activism, and rejoin the wider world. I was less ready than she was. I argued when she took a job across the state and wept when she had to leave my New York flat at the end of the weekend.

In Kate's living room, a portrait of Dr. Martin Luther King Jr. on velvet hung on one wall; on another, a sheet marked with rust-red shapes, like land masses in an uncharted world. One of Kate's West Coast artist friends made the print in collaboration with Mary Lucey, a bold activist living with HIV. The artist mixed the woman's blood with heparin; she'd coated herself in it then lay down and made a print on the sheet. During Kate's trial, I looked at Mary Lucey's map and at MLK and felt I was doing enough to fight injustice. Once we tried to move forward, my mistake became clear: every body contained a world, but loving a single person was not a political cause.

— —

In June 2001, the UN General Assembly held a special session on AIDS—the first such convening devoted to an infectious disease. In the months prior to the meeting, member states worked on the draft text of the declaration that would be launched at the close of the meeting. As with all UN gatherings, considerable work was done in advance, with much of the precise wording hammered out well before the actual event. The draft included a recommendation that intellectual property rights and trade provisions be assessed for their impact on access to essential medications. In a May "Action Alert," Health GAP reported that the Bush administration had argued that such a recommendation was neither "relevant" nor "productive."[39] A longer issue brief detailed concerns about US intervention in planning for the Global Fund. "The United States is opposing bulk procurement of medicines, especially through competitive bidding. The US is also fighting very hard to prevent any participation of generic drug manufacturers in the fund."[40] When it came to the final text of the historic UN Declaration on AIDS, the text walked a fine line. Article Twenty-Six welcomed countries' efforts to secure medicines "consistent with international law" and noted that "the impact of international trade agreements on access...needs to be evaluated further."[41]

In addition to concerns about bulk procurement—a strategy that drove drug prices down—the US government also had concerns about "tiered pricing," a proposed system that set affordable costs for high- and low-income countries. In late July 2001, the *New York Times* quoted from a letter from Bush's US trade representative, Robert Zoellick, to his European counterpart. "The Bush administration is 'opposed to the creation of an international institution or convention to regulate drug prices,' Mr. Zoellick wrote. 'I also would question establishment of a verification process.'" Further, he stated that "we have practical and legal concerns with the concept of maintaining a database on drug prices." Zoellick reportedly wrote that cost was not, in fact, the issue holding back AIDS drugs for Africa. The access gap was "more likely the result of the enormous infrastructure problems plaguing this region, rather than drug prices."[42]

Shortly after the UNGASS meeting on AIDS in New York City ended, Edson, Condoleezza Rice, and the president had traveled to Genoa for the G7/G8 summit. While they bunked at the Jolly Marina Hotel and ventured daily beyond the metal fences erected around the Palazzo Ducale, Sharonann Lynch and Asia Russell bedded down in a nunnery, cadging apples from the nuns after endless days working the press room and inhaling pepper spray in the streets, where the militarized police response to the globalization movement treated every protester as a threat.[43]

On July 20, Kofi Annan had joined the leaders at a press conference about the Global Fund, urging them to offer the funding it needed. "This is a very good beginning. But much, much more is needed."[44] Minutes after he'd finished speaking, the press room had erupted in shouts as news filtered in that a protester, Carlo Giuliani, had been shot and killed, the first fatality in the antiglobalization protests that had been gaining power since the "Battle in Seattle" in 1999.

When news of the killing reached Philadelphia, Kate's living room was bathed in a whitened summer light, and I was not surprised. I sat in the hot, underfurnished room and realized that, ever since the bloodthirsty state ceased to rattle Kate's door, I'd been waiting for it to strike again. I had known—though I had never thought this consciously—that someone would have to die. I was not proud of discovering that I'd moved closer to seeing the world as Kate experienced it, just chagrined that it had taken me so long.

I didn't say that to Edson on the day we met. I did not say much of anything. Edson, who ate only the cookies from the generous catered lunch, ran our interview like a court case or a graduate seminar. He read aloud, at length, from news articles, government documents, and the memoirs of the president and Condoleezza Rice. He handed me pages with highlighted sections and rattled off the names of researchers with whom he'd worked or whose work had influenced his thinking.

When I listened to the recording of our meeting, I heard him thump the table. I also heard my own breathing, heavy and intentional. I had urged Edson to speak with me because I wanted the big picture of the administration's ideas on foreign aid and because my own life had been changed by Bush's actions on AIDS. I hadn't completely stopped making historical events personal, seeing them in terms of what they'd meant for me. I'd only gotten better at seeing what actually mattered, even when that meant seeing a world that was uglier and more violent than I wanted it to be. As he spoke, I'd returned to the time when I lacked those skills and paid accordingly. I began breathing that way to try to calm my racing mind.

But that was not the only reason I took deep, slow breaths while I listened. Over Edson's shoulder, a pair of abstract paintings hung on the wall: black oblongs and lines on a white background. I saw the tops of two buildings, an antenna.

I remembered that too.

CHAPTER 3

FIGHT LIKE A WOMAN

IN JULY 2001, A little more than a year after the Durban AIDS Conference, Milly Katana walked into my hotel room in Kampala, Uganda, carrying a briefcase and grinning, her head canted forward, as though she could not keep up with herself. She gave me a hug, even though we'd never met, and told me that she wanted to rid AIDS from the face of the world.

I was, by then, writing for the newsletter of the International AIDS Vaccine Initiative. The job kept me close to the science of HIV and allowed me to learn new things; I believed in the organization's mission of finding a safe and effective way to prevent or reduce the risk of acquiring the virus. But the office on William Street in lower Manhattan was filled with scientists whose activism, such as it was, was belied by their business suits. I felt removed from the front lines, as I'd encountered them in Durban and New York City. When Anne-christine d'Adesky had secured funding for a women's meeting in Kampala, similar to the one she'd organized in Durban, I'd leaped at the chance to help organize it.

By the time Katana walked into my room at the Hotel Africana on Wampewo Road, she was one of the most prominent Ugandans living with HIV and a member of the National Guidance and Empowerment Network (NGEN+), a group of people living with HIV

(PLHIV) founded by Major Rubaramira Ruranga, a barrel-chested, gravel-voiced military man who'd been diagnosed and publicly disclosed his status in the early 1990s. When Katana was diagnosed five years prior to our meeting, in 1995, she'd been devastated for herself and for her mother, who had "spared everything" from the small salary she earned as a cook at an agricultural college in the Luweero District to send her only daughter to secondary school. "I was very hardworking, very determined. Because I was the only daughter, I behaved more like the boys. There was no difference [like], 'A girl does this, a boy does that,'" Katana told me. Her family—which had lost almost all of its income during the civil war for which Luweero was an epicenter—could not afford college tuition, but Katana had won a government scholarship and moved into Mary Stuart Hall on the campus of Makerere University, the country's most prestigious university. "I was staying with all these children of rich people and I think I had one pair of open[-toed] shoes . . . [M]y mother gave me her blanket to go to school."[1]

Katana had been determined to do as well as, if not better than, the children who'd gone to the "first-world schools" of the country. She was the only woman in her accounting class and rose to become the minister for gender in the university's parliamentary-based government. She'd secured a job at a publishing company even before graduating. By the time she received her diagnosis, she had managed to buy a plot of land but was living in a one-room rented house where she found she could neither eat nor sleep, thinking, "After all the effort my mother had put into educating me, I am going to die."

Katana had gotten tested because she'd left the publishing company and taken a job in the accounting department of Dr. Peter Mugyenyi's Joint Clinical Research Center (JCRC). "I didn't know much about what the organization did . . . I saw so many people coming in and I recall asking my colleague . . . what are all these people doing here?" When her coworker explained they were all lining up to participate in research on AIDS, Katana realized the extent of the epidemic. "When I saw there were so many people who had HIV, I thought maybe I could have it as well." One day, she'd asked a doctor there to draw her blood, though when she looked in the mirror, the face that gazed back—a prominent forehead underneath a cap of close-cropped curls, a dramatic gap in strong, white teeth—looked just fine.

Keen-eyed and anxious, she'd taken note of the string of numbers the doctor used to anonymize her sample, then returned on her own and found her results in the ledger on her own. She hadn't spoken to the doctor again; she also hadn't spoken to the major the first several times she'd gone to his office. "I am a fast walker...I would sit there for five minutes, then run away and disappear," she told me years later. "One day he grabbed me—he is an energetic man—and said, 'Milly, why do you come to my office?'" In response, she'd started to cry.

Katana explained her status, and Ruranga explained that she needed to come and join his nascent organization run by and for people living with HIV. "That," Katana would later say, "started my journey into activism." But still she continued to expect the worst. "I hurriedly built my house, really preparing for my death." She also bought piles of bed linens and towels. Looking ahead to a bleak and imminent future, she thought the linen would "support whoever would be helping me when I can't get myself out of bed." The house was a little box sitting tight beside a giant water-collection tank on a plot of land in Mbuya, a leafy neighborhood to the east of Kampala's small downtown. She put her sheets in a closet and hung a poster of the Makerere University student government from the year she'd been a minister, alongside a photograph of her mother in the compact living room. She was ready to die on her own terms, but she'd go on using her intellect and determination as long as she was able.

On the day that we met, Katana arrived in my room at 10 a.m. As she steered me down the stairs and into her tidy blue Toyota Corsa, which had plastic lace doilies on the backs of the seats, she explained that she had been up since 3 a.m. Power was unreliable, and she woke up when the electricity came on. Besides, there was so much that needed to be done—responding to emails; taking care of family members who were sick, often with HIV, and calling her for help;

phoning the health ministry; and making plans with other NGEN+ members for the weekend van trips out of town. The group's core mission had been to help people living with HIV become each other's safety nets, just as Major Ruranga had done for Milly and so many others. NGEN wanted a group of at least five people living with HIV to exist in every village hit by the epidemic. "People would be abandoned in small rooms and nobody would go in there just to check to see whether the person is still alive or dead," Katana later said. "These members would...be sure that the person is bathed, got a cup of porridge, or organize a bicycle transport to take them to the nearest health facility." On the weekends, the Kampala-based founders drove out of town to talk with members of these groups about nutrition, medications, and "positive living," with a curriculum of their own making that combined materials adapted from American and European networks of people living with HIV and resources from other African PLHIV groups that had undertaken activism as self-preservation.

She also got up early to respond to emails and get work done before dealing with visitors like me. There were, in most African countries, a handful of openly HIV-positive activists who got the calls when someone, whether media or an activist ally, was coming from out of town. In this way, African AIDS was different from American AIDS. Prominent African people living with HIV like Katana were often asked to orient foreigners to their local epidemics and to their countries. In cities like Kampala, this was a practical challenge: there were no grids, no street addresses, just landmarks to navigate by. You could not get someplace unless you already knew, in some detail, how to describe where you were going or had a guide who knew the way.

Some days, solidarity looked an awful lot like hospitality. It was also intertwined with survival, insofar as these activists were, in 2001, often only getting antiretrovirals as a result of a thick network of international connections. In her little Mbuya house, Katana had her medications on her sideboard in a woven basket. They were other people's drugs, the original recipients' names crossed out. She'd gotten them through a group called AIDS Empowerment and Treatment

International (AIDSETI), founded by Hans Binswanger, a World Bank senior employee who himself had HIV.[2] He'd begun to collect and share out the medications left over when a person died or switched to another regimen. There were never enough to go around. Activist groups like NGEN held meetings that considered who should be selected, considering whether candidates had children, how sick they were, and whether they were activists. The ones who were visible and fighting for drugs needed to stay alive until they had won.

As Katana and I drove around Kampala that week, I learned the city's geography and texture. It ranged over a set of seven green hills, with tethered goats and small stands of banana trees punctuating low-slung blocks of stores, facades painted with rainbow-colored ads for paint, shoe polish, and maxi pads. Open-air roadside shopping was organized in blocks: one strip for coffin shops, another for metal gates or wicker beds and chairs. The majority of the city's roads were unpaved; sidewalks were nonexistent. The slums gathered in bowls, as though the mud and brick shacks had tumbled down from the leafy hills, which were, in 2000, not yet decimated by construction. On the slopes of those hills, behind metal gates, the wealthy and the expats lived in compounds that were verdant, sweet scented, fertile, and serene.

In 1999, a trial conducted in Uganda called HIVNET 012 had found that a single dose of the antiretroviral given to a mother while in labor and another given to the infant after birth could dramatically reduce the risk that the baby would be born with HIV.[3] While we traveled between meetings in Kampala, Katana and I talked about a drug called nevirapine, the drug that would reduce their risk of passing HIV to their babies. I told her I thought once women learned about the drug, they would rise up and demand it. This was what the activists averred. Winning access to lifesaving drugs would inspire more demands, more actions, more victories in the fight to rebalance the scales of global equity. In South Africa, the Treatment Action Campaign (TAC) was about to launch a lawsuit against the government, arguing that the failure to launch a national, government-supported program to prevent mother-to-child transmission violated the right to health of women like

Busisiwe Maqungo, who had, in 1999, given birth to a baby girl named Nomasizi. After Nomasizi fell sick and received her HIV diagnosis, Maqungo realized she herself had been tested while pregnant. The clinic had not informed her of her result or of the antiretroviral regimens that could be used to reduce the risk of mother-to-child transmission. Nomasizi had died of AIDS before she reached her first birthday; her mother joined TAC to demand the government change. "I gave birth to an HIV-positive baby who should have been saved," Maqungo wrote in her affidavit. "I will live with it until my last day."[4]

Katana believed wholeheartedly in holding government to account. She was fearless about castigating Ugandan officials for moving too slowly and doing too little. She also knew that up-country women lived far from clinics and delivered their babies at home alone or with traditional birth attendants because the government facilities frequently had no staff, or had staff but no supplies, such as gloves or gauze or medications to stop postpartum hemorrhage. If you had HIV and you admitted as much, no nurse would touch you. A woman wouldn't go to a clinic, even to get nevirapine if it ever became available, if that same clinic would let her die in agony.

"No one is working," Katana said to me. She meant governments of wealthy nations—which had failed to put adequate funds into the Global Fund. She meant her own government too—a critical assessment that put her at odds with much of the Western world, which saw Ugandan president Yoweri Kaguta Museveni as an exemplar of African political leadership on AIDS.

It was an image he'd earned through a highly visible public response urging his country to address the new plague. It began, he said, when Fidel Castro pulled Museveni aside shortly after he'd assumed power and told him that many of the soldiers he'd sent to Cuba for training had tested positive for HIV.[5] The former guerilla fighter needed a healthy military to stay in power; he'd launched a national AIDS education campaign that was, in fact, unlike anything in the region, in terms of the level of visible presidential support and national mobilization. By 2001, the state's tale of what had happened sat between the covers of "The Story of AIDS in Uganda—and

Banana Trees Provided the Shade." I'd get handed that pamphlet at the end of many of interviews during my early reporting trips between 2000 and 2004.[6]

Museveni had demanded that state radio play AIDS-education messages, starting each program with a drumbeat—the traditional sound of alarm. He'd spoken about the virus in every speech and urged faith-based leaders to do the same. He'd promoted condoms and used homegrown metaphors like "zero grazing" to urge people to have a single partner. For those for whom it was possible, he declared it best to avoid sex altogether—to abstain.

All of this activity earned Museveni enormous, deserved credit. It also burnished his sterling reputation in the eyes of the West. He'd built this reputation steadily and deliberately since 1986, hiring a public relations firm run by Ronald Reagan's son-in-law as soon as he took occupancy of the state house, abandoning a dalliance with socialism and barter with North Korea in favor of a wholehearted embrace of International Monetary Fund and World Bank structural-adjustment policies. Uganda's lengthy document explaining how the aid received would lift the country out of poverty had evolved into the Poverty Reduction Strategy Paper that would become a prerequisite for debt relief under the Heavily Indebted Poor Countries program.[7]

Museveni was adept at taking donor ideas, putting them into practice, and making them work so that the donor's own brilliance was reflected back to them. He was also adept at showcasing the impact of homegrown solutions. In the mid-1990s, a range of Ugandan research teams published data that showed declines in HIV prevalence—the percentage of people living with the virus—during the period in which the president had mobilized his people. This included a study of HIV rates among young pregnant Ugandan women attending antenatal clinics in three of the country's urban centers. That study found declines in prevalence between 1990 and 1996—roughly the period when the president had begun his mobilization against AIDS.[8]

In a separate study, researchers asked men and women about condom use and sexual behaviors, and the people said that they had increased condom use and decreased their number of sexual partners. If you put the two sets of information side by side—dropping prevalence and reports of increased fidelity, fewer partners, and greater condom use—it looked like the percentage of the Ugandan population living with HIV was decreasing because the populace had followed the president's advice. In fact, the two sets of information could not be directly linked as cause and effect: the information came from different groups, and the people who reported changes in sexual behavior and condom use were not tested for HIV. "Self-reported" sexual behavior is also a notoriously fiddly data source, since people may say what they believe the interviewer wants to hear or what is socially acceptable.

Nevertheless, the research team concluded that the drop in prevalence and the reported behavior changes supported "the efficacy of AIDS prevention and control interventions."[9] Museveni claimed the victory as his own, and soon enough UNAIDS agreed, issuing a report, *A Measure of Success in Uganda,* validating Uganda's approach and the impact of its prevention program.[10]

These findings concluded that Ugandan prevalence dropped, and that this drop was the result of Museveni's AIDS mobilization. It would be perhaps the single most politicized assertion in the history of the AIDS response in Africa, with implications that spanned decades, propelled billions of dollars of investment, and permeated mainstream understandings about Uganda and HIV, decades after new, better data told a different story. But Museveni was adept at sustaining a story line that captivated Western audiences long after his own citizens had dubbed it fiction.

As Uganda's economy had grown steadily during his first decade in office, so had Western concerns about whether he would accede to the "good governance" conditions of foreign aid and hold free and fair elections.[11] As Uganda funneled money and military support into conflicts in Rwanda and Congo, donors looked the other way and continued to shower praise on Museveni's AIDS response, even when he suggested that his political rival, Dr. Kizza Besigye, had HIV and might be unfit to govern. (At the time, Besigye criticized the president for using HIV status as a political weapon but did not directly address his own status.) The president also used analogies that were, as Katana put it, "very abusive to people living with HIV," such as when he said that people who put their hands into snake holes or termites nests got what they deserved, as though people living with the virus were dangerous vermin.[12] "We have never understood the President. At some points he shows up [as] an image of a champion for the AIDS cause, and in a flash of a second he makes utterances which are totally unbelievable," Katana told me. "At some point we think he is in it for some other reason."

In 2001, the donors praising Museveni also provided 94.4 percent of the country's AIDS budget, while the government bankrolled the military and a ballooning bureaucracy staffed by party loyalists. Donors focused on Ugandan success were undeterred even as the military reportedly displaced and abused civilians in the war-torn north, and "violated the international prohibition against aggressive use of force," in the Democratic Republic of Congo. "By 2000, an AIDS success story was crucial to a wide spectrum of 'stakeholders' who needed to justify further funding of their programmes," concluded Joseph Tumushabe, a Ugandan population scientist who calculated government expenditure on HIV in 2000–2001.[13]

The money that the government did spend on AIDS went for coordination between policymakers and political leaders, a modicum of HIV testing, and almost no medical care. People who received a positive diagnosis at a government-supported testing site could scour the country in vain for a government-funded HIV treatment program that provided free medication. A handful of military personnel did get free antiretrovirals, but it was rumored that Museveni scrutinized the list of service men in need and handpicked a chosen few. In February 2001, when the Indian pharmaceutical manufacturer Cipla announced price reductions, Museveni had not sought to get ahead of the curve, as he once had with his poverty-reduction strategies. He had not demanded access or presented donors with a plan for building clinics for his people. The prices had come down, but the systems by which the drugs would be delivered—the facilities, health staff, and education materials—still required action from the state.

Katana spent three days trying to show me how to help. She took me to meet other women who would help organize the meeting of women living with HIV and to look at the hotel where we'd house the women coming from out of town. She told me, patiently, that we needed a budget and that I would have to make one—I'd never organized a meeting before. She told me, too, that we should have a budget line for a nurse on site who could take care of medical issues if they arose among the participants. I said, "of course," and she told me that the nurse would be a woman named Cissy.

— —

BY THE TIME CISSY was diagnosed with HIV in Kampala, Uganda, in 1991, she was practiced in cheating death. The eldest daughter of a father who belonged to the same extended family as the king of Buganda, the tribe native to the country's central region, she'd grown up amid people who loved her so much they did not even let her know that she was in danger. Ugandan president Milton Obote was intent on destroying the Buganda kingdom, once favored by the British while Uganda was a protectorate. The army looked for the tribe's royalty, who were also its political leaders, and either jailed them or ensured that they "disappeared with no trace," as Cissy later learned.[14] Her father sent his family to live with Cissy's maternal grandparents as a safety precaution. They took pains to keep his children safe, both from the state and from a sense of danger. Her family seldom called her by her name. *Mumbeja*, they said. Princess. But they said it as if joking, lest an agent of the current government overheard.

"We were hiding, but we didn't know the meaning of the word." She remembered being confused about why her male relatives could fetch water off the property when she could not, but mostly she remembered the love and the sense of living off the land. "Everything was so natural. You get it from the garden, you cook it, you eat it. No frying at all. I never saw my grandparents fall sick," she'd recall some years later, when disease had ravaged her country. She wasn't even sure she knew why they'd died. In that house full of happiness, Cissy found ways to break the rules. "We could go out during the night, especially when the moon was high." They'd make noise then, she and her cousins and brothers, pure unbridled sounds of joy. "I felt protected," she recalled, even if she didn't quite understand why *Mumbeja's* uncles called her by this nickname as though it were a joke.[15] When she needed to, though, she remembered the strategy. Sometimes the truth could only be uttered out of the side of your mouth.

"My sister wants to wed," she'd said to the lab technician at the private clinic where she worked. She told her colleague that her sister wanted to check and see if she or her partner had HIV. "Fine," he said, "just bring the blood." Cissy drew her own blood and that of her husband, who'd returned from a business trip looking different, his hair curled in a manner she recognized as a sign of ill health. "I said, 'now what happened to your hair,' and he said, 'I have a terrible headache.'" They stood for a moment on the threshold of their home, and then her husband went inside. "I stayed outside on the verandah. The world was collapsing on me."

"So should I give you the good news first or the bad news?" the young lab technician asked. He liked to call Cissy "Auntie." "The bad news is your sister is infected. The good news is even the man is infected too, so they can go ahead with the wedding." "That time I blacked out," she'd recall. They comforted her as though her grief were for her sister, not herself.

Death had come for her before. There was the gun whose serial number she'd memorized while one of Idi Amin's men trained it on her cousin, a close relative she called by the Ugandan appellation "cousin-brother," in his own living room, as she'd sat beside her sister-in-law. The cousin-brother had died that night in the house, the sister-in-law in the car on the way to the hospital. Cissy, two days shy of her eighteenth birthday and only one year into her nursing degree, would nevertheless wonder her whole life why she hadn't been able to help her sister-in-law survive.

There had been more soldiers, more guns on a compound where she'd fled with an uncle and his family. That time, news had come to her family that Cissy had died. It took her so long to make her way back that by the time she returned, restoring herself from the dead, her father had already purchased the bark cloth shroud in which they intended to bury her.

As a nursing student on the wards, she'd wept with a family the first time a patient died on her watch. The nursing sister in charge had looked her up and down. Did Cissy plan to cry with every person who lost a relative? You couldn't bring back the person who had died, the sister had told her, and there were other ways to grieve besides weeping for every person. You helped the person who was still alive.

She and Katana had met at NGEN+, where they'd also met Lillian Mworeko, a majestic woman with a high forehead and searching eyes. Mworeko had received her own HIV diagnosis on the day that her husband, a biochemist who'd previously tested positive, died. In 1998, she'd found a business card for the major among her late husband's possessions and gone to find him. "I was young. I didn't know what to do," she recalled. Major Ruranga told her about his network. Mworeko went to the meetings and found the group well established, with meetings and fieldwork every weekend. But she was used to arriving when work was already underway. "I was good at catching up and doing things. So it was easy to get in and be accepted and start facilitating," she said.[16]

The first born of seven children, Mworeko grew up in the western part of the country, reared by an expansive, garrulous father and a strict, hardworking mother. Years later, she and her sister still laughed about the time her father had gotten off a bus from his job on a plantation with a parcel of fish but had given all of them away to neighbors by the time he got home. In contrast, her mother was "no nonsense." If a child went to school on a day that she was needed to help at home or in the garden, she didn't eat that night. "It was very rare that I would go to school very early in the morning," she'd later recall. Mworeko was bright enough that she excelled in school even when she arrived halfway through the day. On the days Mworeko arrived on time, she still missed lessons when she left to cook the teachers' lunch, an agreement they'd made since her family could not manage their fees. Like Katana, she earned a scholarship and arrived at a Catholic boarding school without the well-stocked metal trunks of her wealthier fellow students. "I was the only one with a wood suitcase in the whole school," she said.[17]

Katana, Mworeko, and Cissy all had mothers who'd worked hard and enjoyed less education than them; the three young women had gone on from secondary school to higher education—Mworeko had studied to be a teacher—as Museveni moved into the State House. They'd lived through the violence, instability, and terror of the regimes that had come before his ascent to power. They started their professional lives with high expectations, taking nothing for granted, intent on breaking new ground, and invested in doing whatever they could to prevent the country from devolving again into violence. None of them had planned on getting involved in a new war, but when the viral foe emerged, they hadn't had a choice.

One day, Cissy had come home and found her husband sitting despondently in the living room. Why wasn't the television on for the kids, she asked him. "'They should get used to having no TV,' he'd replied. 'They should get used to the hard times coming.' That's what he told me. Then I went in the bedroom. I started crying for my children. Then I said, 'No. Tears are not going to help me. I am going to fight like a woman.'"

She maintained her resolve even after her husband died beside her in the back of a car bound for his homeplace in Rakai District. Her in-laws had thought she was asleep when they began talking about his other family, the second wife. She had not known. "Let us help you, you won't manage, we know the *ka*-salary for nurses," she remembered her relatives saying, using the Lugandan suffix for small. She didn't want their help. "I said, 'I am going to add on the ka-salary.' I went for [a] counseling [certificate]." Armed with another qualification, she started to work with people living with HIV. "Sometimes I could put aside the counseling skills and say, 'You know I have HIV. I was like you, but see me. Just get yourself out of that box.'" She worked two jobs, one in the day and one in the evening, and raised her three children, aged eighteen months to six years, on her own. She hung a picture of the Blessed Virgin Mary on the wall. She worked and prayed. One night, she saw the man named Major Ruranga on television, and then she'd gone to find him.

— —

ON SEPTEMBER 4, 2001, when I met Cissy, she had three T cells. She was considering giving them names. She wore long sleeves because she'd had a violent reaction to nevirapine, the allergy known as Stevens-Johnson syndrome, which blisters the mucus membranes: the skin, the inside of the mouth, the lips, and the "soft parts," as she put it delicately. The skin on the blisters blackens, dies, and peels off; it leaves black patches, like the shadows that clouds make on the ground. She stopped one drug but not the others, even though, as a nurse, she knew this wasn't recommended. The drugs did not work, and her T cells dwindled. She needed a second-line regimen, an alternative, something called Kaletra, and that was expensive. I knew none of this on the day we met, though I'd learn it before we parted ways. That day, I asked her what she needed, and she told me only that she could use some funds for aspirin, antimalarials, and other supplies. She had large eyes and a full, expressive mouth. She looked at me steadily, her gaze warm and patient.

The next day, the women participants in the meeting began to arrive. They did not come at 2 p.m., as they'd been told; they arrived whenever their cramped taxi-van brought them into the taxi park that sat in a jumbled, cacophonous declivity down the hill from Bombo Road. They'd come walking, some of them, others on *boda boda* bicycles, a handkerchief held to their faces against the dust, a single change of clothes or perhaps just a night dress in a black plastic bag or a cheap branded airline tote.

They came smelling of the journey and where they'd started: smoke, sweat, children. Many wore layers of cloth, *kitenge*, one over the other, or *gomesi*, the puffy-shouldered traditional dress belted with a wide, obi-style sash. Someone organized a circle for people to introduce themselves. Just as they had in Durban, each woman in turn said her name, where she'd come from, and how long she had been "living positively," the phrase that NGEN urged its members to utter as though it were medicine.

When the meeting started the next day, a group of women boarded a bus to the International Conference Center on the grounds of the Nile Hotel, which Idi Amin had used as a center for torture and detention, reportedly throwing so many corpses down the elevator shaft that the car eventually could not settle on the ground floor. They listened to the scientific speeches, then milled around in the open hall for tea, conspicuous in their traditional dress. They were foreign even though they were the subject of the conversation.

After tea with the scientists, the women went back to the Hotel Africana to talk in terms they understood. Prominent women living with HIV, including Milly Katana and Beatrice Were, the founder of the National Community of Women Living with HIV/AIDS, led discussions about how the science of mother-to-child transmission intersected with women's lives. The women rose over and over to say that their doctors would not even examine them below their waists; that they had painful sores, discharge, and questions about whether they could have children. Their physicians would not touch them; if a woman came in pregnant, they often yelled at her for being irresponsible, sending her away with nothing but shame.

We talked about what an antiretroviral did in a woman's body and what it did in a baby's body and why it was absurd that this very simple two-dose regimen of nevirapine was not available for everyone who wanted it. The women stood up in turn and named what else was missing, as Katana had known they would: gloves and gauze and sterile instruments and personnel trained in handling difficult pregnancies. Together we tried, clumsily, to find the balance. The pills were essential to fight HIV, but the virus was one of many threats to their well-being.

On Monday night, we had a dance party. Cissy brought her daughters. They wore their school uniforms, had shaved heads, and smiled shyly at us all. An Italian doctor from Nsambya Hospital came and danced, swiveling his groin like Elvis, and the women pulled me aside and said that they were amazed that a doctor would dance with them. I counted the beers that we'd agreed to pay for, haggled with the front desk manager. I'd managed to pull off the role of being in charge. Elated, I grabbed the mic and called out to the women how glad I was to be there with them, shouting a quotation from the Jewish activist Emma Goldman I'd learned at Yiddish school many years before: "If I can't dance, I don't want to be part of your revolution."

The next day, the Tuesday of the conference, was its third full day, and we were going to move on from talking about nevirapine to discuss treatment for women themselves. We'd screen a rough cut of *Pills, Profits, Protest*, the documentary film that d'Adesky was working on with Shanti Avirgan and Ann Rossetti.[18] I pressed play on a big television on a cart, and then, as the film's portentous opening chords began to play to a largely empty room, I went to call the women in from outside. It was teatime, a highlight of the day. On the other side of the wall, stout women in black and white dispensed milk and tea and coffee from tower-sized thermoses and presided over metal platters of samosas, pigs in blankets, and small slices of bone-dry pound cake. Women sat on the grass or in chairs around the cloistered lawn of the inner courtyard, awash with Uganda's abundant, golden late-afternoon sun.

My Ugandan cell phone rang. "You'd better sit down," my friend Leslie Nielsen said. She was a blonde, practical nurse I'd met in New York when she was a nurse at a health center for children with HIV in Harlem. When I'd traveled to Uganda for a reporting trip after Durban, I'd found her at her new job based at JCRC. "I am," I lied. I stood in the door looking out. I tried to see if anyone Leslie and I knew was missing.

"Two planes have hit the World Trade Center and both buildings have both fallen down," she said. And then, because my father worked in the North Tower—a fact that Nielsen did not know—I started screaming. I dropped my phone onto the chair I should have sat on. I kept on screaming. I had not known that the thing people did in movies was a thing people did in real life, and that they did it in order to drown out news they had just heard and did not want to comprehend.

I was not alone for long. Milly and Cissy seized me with a force I'd felt once before, when I was ten years old and a lifeguard had swum out to fetch me from waves pulling me out to sea. Each gripping one of my arms, they steered me through a service door into a back room, all stainless steel and industrial appliances, both to give me privacy and because I was scaring the other women.

They did not let go of me; nor did they stop murmuring as they steered me through the hotel lobby, then up the stairs and into someone's borrowed room. I could scarcely hear them over my own cries. But I know that they did not tell me everything was going to be all right, only that I was going to be all right. There was a difference. You could not always cry for the dead, but you yourself kept going, even when the world as you had known it was unutterably changed. We would know each other all our lives, but even then, when we had just met, I knew that Milly and Cissy knew how to remain upright in their wildest grief. For that reason, I believed them.

CHAPTER 4

THE WORK OF MERCY

SHORTLY AFTER RETURNING FROM the Genoa Group of Eight (G8) meeting in July 2001, Gary Edson convened a Situation Room meeting of all the different US agencies working on global AIDS. He wanted to see who was doing what within the government on AIDS and to solicit input into the form and structure of the nascent, already embattled Global Fund. He'd been shocked by how many people showed up. It was standing room only, and yet each person represented a program working largely independently. What he saw of the US response looked like charity without clarity and most certainly did not meet his preconditions for a strategic action plan of knowing who would do what for whom and by when.[1] He'd taken note of the work to be done coordinating the US response and also of suggestions from his colleagues about structural elements to add to the Fund, like financial and technical bodies to ensure fiscal and scientific accountability. He'd taken those suggestions and used the American position as the Fund's largest donor to ensure that they were taken up at the Fund's initial inception meeting, which Health GAP also came to—appearing without invitation, then insisting on attending.

A few months later, Edson's job changed in ways he never could have imagined. After the September 11 attacks, he was charged with freezing terrorist assets, developing new global terms for travel security, including steps like hardening cockpit doors, and working through the G8 to strengthen export controls for portable surface-to-air missiles.

While the attacks changed the global landscape, they didn't sideline the administration's plans to overhaul aid and invest in African AIDS. Indeed, the attack brought a new rationale. Before, the effort reflected the belief that "Africa could be more than a charity case," Condoleezza Rice would write. "The events of September 11, 2001, added counterterrorism cooperation to that list."[2] In the following years, Bush's foreign aid ventures would frequently be viewed as a post-9/11 effort to counterbalance military incursions—"the sugar with the spice," as Health GAP member Sharonann Lynch liked to say. Indeed, countries in what would become the United States Africa Command, or AFRICOM, for the American military did have strategic value—particularly ones like Uganda, which were prepared to put boots on the ground in neighboring countries deemed vulnerable to Islamic separatists and terrorists.

But the groundwork for an aid overhaul, and scaled-up action on AIDS, had been laid prior to the attacks both within the United States and in global initiatives like the Millennium Development Goals. As 2001 came to an end, Edson saw this global momentum as another source of urgency. The United Nations was planning the first-ever conference on financing for development in Monterrey, Mexico, in March 2002. Officially launched at the G7 meeting, the Global Fund to Fight AIDS, Tuberculosis, and Malaria stood as the sole mechanism for combatting AIDS in sub-Saharan Africa and around the world, and Edson also knew that the upcoming G8 summit in Kananaskis, Canada, would have a strong focus on African countries. The White House needed to "get ahead of the curve," as Edson put it, advancing new ideas about aid rather than defending its critique of the current system; then he needed to continue the work on foreign aid and AIDS.

The planes hadn't prompted the actions Bush would soon take, he said. They'd simply changed the context in which they happened. In the aftermath of 9/11, Edson and colleagues accelerated the pace of work on issues that had been on the radar prior to the attacks in the form of task forces, one-on-one meetings, and a desire for foreign aid reform.[3] The attacks had intensified but not impelled action; I hoped the same could be said about me.

"Start moving," Eric Goemaere told me in Kampala on September 11, 2001. The elfin Belgian Médecins Sans Frontières doctor was the head of a trailblazing South African program in a Cape Town township called Khayelitsha. He explained that you always tried to get as close as you could to the disaster in case there were survivors. My friends tried to help, hurling the contents of my room into my bag. One of them picked up the hotel's insecticide, a towering black can labeled "DOOM." "No," I screamed. It might have been mere minutes or several hours since Milly Katana and Cissy had removed me from the conference hall. I still screamed whenever I spoke. "Not that. That's not mine."

That day, as it turned out, I was right. My father had left for work late and emerged from an R train that skipped his stop without announcement or explanation and discharged its final load of passengers at the base of the burning towers. He'd counted floors for a while, trying to figure out if his office had escaped the impact, waited to break a bill at a newsstand, waited some more for a payphone, and then turned his back to the flaming buildings and walked six miles home.

I was incandescent with relief when I learned that my father had survived. (His colleagues, so close to the point of impact they'd smelled jet fuel running down the exterior, also all made it out alive.) That night and in the days that followed, I became magnanimous, as loose with money as a monarch on a throne.

The "den mother" for the women participants, Sandra Kyagaba, was a petite twenty-something with braids and a blinding smile who stood with her feet planted slightly apart, like an athlete or a sailor on a rolling sea. When, on September 12, Kyagaba stopped me in the Hotel Africana lobby to explain to me that she could not access antiretrovirals (ARVs), I'd told her that I would help pay for them, first with a $500 honorarium for the work she'd done—an exorbitant fee by Ugandan standards—and then with my own money for as long as was needed. I did the same for Cissy, without a moment's hesitation. I was not motivated by or even wholly cognizant of how perilous their health was. HIV can weaken the body from the inside out. Both women were upright, vibrant, and—to my untrained eye—strong. I made my promises because I needed to discharge the gratitude fizzing in my blood, to do something to signal to whoever was watching that I understood and was worthy of my outsized good fortune.

The women of Uganda, the terrorist attacks, and the lifesaving medications were fused in my memory and suffused with something larger perhaps, even divine, that I was loathe to name. The Ugandan women who'd met me days prior gathered and prayed for the salvation of the father of the white woman who'd filled the hallways with her cries. Afterward, I was cracked open and shot through with an unformulated sense of providential intervention. I carried this back to America with me, and it troubled Kate Sorensen as much as my fretful indecision over protesting the inauguration once had. I'd glimpsed the suprastructure of the state, how it preserved privilege and concealed its violence. It was self-indulgent, dangerous to believe there was a reason other than race or class why a life was ever spared. But just then, I—like the men in the White House—was susceptible to a sense of privileged, American exceptionalism and the duty that came with that good fortune.

———   ———

EDSON KNEW THAT IF he wanted to do something innovative, he had to keep it something of a secret. The moment word leaked out that the US government was considering a new investment in foreign aid, he'd be besieged by outside groups and existing agencies, including USAID, clamoring for more money and a seat at the planning table. As a precaution, Edson held his meetings in the White House mess hall, where the clamor of dining and conversation gave his fact-finding an informal cover.

Over the latter portion of 2001, he met with a handful of aid experts, including Al Larson, who worked on economic affairs at the

State Department, Steve Radelet from the Treasury Department, and Clay Lowery from the National Security Council (NSC). Together, the men kicked the tires on the development theory du jour, which held that countries with good governance and sound economic policies used aid to grow their own economies, whereas other countries did not. Edson and his team of experts reckoned that a set of criteria borrowed from other independent institutions, like the anti-corruption group Transparency International and the World Bank Institute, could be used to determine which countries would use foreign aid for growth and that the best approach to aid would apply eligibility criteria to countries and also set guidelines for how the money could be spent. Countries should demonstrate good governance, invest in health and education, and promote economic freedom. Edson also reached out to Robin Cleveland, the program associate director for national security at the Office of Management and Budget (OMB). How, he asked her, could a new approach to aid be set up "without having it be subject to the earmarks that so encumbered USAID." Her answer was swift and simple: add a line to the federal budget. She even supplied the name: the Millennium Challenge Account.

For all his efforts, word of the work at hand leaked out, so he thought, when one of his bosses, Condoleezza Rice, asked him to come to her office to meet with Bono and Jamie Drummond, who'd come with their own ideas for turning aid around. He'd looked at their plan, which relied on countries' World Bank Poverty Reduction Strategy Papers (PRSPs).

The PRSP approach had been pioneered in Uganda by Yoweri Kaguta Museveni. As public health expert and journalist Helen Epstein and the British political scientist Jonathan Fisher have documented, Museveni merged keen intelligence with effervescent charm to win over donors and political allies. He'd retain their support even when his insistence on "one-party democracy" ran counter to their preference for free and fair elections.[4]

Museveni oversaw the development of a Poverty Eradication Action Plan (PEAP) that laid out a nationally owned strategy for lifting

Ugandans out of misery. The World Bank saw the PEAP as evidence that Uganda would make good on its loans and aid, and it became something of a template for the PRSP that the World Bank now required from any country seeking to qualify for debt relief under the Heavily Indebted Poor Countries program. Drummond and Bono liked the PRSPs, as Edson recalled. But he thought they were "not sufficiently rigorous and provided a poor guide for action." The World Bank had no great track record of tying country strategies to real change. It had plowed money into plans that favored corporations, environmental destruction, and austerity measures that undermined any attempt to alleviate poverty. While Uganda would see several years of economic expansion, the poorest of the poor remained in dire straits. Moreover, Edson thought that Bono and Drummond had no objective way of distinguishing a good PRSP from one that would have no impact.

By the time of the meeting with Bono and Drummond, Edson had put together a two-page proposal that outlined what he thought *should* happen; he soon delivered it to Rice. She'd then walked him over to the Oval Office, where they briefed the president. As Edson recalled, he signed off then and there on the concept of what would eventually evolve into the first major US aid agency in four decades. Armed with the green light and with Rice's instrumental leadership and support, he and his team swung into action, identifying the sixteen external criteria that would be used, along with a per capita income threshold, to determine countries' eligibility. The PRSPs didn't make the list, though by Drummond's account he moved to Washington, DC, for six weeks to help develop the new strategy.[5] Edson countered that he'd accommodated all voices, but he and his team took pains to ensure that the vision didn't get watered down.

On March 14, 2002, the president stood in a sun-filled atrium at a meeting of the Inter-American Development Bank, with Bono, World Bank president James Wolfensohn, and Cardinal Theodore McCarrick, the onetime archbishop of Washington, DC, behind him. With the endorsement of the church, a Bretton Woods Institution leader, and the celebrity antipoverty crusader, he announced a "new compact for global development, defined by new accountability for rich and poor nations alike." It was also defined by a major increase in funding. "I have proposed a fifty-percent increase in our core development assistance over the next three budget years. Eventually this will mean a five billion dollar increase over current levels." The president had confidence that the United States could spend that money wisely—and not toss it down a rathole—because of the new aid approach. "These new funds will go into a new Millennium Challenge Account, devoted to nations that govern justly, invest in their people, and encourage economic freedom."[6]

A few weeks later, at the International Conference on Financing for Development in Monterrey, Mexico, participants issued a consensus statement that enshrined the Millennium Challenge Corporation (MCC) principles of prioritizing aid to countries whose approach to governance, economic policies, and investment in health and education met standards set by the Western world. At that same meeting, now assured that it could spend aid in ways that it saw fit, the Bush administration endorsed the Millennium Development Goals on behalf of the United States.[7]

As Edson talked to me about the MCC, his eyes shone. He flipped through pages of printouts slipped from the folders stacked beside him. The passage he was looking for was almost always already highlighted. He read aloud, holding the sheets at the arms-length distance of aging vision, his voice crackling with excitement. Bush's speech at the Inter-American Development Bank was perhaps the finest he had ever heard.

Shortly after lunch though, Edson's glow seemed to fade. We had been talking for over two hours; he'd been doing much of the speaking. He had a right to be tired. But I thought it was more than that. We'd reached the end of the part of the story when everything had still seemed possible and arrived at the moment when reality set in.

As we spoke that day in 2020, the MCC still existed and was held in high regard. The aid approach of transparency, country ownership, and tying assistance to results had gained global currency, with MCC's core principles embodied in the 2005 Paris Declaration on

Aid Effectiveness and echoed—"hook, line and sinker," as Edson said—across the funder landscape. While the principles infused the aid community, practical implementation was uneven. MCC's launch was delayed, then botched. PEPFAR wasn't even an idea at the time that Bush announced the MCC, but the law creating it had moved faster, and money and public support had flowed more freely for the AIDS war than for the MCC. Edson had moved on by then. He'd needed to put his attention to other initiatives, and the staffing, leadership, and launch of the new entity had fallen to others.

In January 2020, then, America was not much closer to a cohesive, strategic national framework for selecting countries and evaluating the impact of its assistance than it had been two decades prior. The HIV-specific effort stood out as a notable success, but America's disease-fighting aid deserved better. Each time the government passed up the chance to reform aid, it reinforced the misconception that pandemics were caused by, and could be remediated by tackling, pathogens alone—and not the politics and uneven distribution of wealth and power that drove them.

When Edson and I finally agreed that it was time to talk about PEPFAR, I felt a sense of guilty satisfaction, like a fan hearing the opening chord of a rocker's greatest hit after a full set of new material. I was ready for some good news. In a way, my jog of pleasure was part of the problem. Lots of people got an endorphin rush off of aid that paid for life-saving pills that they just didn't get from the MCC's cost-benefit analyses and economic rate-of-return calculations for roads or power plants. Jamie Drummond, Bono's close associate and cofounder of the ONE Campaign, explained the difference between MCC and PEPFAR to me in terms of intellect and emotion. "One is a very sober, cold development policy initiative, and the other is a humanitarian response to an AIDS emergency."[8]

But I wasn't a sucker for soft-focus babies and suffering Africans. There was a finer point to my satisfaction. PEPFAR had been an American rejoinder to the Fund, a counterproposal based in part on the proposition that more people could be treated faster by a program that the United States designed and controlled. The moment that the activists began to sketch the lineaments of the "whole new thing," they began to navigate this trade-off between speed and local governance, their arguments shifting, albeit subtly, from cheap AIDS drugs by any means necessary to cheap AIDS drugs via a mechanism that embodied the movement's principles. After PEPFAR was announced, I'd marked that shift and had not been entirely sure that I agreed.

By that time, my susceptibility to the promises of the state had become a problem between me and Kate Sorensen. My father had said little about the day of the attack, save that he admired New York City mayor Rudy Giuliani for putting on a hard hat and heading downtown while the fires were still raging. When I repeated that admiration, she looked at me with blank exhaustion. Men like him, including the president, were not heroes. Not ever. Not even for a day. That kind of heroism was itself a toxic myth. I'd learned a little but not enough, and our relationship ended soon after.

"Let's talk about PEPFAR," I said to Edson. Every time I went back over the story, it was a chance to worry about a shape-shifting question that had stayed with me for nearly twenty years: Could speed in saving lives justify interaction on issues that put those lives at risk? Could a nation that perpetrated plagues effectively do good things? Could the United States of America do something I truly believed in?

—— ——

THE STORY STARTED WITH a plane. In April 2002, just a few weeks after the meeting in Monterrey on international development, Dr. Anthony Fauci, the head of the National Institute of Allergy and Infectious Diseases, and the head of the Department of Health and Human Services, former Wisconsin governor Tommy Thompson, boarded a jet for a whirlwind four-country fact-finding mission on AIDS in Africa. Fauci was charged by President Bush with finding out what could be done on AIDS that would be "transforming." One year prior, in 2001, Fauci had paid a visit to Peter Mugyenyi's AIDS ward in Kampala, Uganda. Then, he'd experienced a terrible sense of déjà vu—as he wrote in the scrupulous notes he kept on the meetings he had and the places he visited as one of the most influential American scientists working on AIDS. Fauci hadn't remained in Mugyenyi's office, as I had. The Ugandan physician ushered his American counterpart into the wing of the building where ranks of beds held people in the end stages of AIDS. Fauci had seen it before. In America, he'd treated the dying before the virus had a name, deducing its presence by the "opportunistic infections"—Kaposi's sarcoma, Pneumocystis carinii pneumonia, mycobacterium avium complex—that took advantage of the compromised immune system.[9]

Mugyenyi, as politically savvy and influential in his native country as Fauci was in his, had walked him around, explaining the types of palliative care he offered for these people who were dying of conditions like the ones Fauci had treated in America and suffering from other afflictions that he'd been able to treat even at the worst of times: florid cases of oral thrush, tuberculosis, and cryptococcal meningitis. What little Mugyenyi had been able to offer had been like "putting a Band-Aid on a hemorrhage," as Fauci would often later say.

One year later, in April 2002, Fauci found more reason for optimism. The two-dose nevirapine regimen that slashed rates of mother-to-child transmission was finally being rolled out as activists in Uganda, South Africa, and numerous other countries had demanded. A politically savvy scientist, Fauci had come back with a proposal that hit the sweet spot between ambitious and affordable. For about $500 million, he reckoned, you could really make a difference. He pitched the plan at a meeting that included the president and his brother Jeb Bush and was delighted when it got the green light.

On Capitol Hill, Senator Bill Frist, a scientifically savvy politician, and Senator Jesse Helms, the notoriously conservative politician, had joined forces to mobilize Republican action on AIDS in Africa and come up with a strikingly similar proposition. Trained as a heart and lung transplant surgeon, Frist arrived in Washington, DC, with a deep faith and an understanding of the toll of untreated AIDS gleaned from medical training and mission trips to Africa. He had a number of like-minded Democratic counterparts, including John Kerry and Joe Biden. Republican allies on AIDS were harder to come by. One afternoon in 2001, Frist, Dr. Kenneth Bernard—who'd joined Frist's office at the end of the Bill Clinton administration—and his legislative director, Allen Moore, attended an event on HIV at the Center for Strategic and International Studies where a woman with HIV and her baby—also infected with the virus—appeared. As Bernard recalled, Frist decided that this woman, or a woman like her, needed to come to visit his compatriot Jesse Helms, an influential Republican lawmaker who believed HIV was a punishment exacted on gays for their immoral, sinful ways. Frist had been quietly working to win Helms over for more than a year; Bono, too, had zeroed in on Helms as an ally in a globally oriented Christian compassion, quoting scripture to him with an Irish lilt, showering his wife with attention at a small dinner, and urging him to expand his vision.[10]

Whether it was that woman or another one, Bernard could not recall—but he and his colleagues arranged for an African woman with HIV to visit Helms's office and for the venerable senator to hold her baby. "Jesse Helms held the baby and started to get emotional and tear up, and then he turned around to Bill Frist and said, 'Bill, this just is wrong. I don't care what you guys do. You need to do something about this, you have my full support.'" It would not do to have these babies dying of the global scourge. Helms agreed to work with Frist to mobilize funding for AIDS in Africa.[11] "We cannot turn away," Helms wrote in a March 24, 2002, editorial. "I know of no more heartbreaking tragedy in the world today than the loss of so many young people to a virus that could be stopped if we simply provided more resources."[12] As he described in the editorial, he and Frist sought an additional $500 million in the emergency supplemental appropriations bill to enable USAID to pay for treatments to prevent vertical transmission.

When the West Wing caught wind of the Helms-Frist proposal to invest in prevention of vertical transmission, Nancy Dorn, the deputy director of the Office of Management and Budget came to Moore and told him that the president wanted to be in the lead on the initiative. She also shared the White House view that $500 million couldn't be spent in a single year—as it would be if the full amount was written into the supplemental appropriations bill.[13] As Moore recalled, she said, "We want to have a White House ceremony next week and make it a presidential initiative, with appropriate recognition to Helms and Frist."[14] Turning the issue over to the White House was easier than reducing the proposed ask from $500 million "no year" funding—available for an indefinite period of time—to a $200 million request for the coming fiscal year. Still, Frist swallowed hard and agreed to reduce the request to $200 million for the coming fiscal year—a step that earned swift condemnation in the press.[15]

Bush's OMB staffer had urged Frist to scale back his ambitions for the coming fiscal year, but shortly after the president announced the Mother and Child HIV Prevention Initiative in a Rose Garden event on June 19, 2002, Bush turned to his deputies and told them he wanted to do more on AIDS. The new money for preventing vertical transmission simply wasn't enough. His deputy chief of staff for policy, Josh Bolten, returned to Fauci and asked him to think bigger, saying, "If money were no object, what would you do?" Bolten meant it. He knew that he "had the President's support and that [he] probably could beat Mitch Daniels [the head of the OMB] in an arm-wrestling confrontation for a few hundred million dollars, or something like that, or maybe even billions."[16]

When Edson and I met, he too recalled the president asking what could be done if there were no financial limits. I knew the scene well, for it featured in all three quasi-official accounts of his AIDS war. I also knew that there had been considerable prior work on the part of senators, including, but not limited to, Helms, Frist, Kerry, and Russ Feingold, and by members of the House of Representatives, including Ron Dellums, Barbara Lee, Nancy Pelosi, Tom Lantos, and Henry Hyde. These legislators and their peers had been urging action and proposing legislation to address AIDS in Africa for years prior.

Indeed, at the precise moment that Bush asked for even more mercy, a well-developed Senate proposal that appeared to fit the bill was already in the works. The path to the Senate bill began in June 2001. On the eve of the UN special session on AIDS, one of those champions, Representative Henry Hyde, an Illinois Republican, introduced a bill calling for a $50 million investment in antiretrovirals, a $15 million Global Fund contribution in 2002, and a $654 million contribution over the 2002–2006 period.

At a June 7, 2001, House International Relations Committee hearing before the bill's introduction, members of Congress sent up warning flares about putting US funding into a "multilateral" pool that could be used for nefarious purposes. "Once you have given to an organization where we lack control, then it is going to be given to Iran, as the World Bank did, and it might be given to the government of Sudan," Representative Brad Sherman, a California Democrat, said. "And then those of us who advocate more expenditures on foreign aid can do nothing more than hope that our constituents become unaware of how their money is being spent."[17]

USAID administrator Andrew Natsios testified at that hearing, offering a warning about the Global Fund that centered on its stated commitment to treat AIDS. "If you look at Kofi Annan's budget, half the budget is for antiretrovirals. If we had them today, we could not distribute them. We could not administer the program because we do not have the doctors, we do not have the roads, we do not have the cold chain," he said. He went on.

> This sounds small, and some people, if you have traveled to rural Africa you know this, this is not a criticism, just a different world. People do not know what watches and clocks are. They do not use western means for telling time. They use the sun. These drugs have to be administered during a certain sequence of time and when you say take it at 10:00, people will say what do you mean by 10:00? They do not use those terms in the villages to describe time. They describe the morning and the afternoon and the evening. So that is a problem.[18]

Natsios repeated his assertion that "Africans can't tell time" to the *Boston Globe*, and it soon became a soundbite synonymous with a racist, wrongheaded view of Africans and their ability to take AIDS drugs. But the full sweep of his remarks that day bespoke a different prejudice that would be more difficult to dismantle. The remark implied that Western AIDS treatment approaches were unalterable. However, the drugs did not have to be taken at a specific hour, just consistently. A person who took them each morning at, say, the time the children left for school or a radio program began or a cow required milking would do as well as someone who set a digital clock to chime. Natsios's implication that only people who owned clocks and wore watches could take the pills signaled that the agency would insist on doing what made sense to its experts—not to the people it served. When I spoke to him some years later, I gleaned another layer of meaning. He'd looked at the requirements for delivering AIDS drugs and the state of the national health systems in the countries that needed them and concluded that providing AIDS meds meant superimposing modern tech onto "old systems," which "given the sophistication of the treatment process," would require, as he put it, "a neocolonial approach."[19]

Reportedly irked by Natsios's assertion, Hyde and his cosponsors introduced the bill and saw it passed in late 2001. After that, it moved languidly toward consideration by the Senate until John Kerry and Frist were ready to propose their own legislation—a development that coincided with the highly secret West Wing mission for outsized mercy.[20]

"We must continue to embrace the new Global Fund for HIV/AIDS, TB and Malaria. This is not a UN fund, or an American fund. It is a new way of doing business," Senator Frist, the Republican physician from Tennessee, declared in his prepared statement for an April 11, 2002, Senate committee hearing called "Capacity to Care in a World Living with AIDS."[21]

The following month, on May 15, Frist, Joe Biden, John Kerry, Jesse Helms, and thirteen other senators introduced the United States Leadership Against HIV/AIDS, Tuberculosis, and Malaria Act of 2002, which authorized a $1 billion contribution to the Global Fund in FY2003 and a $1.4 billion contribution the following year.[22] In order to move to legislation with bicameral support, the senators introduced the Lantos-Hyde bill, then proposed replacing its text with the text of their more ambitious Fund-focused bill, a move that meant the two pieces of legislation would need to be resolved in conference.

The fivefold increase over Bush's $200 million contribution still didn't bring American financing for AIDS to the $2.5 billion threshold, but activists greeted the legislation with cautious optimism. "After two decades of neglect, Congress is finally preparing to roll up its sleeves and confront the global AIDS disaster. This progress is welcome, and long overdue," said Asia Russell of Health GAP.[23]

As the Senate considered the Kerry-Frist bill, though, Dr. Fauci got to work on the plan that Bolten had requested, with Edson taking on the task of subjecting whatever Fauci proposed to "due diligence"—ensuring that it was an actionable strategy. Fauci got the distinct impression that President George W. Bush absolutely wanted to do something big—and that he didn't want it to be multilateral. Fauci had befriended Tommy Thompson, head of the Department of Health and Human Services, and ended up in "a lot of Situation Room meetings where we were talking about what our approach was going to be to the Global Fund." Fauci recalled the United States being willing to contribute up to one-third of the Global Fund's total resources. "But it was very clear in my discussions with the White House staff and then the few times—which turned out to be many times subsequently—that I spoke to the President that he was a little bit reluctant in getting engaged too deeply in multilateral [efforts]," Fauci said. "He always felt that if you wanted to get something done it had to be transforming but it also had to be accountable and whenever you have a bunch of multilateral things he . . . had a little skepticism about that."[24]

Edson swore Fauci to secrecy, while members of the small group of West Wing staff who were in on the plan kept encouraging him to think big. "I knew I had a mandate from the president to think more broadly about the problem and that he was prepared to do something fairly aggressive," Bolten said. "I had also been weathering lobbying from Bono and his folks and his organization at the time."[25] As Fauci recalled, Bush's domestic policy advisor Jay Lefkowitz—who'd help steer the president towards a position on stem cell research—took it a step further, asking Fauci, "What's the moon shot here?"

Time-consuming under any circumstances, the task was nearly impossible to do in secret. In order to work up a public health moon shot and keep up with his day job, Fauci recruited Dr. Mark Dybul, a young researcher and physician in his lab, to help devise the proposal. Both men leaned on the visits they'd made to clinics in recent years. They were taken by the Ugandan example of a "hub-and-spoke" approach, in which central facilities did the lab work and stored the drugs, while more basic, distal sites provided the care. Fauci had seen Mugyenyi's clinic; Dybul had visited Mugyenyi and also gone to Tororo, on the country's easternmost edge, and seen a research project funded by the Centers for Disease Control and Prevention (CDC) that put all the medications and supplies a household needed on the back of a motorcycle ridden by a community health worker with the equivalent of a high school degree. The research project, known as the Home-Based AIDS Care (HBAC) project, was irresistible—the love child of Mother Teresa and Bruce Springsteen—and Dybul would credit it for years to come as a major inspiration.

By July 2002, as the AIDS world began packing its bags for the World AIDS Conference—which had moved from Durban to Barcelona—Fauci and Dybul had a rough sketch of a plan. Both men departed for the meeting, with Fauci assuring Dybul he would present the proposal when the time was right.

I'd left for the conference too, heartbroken over the final end of my relationship with Kate Sorensen a few months prior. We'd split in April, and I'd descended into maddened, hard-drinking sadness. "I'm wracked with grief," I declared to a bemused, blue-eyed man at my best friend's wedding the night before I flew to Barcelona. "Memory is a garden, eventually it becomes ground," he replied, paraphrasing V. S. Naipaul. I looked at him with surprise and curiosity. Perhaps because he didn't ever drink alcohol, Liam Flaherty spoke to me as though I was clear-headed and, for an instant, I was. I'd nearly forgotten that words could be salvation.

—— ——

IN DURBAN, ACTIVIST RAGE and power had fueled a sense of rapid change, of making history. It had been a fever dream. Twenty-four months later, the taste of bile sat at the back of the throat, and no amount of *jamon iberico* or *vino tinto* could wash it away. On the first full day in Barcelona, Milly Katana gave a plenary talk—we'd worked on the speech together. She was intent on shifting from telling a story that centered on herself and her body to taking a professional, intellectual stance. The program had run long, and I sat in the audience in dismay as people walked out while she spoke, an exodus that embodied the meeting's historical moment—after personal testimony, before full-scale response.

The movement was winning in increments, but the revolution was not coming fast enough. Two days prior to the start of the conference, on July 5, 2002, the Constitutional Court of South Africa had ruled in favor of the Treatment Action Campaign and its claim that state failure to make nevirapine for prevention of vertical transmission available nationally was a violation of the right to access health care.[26] With that victory, a woman with HIV would be assured a single dose of nevirapine at the time of delivery, as would her newborn. She would not receive another state-funded antiretroviral until she delivered again. For while the Treatment Action Campaign had won nevirapine, the government—still gripped by AIDS denialism—was far from sponsoring a national treatment program.

The global fight to force drug companies to drive down their prices and back off patent protections for essential medications had secured concessions in the Agreement on Trade-Related Aspects of Intellectual Property Rights that bound nations in the World Trade Organization, but the United States had put up fierce resistance, and few nations had the cheap, essential drugs they needed.

A year after its launch, the Global Fund was still in the early stages of proving its worth, defining its identity and ways of working. It was also caught in a vicious cycle defined by shared mistrust, not shared responsibility. The Fund's funding shortfall and donor-country admonishments to low-income countries to be cautious led to unambitious proposals with treatment targets that were inadequate for national needs. If the countries didn't submit large, ambitious proposals, the Fund looked like it was functioning as planned—letting countries take the lead. But this perception ignored history. Low-income countries were hesitant to submit costly proposals, since decades of yo-yoing aid had conditioned a cautious approach: only ask for aid for programs that might last if the donor went away. The donors were, in some instances, actively urging caution in the midst of carnage, Health GAP thought.

Activists like Asia Russell and Paul Davis worked to push back against donors who urged countries to be realistic in their funding requests, asking for what was feasible, not what was needed to stop the carnage. Russell, who gives rousing speeches with a preacher's cadence and has a shout like a raven's cry, remembered that time as one of seeking to ensure that activist arguments became "the signal in the noise." "It was like a detuned radio and you're trying to tune it," she said. "There were just so many unfounded but seemingly compelling arguments against aggressive scale up. Part of our job was to assault those as systematically as possible."[27] The Fund was also facing the challenge that many countries needed to address both the emergency of AIDS and the long-term project of building health systems. Setting up a funding approach that paid for both at the same time hadn't been done before, and by 2002 the Fund still hadn't figured out what tack to take.

When, on July 9, US Secretary of Health and Human Services Tommy Thompson—Fauci's traveling companion on his whirlwind AIDS junket—took the stage to deliver a speech about America's AIDS response, the bile overflowed. Activists rose up out of their seats. As they walked down the shallow stairs to the stage, Eustacia Smith, Amanda Lugg, Gaelle Krikorian, and Sharonann Lynch juggled placards they'd carried in under their shirts, gripping stacks under their arms, handing them out to other protesters as planned.

At the bottom of the stairs, the activists roared, pointed fingers, and cried, "$10 billion for the Global Fund. Shame, shame, shame." They would not stop, as they sometimes did, after they had made their point, to allow a speaker to continue. The time for negotiated dialogue was over. They drowned Thompson out while his beefy, crew-cut security officers stood behind him on the stage looking on.

Thompson reportedly took the activist action personally, reacting with fury at the activists' disrespect. Fauci calmed him down with stories of all the times he'd drawn activist fire in public, then negotiated with them behind the scenes. This was a performance, he explained, then brokered a meeting between Thompson and the activist groups. The radical call to do more created an ideal backdrop for Fauci to share the proposal he and Dybul had devised.

After the conference, Dybul had retreated to a white-walled, red-tiled convent turned boutique hotel in La Parra, Spain. He'd been summoned from the pool by the proprietor one day, pressed the phone to his ear, and heard Fauci's New York–ese crackling over the line. "Mark, it's Tony. They [the White House team] loved it; we've got to do it."

Dybul handwrote a longer version of the proposal on the plane ride home, then typed it up and, with Fauci, presented it at a meeting that Edson convened in the Situation Room. As Edson recalled, he deemed it intriguing but not nearly detailed enough for him to take to his boss. Edson warned Fauci he'd have to make the case well and thoroughly. Bush had a hunger for mercy; he also had an MBA. The proposal had to stand up to a venture capitalist's scrutiny. When you planned the moon shot, you couldn't eliminate risk, but you asked for every ounce of evidence that the rocket wouldn't turn into a bomb.

Fauci and Dybul went to work on a more detailed revision. There weren't many treatment programs for people with HIV in poor countries—fewer than 50,000 Africans with HIV were on lifelong treatment at the time. So they cobbled together every existing shred of data on the costs of drugs and diagnostics, and approaches to delivering them, in resource-poor settings. They pored over numbers compiled by UNAIDS, the United Nations agency that coordinated efforts on the epidemic, and looked beyond AIDS, pulling data from the Indian Health Service in Alaska, which also used a hub-and-spoke model.

To transfer the hub-and-spoke approach to different countries, the pair mapped the estimated number of people living with HIV and where they were concentrated in each country. They calculated how many hubs and spokes would be needed to bring AIDS drugs to different proportions of those populations, focusing on thirteen sub-Saharan African countries with overwhelmingly high burdens of HIV disease.

When it came to prevention, the plan included information from John Stover, a public health expert who specialized in modeling—calculating the theoretical costs and impacts of various interventions—and provided unpublished estimates of the impact of and price tag for different prevention packages, including condoms, HIV testing, and mass education.[28]

Fauci told me that Edson warned him he was going to have to "iterate" the proposal until it could withstand the rigorous due diligence process that Edson intended to subject it to. Every data point and assumption needed to be tested and vetted, not because the president was unwilling to act but because he was ready to commit substantial resources, and the plan they put together had to be one that delivered results. Fauci, who keeps a meticulous diary, would later tell Edson he reckoned they'd met or spoken ninety or one hundred times over a period of three months—encounters in which the physician and researcher explained what could be done, and Edson explained what else he still needed to know. "When you deal with the White House, it's sort of interesting," Fauci explained to me. "It's like, 'Okay, give us a plan of multiple countries. What happens if you put this country in and pull out these two countries?'" No matter what the questions were, his reply was always the same. "Okay, we'll rework it."

Sometimes, Edson, Fauci, Bolten, Lefkowitz, OMB staffer Robin Cleveland, and Bolten's deputy Kristen Silverberg gathered in person, taking care to gather in rooms in the Old Executive Office Building or in Lefkowitz's office, in order to avoid attention and questions. As the year drew to a close, though, it became clear that at least one meeting needed additional participants before the plan could go to the president. As Fauci recalled, the request came from the Office of Management and Budget. "They joked saying, 'White guy in a suit, we've been listening to you. You've been taking care of AIDS patients for years and years, but they've all been in the United States...You've got to bring me a few people who are actually doing this.'" Given forty-eight hours to assemble the participants, Fauci called Dr. Eric Goosby, a clinician who'd treated AIDS patients in the Bay Area before expanding to work in sub-Saharan Africa; Ugandan Joint Clinical Research Center director Peter Mugyenyi; and Dr. Jean Pape, a debonair Haitian with a well-established research site in Port au Prince. He added Paul Farmer, the saintliest white man working on global AIDS, to this collection of black men in suits.

Mugyenyi told me that he was on the western edge of Uganda at Queen Elizabeth National Park when he got the call;[29] Goosby was walking through an airport in Rwanda.[30] They dropped everything to get to DC—but even at top speed, Mugyenyi arrived in DC too late to join the other experts at Trattoria Sorrento, an Italian restaurant in Bethesda, Maryland, where Fauci briefed them on their mission. It was a dinner that shouldn't have happened. Fauci was, in a way, tampering with witnesses. But over his usual—*arrabbiata* and fried calamari—the doctor who knew the politics of public health as well as anyone explained the stakes.[31] He wouldn't leave anything to chance.

The next day, the experts endured hours of questions about what was possible from a group including the West Wing team; Robin Cleveland; and Nils Daulaire, a physician who headed the DC-based Global Health Council. The physicians offered evidence and images of healthy Black bodies as proof that treatment worked in poor people and impoverished settings. Here was a skeleton, here a man with a wide smile and smooth skin. They were the same person.

"Don't give up, stick to your guns," Joe O'Neill, the White House AIDS czar told Peter Mugyenyi during a coffee break. (O'Neill was the only member of the White House team who was a physician regularly seeing patients and played an instrumental role in the creation of the President's Emergency Plan for AIDS Relief [PEPFAR], though he is the only one of its architects who has not done public interviews about the subject.) Mugyenyi didn't give up, insisting in his slightly high-pitched, assured voice that his clients could and did take ARVs; that his clinic could and did measure their immune health, side effects, and drug resistance. Mugyenyi had long accepted that northern nations saw proof that Black Africans could take medications as a prerequisite for generosity. If he didn't question the premise, he also refused to give quarter in a "due diligence" session so rigorous that it smacked of skepticism. Mugyenyi recalled that one of the participants came to his hotel that evening to apologize and explain that they'd had to be thorough in order to make sure that the program would pass muster with their boss, who was deeply and personally committed to taking action.

"That meeting gave us the final bits of ammunition that we needed," Edson told me. "It went right into the decision memo that I wrote for the president."[32]

By late November, the proposal that Edson had put through its paces was sound enough to take to the president. It contained a series of options that Fauci classified in terms of cars: a Mercedes, an Oldsmobile, a budget Chevrolet.[33] The vehicles in this runaway American dream stood in for price tags, which in turn stood in for different proportions of the population to be treated with antiretrovirals.

The ambition of the proposals was exciting—it also had an analog in a bill making its way through Congress. Weeks before the meeting that informed the White House decision memo, the House/Senate conference to reconcile the two AIDS bills swung into action. The process hit snags right away. One congressional aide would later say that each chamber expected to prevail and so delayed starting discussions in earnest. "There was a presumption on the Senate side that the House should just accept the Senate bill and pass it—and there was a presumption on the House side that our bill was smaller, cleaner, and more feasible. So neither side began talking in earnest, negotiating in earnest, until the very tail end of the session." Jurisdictional concerns reportedly abounded—different congressional committees wanted oversight; USAID and CDC could not agree on who should do what, even though both proposals carried recommendations for a neutral, high-level coordinator position. In the Kerry-Frist bill, the position would hold the rank of ambassador and sit at the Department of State. When Republicans gained control of the Senate in late 2002, that shook things up even more.[34]

By the time the Kerry-Frist bill died in conference at the end of the 107th session, Paul Davis had realized he wasn't getting any traction among "Congress critters" for a major contribution for the Global Fund. In the preceding months, the United States had begun what felt like an inexorable march to war. Each passing day brought new assertions of Iraqi menace, with claims from weapons inspectors that there was no evidence of concealed wrongdoing.

In September 2002, the White House released a new National Security Strategy (NSS) that stated, "While the United States will constantly strive to enlist the support of the international community, we will not hesitate to act alone," including "preemptively" where needed.[35] Elaborated throughout the document, that assertion of the right to use preemptive force, which would come to be called the "Bush Doctrine," was to some extent a more explicit statement of a preexisting interventionist stance that sought to consolidate America's post–Cold War domination. But it raised additional alarms by marking "a potentially major shift by arguing not for pre-emptive military strikes (when an attack is imminent) but preventive war," as one foreign policy expert said at the time.[36]

While the Bush Doctrine dominated discussion of the NSS, the same document also elevated development and foreign aid as part of security strategy with unusual clarity about what a "smart power" agenda should look like—putting the traditional "soft power" development agenda on par with national security. With a blind but excoriating takedown of USAID, the NSS embraced the principles of the Millennium Challenge Account: outcomes not inputs, shared accountability for results and sound economic policies, investment in the people, and a focus on results.

Davis wanted the Global Fund, but he wanted AIDS drugs for Africa just as much. Working with Paul Zeitz of the Global AIDS Alliance, Salih Booker, and a range of faith-based and Black American groups, Health GAP launched a call for a comprehensive presidential AIDS initiative and planned a march and civil disobedience to call attention to their demands.[37] As the groups assembled their position, the Congressional Black Caucus dispatched a letter to the president asking for a major initiative on African AIDS.[38] By the time they'd sent the letter, though, the proposal for PEPFAR had been presented to the president.

On December 4, the day of the White House Hanukkah party, Lefkowitz, an observant Jew, had accompanied the president to a meeting with select Jewish leaders who'd praised the president's moral rectitude, telling him that he would have bombed the tracks leading to the death camps—a step Franklin D. Roosevelt had failed to take. Lefkowitz would always remember how they'd left that meeting and walked straight to the Oval Office for the final PEPFAR discussion, how the president had looked around the room and declared that there was no choice but to act.[39] He'd given the green light to the most ambitious proposal, brushing aside some consternation from OMB head Mitch Daniels. The size of the effort was no longer in question. But the president grabbed Edson before he'd left the room. Signing off on the proposal had been easy, he said. Now came the hard thing. "You understand now you have to make this happen."

Almost no one outside the small rooms the team from the White House and the National Institute of Allergy and Infectious Diseases used for its meetings had any inkling of what was coming. But many people knew what was needed. On November 26, 2002, I marched with hundreds of other people down a windy DC street. "Bush Junior, Bush Senior, which one dealt with AIDS? Neither," I shouted until my throat was raw, trying to keep the body bag prop in my arms from floating away in the wind. I set it down before the wrought iron fence of the White House so that I could chain myself to the people I stood beside, getting arrested for the second time in my life.

By the time I was arrested, the OMB meeting had vetted and signed off on the ambitious AIDS plan. When I asked Fauci about the role of activists in it all, I let a hint of pique creep into my voice.

"The thing is, so many people think they were involved and they had no idea. They were talking in vagaries," Fauci replied. He corrected himself. "I don't mean vagaries." And then, as though he actually did mean to use that word, he said that the activists had had only questions. "Like, 'We really need to do something. What can we be doing?'"

When he said that, I thought of Bush's 2003 State of the Union. How he had lingered on the cost of drugs—now just $300 a year—as though the price had fallen due to gravity and not the tireless work of people who did not believe that markets meant salvation. Fauci had been able to find the hub-and-spoke model because Peter Mugyenyi risked arrest importing generic antiretrovirals into Uganda. Fauci and Dybul had been able to use the cost of generic medications in Mugyenyi's calculations because of the Treatment Action Campaign and leaders like Busisiwe Maqungo and her fellow TAC comrades, including Siphokazi Mthathi, Vuyiseka Dubula, Zackie Achmat, and Mark Heywood. Mugyenyi's hub-and-spoke model had clients who came for their medications and adhered to their regimens because of Milly Katana, Lillian Mworeko, Cissy, the Major, and many other Ugandans who refused to hide their HIV status. Yvette Raphael had used her body as proof, taking the medications to demonstrate that they were not poison, to show her friends who could not afford them that their children would not go uncared for when they were gone. They had contributed far more than questions.

Still, the scale and specificity of Bush's AIDS war had been astonishing. On January 28, 2003, when Bush announced his AIDS initiative, the camera cut to Peter Mugyenyi, seated alongside Laura Bush, clapping with abandon. I too wanted to applaud; instead, I began to cry. I was not supposed to like anything this man said. And when he went on, I didn't.

"This nation can lead the world in sparing innocent people from a plague of nature," Bush said after he'd called for $15 billion for a "work of mercy" to treat and prevent HIV in Africa. "And this nation is leading the world in confronting and defeating the man-made evil of international terrorism." Before I'd had time to absorb the promise he'd made to save two million lives, he'd moved on to the logic for claiming countless more.

This was why I had sat down to watch the speech in the first place. Congress had voted to authorize use of force three months prior, but America had not yet gone to war. Across the country and around the world, people filled the streets in an effort to prevent it from happening. That month, people had filled the streets in Tokyo, Moscow, Paris, London, Dublin, Montreal, Ottawa, Toronto, Cologne, Bonn, Gothenburg. Florence, Oslo, Rotterdam, Istanbul, and Cairo. In Seattle, an entire five-mile route filled with people. In San Francisco, the crowd had been 50,000 strong. That very day, January 28, protesters had swarmed the Davenport Naval Base in Auckland. But the Kiwi naval ship HMNZS *Te Mana* weighed anchor and, bound for the Persian Gulf, steamed away. US troops were already moving too. A vast and lethal mechanics was grinding, and it paid the protests—the biggest were yet to come, including a record-breaking three million people in Rome—no mind.

In my railroad flat in downtown Brooklyn, I had cable. Before the Twin Towers fell, I hadn't needed it. My State Street apartment had a sightline over lower Manhattan. I had once been able to see the towering antenna atop the North Tower. Now, the firehouse right next door had a wooden box filled with plastic flowers and pictures of the fallen. At night, when the trucks slid out with their sirens off, the red and white lights spinning on my bedroom ceiling looked like harbingers of a carnival, not an emergency. "If you see something, say something," the subway signs advised. I'd watched that night because, whatever happened, I would be able to say I had been paying attention.

Next, the president marched through the rubble of the past two years. He did not spare a scene: the two towers, the western wall of the Pentagon, and the field in Pennsylvania. I saw then that he had brought the angel with him. "Where we perceive a chain of events, he sees one single catastrophe which keeps piling wreckage upon wreckage and hurls it in front of his feet," philosopher Walter Benjamin wrote. The angel of history cannot close his wings for all the debris that's piled up behind them. Bush placed all the wreckage cleared from the downtown site New Yorkers called "the pile" behind that angel's wings. He reminded his audience of past triumphs over "Hitlerism, militarism and communism," soared over the Korean Peninsula, and then alit on this conclusion: America could "not allow an even greater threat to rise up in Iraq."

He had the terrorists on the run, he said. They were "one by one... learning the meaning of American justice." *One by one*—so intimate, so clear. Details that would be revealed in time were not yet known. Yet truth shone through the gaps. If the details of the rendition, detention, and interrogation program were still opaque, its existence manifested every day with roundups in New York City, Washington, DC, and other metropoles. Those people went somewhere. They went to Leavenworth, Kansas; Kearny, New Jersey; and Oakdale, Louisiana. To know that was enough. Enough to feel the use of private contractors, water boarding, and extraordinary renditions to countries not bound, as America purported to be, by the conventions of international law.

Perhaps there was no other virus that Bush could have chosen as a foe. HIV was a pathogen that seeded itself in moments of proximity, if not intimacy, between two people. It became an epidemic due to the violent forces of the state. A state set on unleashing intimate violence in the war on terror could not find a more appropriate viral foe to combat with healing.

In the years to come, the things later revealed about PEPFAR would become confused with the things President Bush said that night, as though he had, right away, stated that the money could only purchase branded drugs, that it could only go to groups that repudiated sex work, and that each country, regardless of its own priorities, would have to spend a specified allotment on abstinence-until-marriage education. As though he had been more explicit about the relationship between the war on AIDS and the war he was soon to launch in Iraq. People would argue that he'd launched the former as a compassionate counterweight to the latter, that he had, in some way, said as much.

He didn't say any of those things the night the new world began. He spoke just a handful of sentences, made a few scant promises. That night, what a person loved or hated was primarily what he or she imagined or believed the president's AIDS war would be. He made you, against your will, imagine it, so that from that first moment, everyone who watched and reacted was enlisted in its creation.

He needed this help. A president can ask for many things, but even the commander in chief cannot have money for everything. After John F. Kennedy's moon shot speech in Texas—the finest piece of American aspirational oratory tied to a congressional budget request in history—Dwight Eisenhower reportedly huffed that spending $40 billion to get to the moon was "just nuts." Kennedy had to make the pitch again, at the United Nations, before American lawmakers would give him the money.[40]

Bush, that night, had laid out his vision for one war that would maim and another that would heal. He would have to work harder for the AIDS war than for the Iraqi invasion, for foreign aid was still a rathole to many fiscal conservatives, and Africa was very far away. He needed the lawmakers in the Capitol Building, and the activists who'd gotten arrested in front of the White House, and the thousands of people who had, for the past several years, sought to prove that it was possible to treat AIDS in Africa. He needed people to come down on his side. By not filling in the details, he forced people to imagine them. To put themselves into the picture, to ask "what if" questions whose answers might repel. This made it very personal indeed. Starting the next day, if you worked on AIDS in Africa, you had to decide not just what you believed about the issue but whether you believed—or could trust—the man behind the podium.

CHAPTER 5

THE COST OF VICTORY

O N JANUARY 28, 2003, Bush sketched out a vision for fighting AIDS that was ambitious, unprecedented, and likely to be embraced by the Christian conservatives who were his influential political base. Jesse Helms had already prayed with Bono; Senator Dick Durbin had carried the photo of Bernadette, a Ugandan granny whom he'd met on one of Sandy Thurman's AIDS-in-Africa tours, onto the Senate floor.[1] Shepherd and Anita Smith, communications professionals turned Evangelical AIDS counselors and congressional advisors, had persuaded congregations that they could embrace those with HIV within their flocks, gently counseling one group that the virus would not spread as giardia had in the Sunday school.[2] The Smiths had, along with fellow Evangelical leaders Rick Warren of Saddleback Church and Franklin Graham, founder of Samaritan's Purse, carried stories from the missionaries returned from African countries who were seeing something really, really bad. Graham had prayed for those AIDS orphans and the women who carried them, their bodies emaciated and drawn.

"In ten or twenty years, [the AIDS proposal] will be the most significant thing the president said tonight," Senator Bill Frist recalled telling CNN when interviewed immediately after the speech. Frist had been the sole congressman in the vermillion-walled Red

Room at an intimate White House dinner a few weeks prior. That night, President George W. Bush scraped his chair back from the table and told the senator and his wife, Kofi Annan and his wife, the president's pastor, and a handful of advisors, "I can't tell you the details but I am going to make you proud." Next, Frist said, Bush's pastor rose and praised the coming work of mercy.[3]

On January 29, with the details revealed, Bush's team set about turning that good will into support for legislation that enshrined the specifics of the most ambitious of the proposed plans, which called for two million people on antiretroviral drugs, seven million infections averted, and care for ten million people living with the virus. The "2-7-10" goals set the president's proposal apart from the legislation that had died in conference the year before. So did the $15 billion price tag and the all-important presidential imprimatur. It was a bigger investment with a more powerful champion; it was a grander version of the legislators' vision.

But when Jay Lefkowitz, the domestic policy advisor, embarked on the task of turning the proposal into a law, he discovered that it would not be as easy as the West Wing had hoped.[4] Lefkowitz offered Allen Moore, Frist's legislative affairs director, a draft bill that was less than ten pages long. To Moore, the slim proposed text didn't capture "the enormous effort" that had gone into drafting the Kerry-Frist bill—which ran to well over one hundred pages—over the past two years. Moore recalled telling Lefkowitz, "Is this [draft bill] enough legally? Probably. Is this enough politically, procedurally, institutionally? No."[5] The senator's office politely but firmly declined to introduce the White House draft legislation.

The day after the State of the Union, the president called Lefkowitz, a friendly, precise polymath who'd helped steer Bush toward his position on stem cell research, into the Oval Office. He needed to get the bill through Congress and to the president for signing in time for the next Group of 8 (G8) summit in June. Lefkowitz left with his own marching orders and with the president's question ringing in his ears: What could he do to help? That day, and in the days that followed, Bush peppered Lefkowitz with questions: Whom should he call? Which meetings needed to happen? What could he do as the president to move this forward? "He was willing to be his own staffer on this issue," Lefkowitz marveled.[6]

Lefkowitz offered suggestions, and Bush acted on them, but after two weeks, there was little progress to report. Lefkowitz recalled that even after Bush reached out to Senator Richard Lugar, the chair of the Foreign Relations Committee and a staunch proponent of foreign aid, he could not get traction for a Senate-led legislative process. Backing the president's bill meant stepping away from a prior bipartisan effort, a move that was easier for Republicans than Democrats. In mid-February, news broke that Senator Frist, who had become the Republican majority leader, was withdrawing support for S2069—the bill he'd cosponsored with Senator John Kerry, and throwing his weight behind the White House draft.[7] The same article reported that Lugar, who had resumed chairmanship of the Foreign Relations Committee after a sixteen-year gap, planned to introduce a bipartisan alternative.

According to Frist, Moore, and aides to Biden and Lugar, none of the lawmakers opposed the effort; instead, they viewed the outcome as inevitable, given that the president had asked for it, and wanted to see the legislative process done right. For his part, Lefkowitz thought that Kerry and Biden in particular did not want to see the president supplant their bill, and the credit they'd receive. ("Poetic justice," Bill Clinton's AIDS czar Sandra Thurman would say, still fuming that Clinton hadn't done more when he'd had the opportunity.)[8]

"I'm just a bill, yes I'm only a bill, sitting here on Capitol Hill." Lefkowitz thought of the ditty from the 1976 *Schoolhouse Rock!* cartoon, which had run in the breaks between *The Jetsons* and *The Flintstones* on weekend mornings. He gave up on the Senate—"We went hard," he'd later say with bemused chagrin—and walked his request over to the House. *Let's get this done*, he remembered imploring. *If you introduce it, the White House will support you.* Representatives Tom Lantos and Henry Hyde, along with Barbara Lee and Nancy Pelosi, had all been longtime champions of legislation to expand spending on AIDS. As with their counterparts in the Senate, aides to

Lantos and Hyde do not recall needing any persuasion. Instead, it seemed that the president had finally come around to their legislative agenda. These divergent points of views on who drove the agenda worked in favor of the time line that Lefkowitz knew he needed to meet in order to deliver a bill to the president for signing in advance of the June 2003 G8 summit. The president's signature initiative would move swiftly in part because of congressional leaders who saw it as their own. Lefkowitz also knew he'd need that commitment when the bill emerged from the House of Representatives. Swift passage depended on the Senate accepting the House version with changes. A conference process to reconcile different versions would chew up precious time.

In the House, support came easily—at first. "Hell, I'd spend fifteen billion dollars," Representative Chris Smith said at a House International Relations Committee meeting. Perhaps he had not used those words, but Lantos staffer Dr. Pearl-Alice Marsh remembered the jocular enthusiasm and how, after that, her boss, Peter Yeo, Lantos's chief of staff, had turned to her and said, "Go write that bill."[9]

Almost easy—but not quite. Previous American presidential initiatives had focused on babies, who were configured as "innocent" victims in contrast to people who acquired HIV through sex or drug use. (Even the single dose of nevirapine administered to the woman with HIV had the purpose of protecting the newborn.) But the new proposal, with its expanded mandate of adult treatment, forced a reckoning with how these adults acquired the virus in the first place. For some, it was through sharing needles during drug use. For the majority of people in the African countries where the bulk of the money would flow, HIV was passed on through sex.

To advocate for nevirapine to prevent vertical transmission, one did not have to talk about sex, only the consequences of sex for reproduction. That was why the Bush administration had started with its nevirapine investment and why Sandra Thurman always took members of Congress to orphanages first. "That was the safest course to follow," Dick Durbin, champion of Bernadette the Ugandan granny, told the *New York Times* days after the president's new proposal. The prior focus on women and the contents of their wombs "was not politically charged." Durbin warned that this new initiative would lead to charged areas like "gay sex or use of condoms."[10]

But there was no immaculate conception on this earth. HIV was inseparable from its modes of transmission, which included sex and needle sharing. Any honest, specific, and scientifically accurate conversation about the virus eventually ended up at these inconvenient human truths: not all sex happened within marriage between men and women living in the genders assigned at birth, and not all fucking was undertaken to make a family. Women did not always want the children they conceived; sometimes they did not want to conceive at all. Same sex couples loved each other and had sex in the context of committed relationships. Sometimes, though, both gay and straight people had sex for sheer pleasure, with strangers or friends. By the time Durbin had sounded the alarm, the discussion about the president's proposal had entered the danger zone, centering not on gay men or condoms but on the possibility that this new money might somehow end up subsidizing contraception or abortion.

"Not even a nickel," Austin Ruse, head of the Center for Family and Human Rights, emphasized on January 29, the day after the State of the Union, in an email to subscribers to a special edition of his Friday fax—a weekly antiabortion, pro-abstinence jeremiad. He and his army of the faithful needed to watch the process closely to be sure that "pro-abortion and abortion providers do not get any of this money."[11]

Ruse had little reason to worry. The Helms Amendment—which bore the name of the man who'd wept with Bono over scripture—already prohibited the use of US foreign assistance funds to pay for abortion. There was, too, the Mexico City Policy (MCP), which had, for nearly two decades, been enacted by every Republican president since Ronald Reagan. The MCP specifically limited the activities of foreign groups receiving US funding from the family-planning foreign aid budget. The MCP stipulated that foreign organizations receiving US family-planning funds could not provide, speak about, refer for, or advocate for abortion.[12] Women's sexual and reproductive health advocates argued that safe abortion and postabortion care were critical components of basic women's health, and many programs around the world included it in their offerings.[13] Under the MCP, they were ineligible for US family-planning funding.

In 2003, the Mexico City Policy did not apply to other US foreign aid for health. Foreign groups receiving American funding for immunizations, malaria, or tuberculosis prevention, for example, were not bound by its prohibitions. But those other US health programs were also highly unlikely to offer women contraception. Ever since the late 1960s, the United States and its development agency, USAID, had worked diligently to cleave contraceptive programs from all other health services, demanding that ministries of health create separate offices and programs to deal with the pill packs beloved by neo-Malthusian white men who saw population control as the path to economic growth.[14]

Those men loved pill packs, IUDs, and, for a time, abortion. Rei Ravenholt, USAID's lead on population from 1968 to 1975, carried in his pockets cannulas used for an early-termination process called menstrual extraction, reportedly using them to stir his cocktails. These men did not love any other women's health service though and feared dilution of their dollars if funding for contraception and cannulas was diverted to breast and pelvic exams or other health care for women's bodies. Population control was the top priority for these men, who were led by George H. W. Bush, who successfully implored the United Nations to launch a family-planning fund and secured seed funding from the American government—zealotry for which he was rewarded, by his fellow lawmakers, with the nickname Rubbers.[15]

Rubbers's son's AIDS effort would send money into countries that had, for decades, lived with a US-constructed firewall between family planning and all other health services, a "vertical" programming approach that cleaved women's bodies into pieces like a magician's box. The approach didn't just segment services; it affected training for providers and procurement of commodities. The people who knew how to counsel about contraception and menstrual extraction worked in one place, with one set of supplies; all other health work went on elsewhere. It was a convenient reinforcement of and cover for male doctors' reluctance to address women's health holistically. "If you tell a doctor you have an ulcer, they ask you what color it is, but they are reluctant to examine you," a participant at the Ugandan Focus on Women conference had said, the women around her nodding vigorously. They were responsible for describing lesions, sores, and discharge from their vulvas. "By the time you have a diagnosis, it's too late," another woman said.

Nevertheless, when Jay Lefkowitz's phone started ringing over the weekend after the State of the Union address, the primary concern of the white men on the other end of the line—including Senator Sam Brownback and Representative Chris Smith—was expanding the Mexico City Policy to the new initiative. The president had pledged to spend unprecedented funds to put pills in the hands of women, some of whom were, at that moment, too weak to walk, too sick to produce milk. Lefkowitz spent hours on the phone with the Republicans who wanted to be assured, before they threw their weight behind the program, that if those women got the pills and got up off of their beds or palates on the floor, they would not, under any circumstances, have an easier time getting an abortion as a result of the funding that had paid for their return to health.

Soon enough, the condom question Durbin had warned about would emerge. But in those first days, many of the moral conservatives—whose stalwart support for expanded American action on AIDS was needed to win over fellow Republicans—required clarity above all about where the new program stood on women's rights to control their fertility.

There could be no question where the president stood. Bush Junior had already cut funding from the United Nations Population Fund (UNFPA)—against the recommendations of an expert committee—and diverted it to USAID because of allegations that the UN funds in China paid for coercive sterilization and abortion.[16] Nor was there any question about his broader stance on the provision of comprehensive, age-appropriate sex education. He had ramped up funding for abstinence-until-marriage education programs in the United States, despite the absence of any evidence that these programs, which omitted information about how to have safe, pleasurable sex outside wedlock, reduced rates of pregnancy or sexually transmitted infections over the long term. The Centers for Disease Control and Prevention (CDC) had edited the condom fact sheet on its website to suggest, erroneously, that they were not effective in HIV prevention.[17] The National Institutes of Health (NIH) teams that reviewed and approved applications for research were, as the debates about the President's Emergency Plan for AIDS Relief (PEPFAR) unfolded, receiving regular phone calls from government watchdogs who wanted to track the research dollars paying for studies on sex workers, gay men, condoms, and sex education.[18]

After the weekend of marathon phone calls, Lefkowitz walked into the Oval Office and told the president that he faced a "binary" decision about whether or not the program would fund groups like Doctors Without Borders, which were ready and willing to provide antiretrovirals and would not submit to the policy's restrictions. The president thought the choice was clear, Lefkowitz recalled. It was a medical mission that needed to move fast. If expanding the MCP meant losing a provider who might be the only clinic for miles around, that ran counter to the mission. Bush was certain about the way forward. The President's Emergency Plan for AIDS Relief, which sought the largest disease-specific foreign aid investment in American history, would not be subjected to this policy, a decision Lefkowitz communicated in a West Wing memo circulated on February 10.[19]

While the decision showed a remarkable clarity of vision about the program's purpose, it also demonstrated an all-too-familiar reductionist approach to cisgender women living with HIV.[20] No provider competent in providing antiretrovirals could be excluded. But no truly competent provider seeing women of childbearing age—with or without HIV—would omit sexual and reproductive health from conversations with their clients. Like all women who desired children, women living with HIV wanted healthy children. For many, this meant having the ability to space pregnancies and the option of terminating an unplanned pregnancy. But it also meant preserving the right to have children at all. Many women with HIV in both high- and low-income countries alike faced sharp criticism from health providers if they ventured to ask about options for having children—even though many longed to and many had done so safely. A woman with a known HIV status who delivered in a hospital risked forced or coerced sterilization.[21] Choice was of the utmost importance, and true choice meant programs that offered support and services for women who wanted to prevent pregnancies or needed to terminate them, as well as those who wanted to conceive and deliver. It was a complex, deeply personal reality that required programs that "put the woman at the center," as Lillian Mworeko and other reproductive health advocates liked to say.

The White House decision on the Mexico City Policy didn't stem from this analysis. The president and his aides were intent on scaling up access to antiretrovirals with speed, and the existence of a vast and durable web of restrictions, from legislation to executive orders to USAID policies, made it highly unlikely that any single American-funded program would ever provide comprehensive women's health care.

That web didn't look like a safety net to the conservatives asked to move the bill forward in the house. Not to Chris Smith and not to Henry Hyde, who knew that the Democrats would also never accede to writing a Mexico City–like provision into the new legislation. More needed to be done to ensure that not one nickel went astray. Hyde's aide, Sam Stratman, and Lantos's chief of staff, Peter Yeo—who'd grown up doing clinic defense with his mother, a pro-choice reverend and women's health clinic manager—found a way around the impasse.[22] They'd write a bill that didn't enshrine Mexico City but did specify that not one nickel of the new funds could be used for contraception. They'd trade comprehensive women's health programming for real money to fight AIDS. Pearl-Alice Marsh, the Lantos staffer charged with writing the bill, recalled the agreement in blunt terms. "The bugaboo was the $15 billion. The quid pro quo was taking family planning out of the bill."[23]

A descendant of African American loggers whose presence in an Oregon company town had violated the state's racial exclusion laws, Pearl-Alice Marsh was raised knowing that laws could negate a person's right to exist.[24] By the time she'd become the first Black woman to earn a PhD in political science from the University of California, Berkeley, she'd developed a conviction that the solution lay in the people making laws and policies themselves. She'd done her field research in South Africa, studying labor unions and their role in anti-apartheid organizing; in California, she'd watched Berkeley activists mobilized "within hours" of the South African government's announcement that Berkeley's sister city, Oukasie, was to be bulldozed. "Telephone calls went directly from the Berkeley City Hall to the South African Embassy in Washington," as part of a concerted, multipronged, and ultimately successful effort to stop the razing. Marsh called this kind of work "grassroots statecraft," and she arrived on Capitol Hill convinced that people who were not elected officials had a critical role to play in shaping policy and programs.[25]

With the green light to write the bill, Marsh commandeered a House of Representatives conference room and put her theory of grassroots statecraft into action, issuing an open call to AIDS activist and advocacy groups to offer input. She also convened a small group of Hill staffers, including Christos Tsentas from the office of Congresswoman Barbara Lee and Naomi Seiler from Congressman Henry Waxman's office, to work on the drafting, making sure to keep high-quality liquor stashed in a drawer in her desk for the end of marathon sessions in her office—which she dubbed "Pearl's *Shebeen*," a reference to the bars in the South African townships where she'd researched her PhD.

As the advocacy groups responded, often organizing into working groups on different sections, women's groups tried, and failed, to get consensus that comprehensive sexual and reproductive health needed to be in the legislation. "It was a very small crowd of us...and I remember a lot of upset feelings even amongst each other about what was being negotiated away in the midst of this," recalled Heather

Boonstra, a policy analyst and strategist at the Guttmacher Institute, a reproductive rights organization.[26] Adrienne Germain, a founder of the International Women's Health Coalition, had done groundbreaking work to break down silos and support clinics that offered comprehensive women's health care under one roof. After Bush's announcement, she urged her reproductive health colleagues to pay attention to AIDS—often viewed as a world apart. As much as she urged close collaboration, Germain also found herself facing off with male AIDS activists who insisted that securing antiretroviral treatment to save lives was a priority above all others. The ferocity of those arguments remained with her for decades.[27]

The treatment-focused AIDS activists didn't disagree with the women's-health-focused groups, but, like the Democrats on the Hill, they were willing to compromise to get what they wanted most. They also didn't believe that the Bush administration intended to make good on the president's generous pledge. On the night of the State of the Union, Paul Zeitz, a gregarious, passionately idealistic physician turned activist and founder of the DC-based Global AIDS Alliance, announced a press conference with the Congressional Black Caucus and Health GAP on the new initiative for the following day. At that event, Congresswoman Barbara Lee warned that she'd "be examining the President's budget request very closely" to see if it matched his promises.[28]

Six days later, Lee's skepticism was born out. On February 4, the White House FY2004 budget request—Lee called it "the worst budget in decades" for its slashing of benefits and soaring defense spending—sought a total of $2 billion for global AIDS.[29] Of that, $200 million would go to the Global Fund—the same grievously low amount that the United States had pledged two years prior. The balance of $1.8 billion was 60 percent of the $3 billion per year that simple math dictated for the president to make good on his $15 billion, five-year proposal. What's more, the funding request appeared to take some of the AIDS monies from the foreign aid accounts for maternal and child health, instead of allocating new money, as he'd promised. The United States also hadn't significantly shifted its pro-patent stance.[30] Overall, Bush's work of mercy looked an awful lot like a cynical, pro-corporate maneuver to put money into drug companies' coffers.

Cynical or not, the proposed initiative promised money for exactly what the activists had been demanding for the past eight years. This meant they'd be critical, skeptical, and downright vicious about the proposal—but they wouldn't oppose it directly, no matter what caveats or restrictions applied. The AIDS activists argued that money for treatment was too important to pass up for any principle or service—a logic strikingly similar to that of the White House.

"Democrats pay for Republican policy change," Katy Talento crowed to me sixteen years later with unabated glee.[31] A Republican congressional staffer with a Harvard public health degree, she was instrumental in setting the conservative agenda on the first PEPFAR and its subsequent reauthorizations. With her no-nonsense patter and thin, determined mouth, Talento reminded me of the southern women I'd so admired in North Carolina churches when I was younger. Talento married deeply held Christian faith with a sharp scientific mind, a healthy appetite for expletives, and a Beltway insider's understanding of how to get things done on Capitol Hill.

When we spoke, she'd sometimes tell me about a time she'd used "demagogue-ish language" to make a point—and I'd think of her essays, like the one that asserted that hormonal contraceptives "break" women's "perfectly-functioning fertility."[32] She deplored "safe sex" education that taught people how to have hot, low-risk encounters and took pains to compile reports on what she considered dubious federally funded programs, including her bête noire, "flirting classes."[33]

Scientific evidence about the risks and benefits of contraceptives and of age-appropriate comprehensive sexuality education contradicted Talento's demagoguery.[34] But some of her observations also rang true. In the years prior to PEPFAR, Talento had made it her business to understand what the US government was paying for when it came to AIDS prevention and treatment at home and overseas. She'd surveyed USAID-funded condom promotion and billboard-based behavior-change campaigns in Africa and decided they were a waste of money.

Rising rates of HIV infections seemed to support this assessment—especially for women. At the end of 2003, UNAIDS would report that women in sub-Saharan Africa were more likely to have HIV than men. Fifteen- to twenty-four-year-old women were two and a half times as likely to have HIV, compared to male counterparts of the same age. Of the estimated twenty-three million adults living with HIV in sub-Saharan Africa, roughly thirteen million—more than half—were women.[35]

Scientists advanced biological explanations for this gender gap: women's genital anatomy was thought to be more susceptible to HIV, especially during adolescence. But there were many other reasons why women were at substantial risk—and this included the fact that condoms were not always an available or desirable option.

Many did not have control over when or with whom they had sex and risked being accused of infidelity or even having HIV if they suggested using a condom. Many women wanted to have children; condoms would not allow them to conceive. Billboards and bowls of latex were absolutely insufficient for changing deep-rooted community norms. Still, I and many others believed that condoms should be everywhere: even if they weren't sufficient to eliminate HIV risk for everyone, they could—with the right programming—help some people, while starting a conversation among many others. Talento and I disagreed on this, but on the day she explained how Democrats got their money by agreeing to Republican demands, I liked her very much indeed, for it was as succinct a summary of the bargains that begat PEPFAR as any I had ever heard. I liked her even though Talento (then Katy French) had been one of the reasons why the deal that Hill staffers Yeo and Stratman brokered over excluding contraception was not the end of the negotiations but the very beginning.

— —

HR1298, THE BILL THAT emerged from the *shebeen*, was scheduled for markup on March 20. But on the eve of that meeting, the staff of Representative Joe Pitts, the chair of the Pro-Life Caucus, blasted a message out. Pitts "OPPOSES this bill, and cannot support it in its current form," the memo ran, then detailed the principal objections: the proposed $1.1 billion earmark for the Global Fund, which funded "UNFPA, North Korea and Sudan"; the lack of clarity that abstinence "works better than social marketing of condoms"; the absence of a conscience provision that would allow faith-based groups to get the funding even if they disagreed with condoms; and the need for binding language on the percentages of funds allocated for prevention, treatment, and care and a way to ensure that "groups that support prostitution [would] not be our surrogates for AIDS help in Africa."[36]

Talento had enumerated many of the same priorities in a document she called "Republican Principles," which she'd hammered out on the afternoon of January 29, while the night before was still fresh in her mind. She'd watched the speech at home—she "hated watch parties"—and burst into tears. An American president had finally acknowledged the importance of treatment. Antiretrovirals worked. They saved lives. It was simple, evidence-based, and a far cry from condom campaigns and billboards that sought to "end AIDS." In her memo, antiretrovirals were the top priority. To that end, she wanted a "treatment floor"—a minimum amount of the new money earmarked for treatment. But if she wanted the bulk of the money spent on antiretrovirals, she wanted assurances that the other money wouldn't be spent on airfares and international meetings—another one of her gripes with US foreign aid—or to abortion, which ran counter to her faith. A program that saved lives with AIDS drugs and also paid for pregnancy termination was, to her mind, "one giant hypocritical nullification of the program's purpose." (Reproductive health and rights advocates countered that treating a woman with HIV without ensuring she had access to the full range of reproductive health services needed to prevent maternal mortality was a similar nullification.)

Talento advanced an agenda similar to that of Representative Pitts: cut the money for the Global Fund, push money to faith-based groups, and explicitly fund programs that focused on abstinence and fidelity. Senator Judd Gregg, Talento's boss, had helped to scuttle efforts to reconcile the Hill and Senate AIDS bills in conference in

2002, with Talento urging him on. She thought that the legislation, which proposed more than $1 billion for the Global Fund and endorsed treatment without specifying any targets, was ripe for exploitation by USAID contractors who'd be able to pay for programs other than testing and treatment. The Kerry-Frist bill that passed the Senate also contained an extensive, forward-thinking section on HIV prevention in girls and women that encompassed everything from microfinance (small loans) to microbicides (experimental products that a woman could use to reduce her risk of HIV, unlike male condoms, which required male cooperation).

Concerns about the House draft reverberated in the White House. The week before the scheduled March 20 markup in the House International Relations Committee, Lefkowitz was summoned to the Senate Values Action Team, which sought assurances that the White House would only back legislation that included the provisions about funding faith-based groups, elevating abstinence, and limiting contributions to the Global Fund. He also met with Shepherd Smith and Dr. Edward "Ted" Green, who came to make sure that Lefkowitz and his colleagues appreciated what had happened in Uganda with the Abstain, Be Faithful, Use a Condom, or ABC, strategy that had won President Museveni so much acclaim.

Lefkowitz was, in fact, well aware of ABC—as was Gary Edson. During the months when Anthony Fauci and Mark Dybul had mined data and crunched numbers, Lefkowitz had talked to as many experts as he could about HIV programs. In a block of time he tried to reserve each week, he'd talk to experts he'd invited to the White House—everyone from Tracy Kidder, author of the book chronicling Paul Farmer's work in Haiti, to experts familiar with the ABC program in Uganda. He'd been persuaded of its value long before Smith and Green arrived in his office. But Smith and Green wanted the meeting anyway—neither man left much to chance.[37]

By the time Bush gave his 2003 State of the Union, the Smiths were a pair of the most influential Evangelical AIDS experts in the world, though there hadn't been much competition for that position when they'd started doing domestically focused work in the late

1980s, founding an organization called Americans for a Sound AIDS Policy and providing what amounted to a two-person hotline for churches and conservative elected officials who called with questions about what to do when a congregant or constituent tested positive for the highly stigmatized virus. The Smiths would often travel to the community in question, urging families and church groups to create spaces of acceptance. If their antistigma work aligned with the messages of the people-living-with-HIV-led activist movement, their stance on HIV testing didn't. The Smiths felt strongly that testing should be widespread and routine, as it was in many other public health emergencies. People with HIV countered that forcing people to learn their status only worked when human rights were also in place. As long as a positive test result could cost a person his job, insurance, partner, or community support, no one should be required to receive a diagnosis. The Smiths also argued that condoms did not belong at the top of the hierarchy of prevention. They worked, but not all the time. People should know that and be urged to abstain.[38] While technically true—complete abstinence is more effective than condoms at reducing risk of sexual transmission of HIV—this argument was, to people who viewed sex as an inevitable and even enjoyable part of human life, akin to warning that seat belts could cause bruising if a car came to a sudden halt, so people ought to be told to walk everywhere if they truly wanted to be safe.

At first glance, the Smiths had little in common with Ted Green, a onetime conscientious objector and medical anthropologist who'd spent two years in the Amazon rainforest in Suriname. But they were linked by their enthusiasm for President Yoweri Museveni's purportedly effective HIV-prevention strategy. The Smiths had encountered it when they'd visited Uganda on one of their many mission trips to Africa. There and in Zambia, they'd begun working with churches to set up centers for counseling and care that could, as AIDS drugs became available, begin to offer treatment. In this work, they tapped into the large network of faith-based institutions that provided medical care of a quality not offered by the states in East and Southern Africa. These institutions were often embedded in and trusted by the communities they served. When they'd gone to Uganda, they'd encountered church groups doing their part to fight AIDS, including spreading the messages that, as they saw it, put the hierarchy of prevention in its proper order: abstain, be faithful, use a condom.

Green had gone to Uganda as an advisor to USAID and become enamored of the national mobilization of faith-based leaders, the zero-grazing messages, and the drumbeat on the radio. The author of a volume focused on the value of "indigenous" medical wisdom, Green thought in terms of local and imported public health approaches. In Uganda, he saw an alternative to the condom-first, US-funded messages and the state silence in other parts of Africa. He'd been sufficiently impressed that he had, in 1998, helped to write the National Health Education Strategy on HIV/AIDS for the AIDS Control Program.

It was Green who'd named the Ugandan prevention strategy "ABC." It was a basic name for a hugely complex approach. The notion of abstaining until marriage depended on a person's being able to choose when she had sex and with whom. But in a contemporaneous study in Burkina Faso, Ghana, Malawi, and Uganda on the prevalence of "coercive first sex," many twelve- to nineteen-year-old girls explained they hadn't been given a choice: 23 percent of Ugandans and 38 percent of Malawians were "not willing at all" the first time they'd had sex. Whether they'd wanted to abstain until marriage or not was beside the point.[39] In many instances, women's husbands held the decision rights over their bodies and their shared property, including livestock and land. A woman could be faithful herself, but she could not guarantee her partner would do the same. In studies of "married" adolescent girls—women's health activists railed that use of that word, "married," lent propriety to the practice of placing girls just out of puberty in much older men's beds, care, and homes—being in a partnership was a risk factor for HIV. "Early marriage increases coital frequency, decreases condom use, and virtually eliminates girls' ability to abstain from sex," a researcher wrote of findings that unmarried Kenyan and Zambian girls were more likely to be HIV-free.[40]

Lefkowitz told me that the White House supported ABC and wanted to see it as a central component of the proposed plan, and Austin Ruse's fax alert suggests that conservative allies had an inside track on some of this analysis. But as late as March 2003, the White House hadn't articulated a position on HIV prevention. Bush hadn't mentioned specific strategies in the State of the Union, and on the White House Fact Sheet released the following day, the only prevention strategy named was HIV testing (which doesn't prevent HIV at all, though it can prompt a person to take steps that do). Fauci and Dybul hadn't elevated abstinence in the prevention strategy they'd derived from John Stover. "We had nothing special about abstinence and being faithful in the original," Dybul said. "If you look at John Stover's list of prevention interventions it is one in a series of interventions... it was all in there, the full package was all part of it."[41]

Whatever the president thought, the conservatives were crystal clear about the terms of their cooperation. When Lefkowitz paid his visit to the Values Action Team, lawmakers asked for assurances that the bill would address their concerns. In the House and the Senate, legislators muttered about drafting alternate bills—which would, if introduced, slow the process down.[42] Lefkowitz acted on the concerns and stalled the markup scheduled to begin on March 20. That night, at 10:15 p.m., President Bush addressed the nation from the Oval Office, his twin daughters' picture on the sideboard behind him, and said, "On my orders, coalition forces have begun striking targets of military importance to undermine Saddam Hussein's ability to wage war."

— —

I DIDN'T KNOW THE details of these backroom meetings in 2003, but I knew enough about Uganda and HIV prevention to be concerned with positions taken by both the Right and the Left. I worked for an organization devoted to finding an AIDS vaccine. Participants in the trials that evaluated these vaccines received state-of-the-art counseling about risk reduction through monogamy and partner reduction, generous supplies of condoms, and treatment for sexually transmitted infections. Yet, in every trial, in every country, people still acquired HIV. Condoms were not sufficient; people had sex and either couldn't or didn't want to wear them. The liberal argument that ABC should be replaced with a condom-forward sex-education strategy like the one that had worked in the United States didn't ring any truer than the notion that HIV would disappear on the basis of Museveni's exhortation that people adopt a "zero-grazing" approach to sexual partners—a cattle ranching metaphor for monogamy. Christian conservatives espoused views that, when implemented, stripped women of their bodily autonomy; yet faith-based groups were pillars of health provision and community support in many countries. Condoms were not the solution, churches were not the enemy—but in a country embroiled in culture wars with life-or-death consequences for queers, women, and many other groups, it was hard to find a middle ground.

For a time, I was also troubled by the way that Americans seemed to assume that the Ugandans themselves had no hand in promoting this agenda. Green, in particular, was accused of co-opting a Ugandan approach and position; yet it was abundantly clear that the president and First Lady were themselves invested in the reputation-bolstering narrative. Here, I need not have worried. Their agency was soon on full display.

On April 2, 2003, the House International Relations Committee finally started markup on HR1298.[43] The same day, Janet Museveni faxed a letter to the ranking member of the Senate, Dick Lugar, to explain her country's prevention program. "I feel I should shed some light on the issue of preventive measures against HIV/AIDS, since I have had firsthand experience in activities in behavior change for over a decade. My experience has led me to conclude that, when dealing with young people especially, it is vitally important to emphasize abstinence as the first line of defense, so to speak." She believed this to be the case because she thought that explaining abstinence allowed humans to use their conscience to preserve their health. "I believe that we humans have an innate mechanism called conscience, which convicts us concerning what is wrong and what is right, or what is good for our survival and what is harmful." She quoted biblical proverbs to make her case and said that while condoms were available, in her experience, conscience, well applied, was the better prophylactic.[44]

Mrs. Museveni, a devout born-again Christian, might have been kept abreast of developments by Rosa Whitaker, the principal at the latest US-based communications firm that her husband had retained. More information might have come from Bush advisor Jendayi Frazer—a close personal friend of the Musevenis who'd spent the Christmas after September 11 at their cattle ranch.[45] With close personal ties between the two state houses, the First Lady knew that her intervention would help American legislation pass with the religiously infused messages intact. And, in fact, it did.

On May 1, HR1298 finally went to the House floor, trailed by a flurry of fax blitzes from the Eagle Forum and internal memos circulated among Republicans urging support for "pro-science based, pro-family amendments."[46] Once it reached the floor, the discussion went as Peter Yeo had known it would. Representatives Smith and Pitts reintroduced their amendments on abstinence, the conscience clause, and a requirement that groups receiving the money repudiate sex work, also called "the antiprostitution pledge." Each of them passed. The legislation also contained a set of "sense of Congress" earmarks, allocating 55 percent of the funds to treatment, 20 percent to prevention, 15 percent to palliative care, and 10 percent to orphans and vulnerable children. The legislation also stated that 33 percent of prevention funds were to be spent on abstinence-only education. The bill was larded with mentions of faith-based groups and the model prevention program in Uganda. At 3:36 p.m. Eastern time, HR1298 passed the House of Representatives.[47] That day, Bush landed on the deck of the aircraft carrier of the *Abraham Lincoln* and, in his flight suit, addressed the nation before a banner reading, "Mission Accomplished."[48]

He was wrong about the war on terror, right about the war on the virus. Once HR1298—the Global Leadership Against HIV/AIDS, Tuberculosis, and Malaria Act—passed out of the House, Frist's staff began working "to come up with a fix to several problem areas," Frist's legislative director Allen Moore said, "particularly the language relating to abstinence-until-marriage." They labored over the text, trying to come up with edits that the House would accept without sending the bill into conference. But the White House urged Frist to move to accept the House-passed bill without changes in order to meet the president's ambitious time line. When that request came, Frist's team realized they were out of time and that the new Senate majority leader would need to persuade his colleagues to sign on to a "no-amendment" strategy, in which Republicans did not submit amendments to or vote for Democratic amendments to the legislation. If they worked together, the bill would pass. "This was a tough decision," Frist said. "It was controversial." But the money on the table made it worth it.[49]

In the White House, Jay Lefkowitz knew that this was a critical moment, and so he too took pains to ensure that the president's party endorsed the no-amendment strategy. To see his "endgame" through, he turned to Bono, the U2 front man who'd used charm, Christian faith, and considerable intellect to compel American political action. Bono had become something of a regular at the White House, comfortable enough that he left a doodle in Lefkowitz's office one day when he'd stopped by and the domestic policy advisor wasn't around. Now Lefkowitz reached out to the rocker. "I have the house wired," he recalled saying. "But I am going to need your help on the Senate floor. And he [Bono] said, 'I'm on it.' "[50] Along with activist and Kennedy family scion Bobby Shriver, Bono urged left and centrist senators with whom Bush had little pull to go along with the no-amendment strategy.[51]

AIDS activists had not fought too hard against the strategy, behaving as Talento knew they would. They wanted the money; if amendments were allowed to be introduced, the Mexico City Policy might reappear. At best the fragile compromise would be lost and work on a consensus version of the bill would begin; at worst, it might get adopted and written into law. The sheer amount of money on the table and the size and specificity of the treatment targets were too important to turn away from—PEPFAR would be born on the back of a compromise that would, in the coming years, be repeated again and again.

Still, when HR1298, formally known as the United States Leadership Against HIV/AIDS, Tuberculosis, and Malaria bill, arrived in the Senate of the 108th Congress on May 15, 2003, the passage was not swift. Knowing that their amendments would be defeated, the Democrats still took pains to introduce unresolved issues. (Republican senator Rick Santorum would also break with his party and introduce an amendment, much to his colleagues' chagrin.) The debates went on for hours, past midnight and until dawn, revolving again and again around Uganda and, more specifically, one supremely powerful Ugandan woman, the First Lady Janet Museveni.

"She said very clearly and directly this is about a change of culture," Senator Brownback said, speaking of a meeting he'd had with "Mama" Museveni, who'd flown to the capital that week. "About pushing a model of ABC which started with abstinence and being faithful." "When I met with the First Lady of Uganda Tuesday, she told me how this approach of emphasizing abstinence was a return to traditional African values that is working well," said Senator Lamar Alexander.

Republicans were not the only ones who relied, for their arguments, on the Ugandan head of state and his wife. "I was sitting with President Museveni when he got his first real briefing, by USAID officials, on the calamity of AIDS in his country," Senator Patrick Leahy offered. "At that time, he switched from opposing the use of condoms as an acceptable way to protect against AIDS to supporting it." Leahy made his remarks in the context of supporting an amendment, offered by Dianne Feinstein, which sought to strike the abstinence earmark, retaining Uganda as a model but allowing programs to make their own determination on how much to spend on each component of ABC.

In the dark hours of a new day, the senator from New York State stood and took the floor. "I am concerned that abstinence is not a prevention tool realistically available to many girls and women throughout Africa. So many of the prevention tools are controlled by men, and by customs and traditions, in communities where the expectation may very well be for a young girl to be married at a very young age," Hillary Clinton said. She offered an amendment that would focus on women's empowerment, on expanding access to prevention products like microbicides, an experimental category of substances being designed to reduce HIV risk via a gel or film, used the same way as a spermicide. Microbicides had been as foreign as ABC to the Ugandan women at the Focus on Women conference, but they'd thrilled to the concept, first advanced by a Jewish South African antiapartheid physician named Zena Stein.[52] That was what they needed—a way to protect themselves that did not require male acquiescence or cooperation.

Clinton said that gender-based violence, pre- and postnatal care, and prevention of cervical cancer needed to be considered. "When we are talking about women's health and looking at all of the problems women have, it is important that we not focus just on HIV/AIDS, as though that is some separate, abstract problem that can be removed from cervical cancer and sexually transmitted diseases and other problems that women suffer from so grievously, not only in Africa but in many countries around the world."

She said that she knew the majority did not want amendments, that the bill needed to move. She hoped, though, that this language could be added in during the appropriations process. And she asked, now, for a voice vote to gauge support for the amendment that "specifically stands up for the girls and women of Africa." The vote was held, as requested. Senator Clinton's amendment failed.

Ted Kennedy also offered an amendment aimed at stripping away the law's provision that all drugs purchased for the program had to be approved by the US Food and Drug Administration (FDA). The FDA had not approved any generic antiretrovirals, so this provision meant the money would go for the pharmaceutical company's branded drugs. Proponents of the provision said it was a matter of common sense, ensuring American taxpayer dollars didn't buy shoddy drugs. Kennedy pointed out that the obligation was to stretch the money as far as possible, to buy the cheapest drugs available that had been approved by the World Health Organization. His amendment, like Clinton's, failed.[53] Shortly after both offered their amendments, HR1298 passed in the Senate.

The president had what he wanted—a bill ready to sign into law that created the largest disease-specific foreign-assistance program in US—and global—history. The bill also authorized a $1 billion contribution to the Global Fund, which, if realized, would make the United States the largest contributor to the multilateral fund as well. The legislation stipulated that the United States could only cover up to 33 percent of the Fund's total budget—for every dollar America put in, two more had to be raised from other sources. With that, America became both the Global Fund's largest single donor and the funder and architect of the largest disease-specific health initiative in world history.[54]

On Monday, May 19, the bill was back in the House for consideration of the scant handful of textual changes resulting from the Senate's marathon debate.[55] It passed handily and went to the White House on May 23—the same day that Representatives Nancy Pelosi and Henry Waxman wrote to Bush's AIDS czar, Joe O'Neill, raising concerns "about the influence of politics in HIV/AIDS policy" in America. The pair said they'd been impelled to act by reports that the CDC and the NIH were subjected to White House–endorsed approaches to scouring scientific grants for watchwords like "sex worker" and "gay"—an approach that the dean of the Bloomberg School of Public Health at Johns Hopkins University said had created "a pernicious sense of insecurity" among scientists.[56]

The bill's passage had created its own sense of insecurity—particularly at USAID, which could not ignore the rebuke to its leadership codified in the law: the entity that would implement the President's Emergency Plan for AIDS Relief—which would, in time, be called the Office of the Global AIDS Coordinator—would be housed at the State Department, headed by an ambassador-level appointee. That global AIDS ambassador would report to the secretary of state and answer to the president. USAID, the CDC, the Department of Defense, and the embassies in countries would work together to make and implement the AIDS ambassador's plan.

To underscore this point, on May 27, 2003, roughly three and a half months after the State of the Union, Bush left the White House and traveled in his motorcade to the Dean Acheson Auditorium in the State Department building to sign into law HR1298, now known as the United States Leadership Against HIV/AIDS, Tuberculosis, and Malaria Act of 2003. Dr. Pearl-Alice Marsh and the other denizens of the *shebeen* were there in the front row.[57]

This was lawmaking at lightning speed, a triumph of trade-offs: an enormous amount of money for treatment in exchange for fine print that, in some cases, increased people's risk of HIV. This new US-run effort allowed the United States to impose conditions that it could not apply to recipients of Global Fund grants, including the requirement that recipients of bilateral funding sign a pledge repudiating sex work—a provision anathema to sex workers and their allies, for whom the pledge negated their work to organize and lead public health programs that worked for their communities. While the final forty-page law did leave the door open for prevention activities for people who use drugs, it contained no mention of "gay" or "homosexual" people at risk of HIV.[58] The law also contained the abstinence-until-marriage earmark on prevention funding and stipulated that the funds could only purchase medications approved by the US Food and Drug Administration, which effectively meant it could only buy costly, brand-name drugs. (To underscore this point, the section of the law that quoted from Bush's State of the Union was edited to remove his statement that the drugs cost less than a dollar a day. A set of asterisks sat on the page where the president had named generic prices.)

Some compromises that hobbled the program's ability to offer evidence-based prevention and treatment would be quickly reversed, while others would endure and become defining traits of an American war that saved many people from dying of AIDS, without adequately attending to the factors that led others to acquire HIV.

You could love, hate, or tolerate the law, but trying to use its text to understand PEPFAR was like using an architect's blueprint as a substitute for standing inside a cathedral. You had to get close, get inside to apprehend its scale and power and to imagine what was possible. From the moment that Bush signed PEPFAR into law, the personalities, passions, and strategic acumen of the people who would be spending the money began to matter very much indeed.

Bush's decision to hold the signing ceremony at the State Department was a signal about his intention that this program's leadership would stand apart from USAID, a message about where the power would sit, legible to anyone who was watching.[59] But if this was the first time you'd noticed that this new program would shift the center of power in foreign aid for global health in unimaginable ways, then you were already too late.

Months before, in the weeks when America was not yet in another war in Iraq, while the AIDS activists had both argued that the promised funds should flow to the Global Fund and sought to make the proposed bill as strong as it could be, and as the Republicans had agonized over whether it reflected their morality, Americans who worked for USAID, CDC, and the Department of Defense—people who knew what they would do with the money—were all getting into position. For them, there had never been any doubt at all about whether this was going to be real or not. The question had always been not "if?" but "how?"

One of those people was Dr. Deborah Birx, a US Army colonel, doctor, and immunologist and the head of the US Military HIV Vaccine Research Program. She saw the opportunity on the night of the State of the Union. All the machinations on Mexico City, the odes to condoms, and the white men parroting the wisdom of "Mama" Museveni were, while not irrelevant, hardly the primary matter at hand. She had never been easily distracted. "Won't you get pregnant?" the military had asked her years ago during a job interview, flagrantly violating employment law. "Oh no," she'd said in her helium voice, shaking her head of blonde curls. "My husband and I only have oral sex." She'd flashed her brilliant smile and known they wouldn't ask more.

In the first week of February, she got into her car, a binder of slides beside her, and headed to the home of AIDS czar Joe O'Neill. When she wanted to get something done, she stopped at nothing—and she wanted something from this program, which did not even have a name. In the early February chill, Deborah Birx started her engine.[60]

CHAPTER 6

STRETCHING THE WEEK

I N DECEMBER 2003, WHEN Cissy moved into my apartment, I
didn't know exactly why she was there. I was delighted to have her
warm, loving presence in my home, and it seemed natural that someone from Uganda would come to New York when they had a chance
to do so. I listened with half an ear as she explained that Milly Katana
had, after cashing in all of her frequent flier miles, only been able to
get her a ticket as far as Brussels and had then loaned her the money
for the next leg of the journey. While I eyed her luggage and considered whether I owned enough towels for both of us, she told me that
her job had given her a loan against her salary, which she had used to
repay Milly, and emphasized how remarkably flexible her employer
had been. I nodded knowingly and shooed my cats—who horrified
her—off the lumpy futon that would be her bed.

After a total of about six months in different African countries, I
thought I recognized this as a story about the elaborate logistics of
everyday life that I had encountered there. Everything took time,
multiple hands, patience. I did not wonder why Cissy had left her
job and three children, or if I did, it was not with any level of alarm.
This was likely how Cissy wanted me to react. She told stories that
took care of the listener. The adolescents she worked with thought
she was young like they were; they dubbed her "Sweet Sixteen."

When she had finished explaining Milly's miles and the salary loan like it was all serendipity, she beamed her solar smile at me and then asked, almost as an afterthought, if I could help her find a doctor.

On December 12, 2003, I went to a Bronx clinic with Cissy and Cindra Feuer, my former colleague from *HIV Plus*. That night, Cissy went to stay with Feuer, and I returned to my narrow railroad flat, and looked at the futon pressed up against the exposed brick wall in the space I called my living room, where Cissy had lain motionless, for hours at a time, watching a Christian cable channel she'd found—a static camera trained on an altar that remained empty for hours at a time. Now I knew what she was doing in New York and why she seldom stirred. I was chastened. How could I have missed it?

In the ten months since President George W. Bush had made his announcement, I often found myself unsure of what I was seeing or being told. Most, if not all, of the activists I knew reacted with fury and skepticism at the president's proposal and, later, the law. Yes, there was expanded funding for the Global Fund, but the law also created the new alternative, bilateral mechanism that put power in the hands of the US government.

I disliked the provisions as much as anyone in my activist circle, but I wasn't certain that I understood or agreed with the critique of the entire initiative. Around the time that Cissy arrived, a coalition that included Health GAP and many other activist groups issued a 2003 "Year in Review" report contrasting the "up-and-running, multilateral but chronically underfunded" Global Fund with the "showy, limited, still-on-the-drawing-board" bilateral American effort.[1] The Fund had indeed been up and running for longer, but as the authors noted, it was undergoing growing pains, and I wasn't sure that all of them could be fixed by funding alone. Kate Sorensen and I had split for many reasons, including my stubborn susceptibility to stories about American valor. When I looked at PEPFAR, it wasn't clear to me that the American plan was all for show or that the activists knew with certainty that the Fund would be faster or better at treating people with HIV.

In the past three years, since leaving *HIV Plus*, I'd gained confidence in my own reporting skills and clarity about the work I liked to do. I'd worked with Milly Katana to help secure a small grant for an advocacy organization focused on advocacy by and for Ugandan women living with HIV. I was helping, without always waiting for someone to tell me what to do. Privately, I let myself nurture what I felt was a contrarian view of PEPFAR and began to develop a plan to see for myself.

By the time Cissy arrived in Brooklyn, I'd completed an application for a Fulbright journalism grant that would allow me to move to Uganda and watch what happened when, as I wrote, "the world changed." I also started asking people outside my close activist circle what they thought. On December 12, at home in the apartment without Cissy, I cracked the window onto the alley—Cissy slept under all the blankets and towels I gave her, plus her coat, and kept the windows shut—and placed a phone call to Dr. Deborah Birx to find out if there was a reason for the optimism that I felt, with a twinge of shame, in my gut about the president's new plan.

For the first but by no means the last time, she seemed to know exactly what I was thinking. "It's almost like when Kennedy said we're going to go to the moon," she said in her fluting, flat-voweled voice. "I know that I thought and others thought that this problem is so great, and we were just whittling around the edges. Now we have enough money to stop whittling and really make a difference."[2]

I'd met Birx, then head of the US Military HIV Vaccine Research Program, a few years prior at the government-convened vaccine research meetings that my employer, IAVI, would dispatch me to cover for its newsletter. She often wore drab-green military sweaters with epaulets and always ate her lunch out of a Tupperware container she'd brought from home—a habit she'd picked up after a violent allergic reaction to kiwi in an airplane meal caused an emergency landing.

Birx wore her rank and vulnerability with equal ease. For our interview, she'd given me two numbers to reach her on—her cell phone and the landline for her parents' home in Mechanicsburg, Pennsylvania. During that December interview, she told me she was there with her ninety-eight-year-old grandfather. Sherman Sparks was just six years into retirement from the country store he and his wife had run for seventy-odd years at a crossroads in northern Baltimore County.[3] She told me she might have to pause our interview to plan dinner with her husband on the other line.

In a stolid scientific community, Birx stood out as one of the few people I interviewed regularly who suffused speech with emotion. That evening, she was buoyant. "It's so exciting. This is our time." She added, "I'm hearing that money for this first year is really quite good." She spoke as though she'd been following along from a distance. I'd figure out later that by the time we spoke, she was delighted because she had secured PEPFAR money for the Department of Defense, her own program. I didn't know this, though. I was still learning how to ask questions, to listen. That night, for the second time in as many weeks, I listened to a woman describe what sounded like logistical and technical details and failed to discern the truth, which was that a pitched battle with highly personal stakes was underway.

— —

EARLIER THAT DAY, CISSY and I had taken the C train to 181st Street, exiting into the plastic festivity of the holiday bazaar on Juan Carlos Duarte Boulevard. It was frigid. Cissy wore a blue padded coat, a voluminous acrylic scarf striped with different shades of blue, and two pairs of leggings beneath her velvet pants. As we walked to the crosstown bus stop that would take us into the Bronx, I adjusted my speed to her slow, precise gait—something like a bride going down the aisle. Step, pause, step, pause. She moistened her lips before she spoke, her smile genuine and taut at the same time. It wasn't the layers on her legs or a quintessential Ugandan tempo that set the pace but—though I did not realize it then—pain.

When Cissy had asked for some advice about a doctor, I'd turned to Feuer, who'd once worked as a case manager at Housing Works. She'd made phone calls and secured an appointment with Dr. Barbara Zeller, the HIV clinician and activist who was also married to Health GAP founder Dr. Alan Berkman.[4] "Look south!" Feuer and I cried when the eastbound bus crossed Washington Heights Bridge.

"You can see all the way to the bottom of Manhattan." Dutifully, Cissy looked, then turned back and made a circle around her head with a finger. She'd been searching for the harbor's patron saint of weary travelers. "Where is the lady with the crown?"

Dr. Zeller's office was also ready for the holidays. Tinsel boas and small stockings adorned the walls; a wreath on the door hung alongside the year-round decor: children's drawings of trees, a sign that read, "The Street Ends Here." Zeller herself was a small woman with a puff of gray curly hair and the chunky jewelry and loose-tailored raiment of an Upper West Side liberal. A stalwart activist and skilled clinician, she was the first port of call on the underground railroad of doctors who treated people with HIV for free, regardless of where they came from or how long they'd be staying. Feuer and I left the room while Dr. Zeller examined Cissy. Then we came back, perching on the crinkling paper of the exam table, and I began to understand why Cissy had come to America.

We listened as Zeller spoke to a colleague on the phone. She said she'd never seen a case quite like what Cissy presented; she used the word "exuberant" in a way I had never heard—as it related to flesh, not the sense of joy. As Zeller and Cissy discussed the unsuccessful treatments she'd tried, Cissy's medical knowledge came through. She said "bid" for "twice a day" and switched between brand and generic names. When she rolled up her sleeve for a blood draw, she frowned and rolled her eyes at her forearm. Zeller asked, "Did you bring your veins to the US?" then retied the rubber tie even tighter.

Cissy had an AIDS-related ailment for which antiretrovirals (ARVs) were not the remedy. She required another drug that was rarely in stock in Uganda and, when available, was exorbitantly priced. She had lived with the un- and undertreated condition for as long as she could, taking her antiretrovirals all the while, but the symptoms had become unbearable, beyond what even she could handle with prayer and stoicism. Milly Katana and her coworkers had sent her to New York because if she did not come, she was likely to die. If Cissy hadn't told me this, it was in part because I hadn't asked. I had assumed that as long as she was able to buy antiretrovirals with money that I'd given her and that other family members also supplied, she would be okay.

I also did not ask Birx how much of the money, about which she was so enthusiastic, she had obtained. If I had been able to pose that question to Birx, I would have learned that the program that the activists treated as a false promise and a political ploy had taken shape with what was, by Washington, DC, standards, blistering speed. I might have also gotten an inkling that the structure of the program designed to wage war on the virus had engendered a war for resources among the eligible American agencies that would go on for as long as the program did, defining and undermining this singular, purpose-built effort to control a modern plague.

— —

PEPFAR's structure is its Achilles heel, its stroke of genius, and the single greatest workaround for a problematic foreign aid structure in American history. Under the design devised in the West Wing and enshrined in the legislation, each of the American agencies working on AIDS in each of the countries targeted for PEPFAR funding—the Centers for Disease Control and Prevention (CDC), the Department of Defense, USAID, the Peace Corps, and the American Embassy—would be coordinated by the Office of the US Global AIDS Coordinator (OGAC), housed in the State Department and headed by an ambassador-level appointee.[5]

When I spoke to Jay Lefkowitz and Gary Edson, two of the program's chief architects, they offered affirmative explanations for the structure, which had also been proposed in the Kerry-Frist bill in 2002. The State Department placement offered prestige and protection. Secretary of State Colin Powell was a staunch supporter of work on AIDS and broader American support for Africa. The ambassador-level position afforded independence, autonomy, and a direct line to the Oval Office. But they also placed the new AIDS initiative in the State Department because they felt there was nowhere else for it to go. Neither USAID nor the CDC, nor its parent agency, the Department of Health and Human Services (HHS), could be trusted to lead with a neutral, even hand. Had HHS or CDC been put in charge, "they would have thought they were turning into the WHO," Lefkowitz said to me, referring to the World Health Organization.

USAID had never delivered medical services on a meaningful scale and had spent years cleaving its family-planning and immunization programs off broader health programs in the countries it served. Moreover, the agencies seldom had shared turf in foreign countries. USAID had offices, CDC dispatched teams. By the advent of PEPFAR, this had changed, but only recently, with the CDC's expansion into Africa-based AIDS.

Prior to 1999, the CDC ran research programs overseas; any programmatic activities were funded and therefore managed by USAID—a subgranting approach that had also been used in the American contribution to smallpox eradication launched in 1966. The agencies had only ventured into working as peers in the context of Bill Clinton's LIFE initiative and George W. Bush's subsequent mother-to-child transmission prevention program.

Sometimes, it had gone well, but often the agencies squabbled on the ground. When Eugene McCray assumed leadership of the CDC's Global AIDS Program in 1999, he traveled to African countries to set up partnerships with governments to measure the epidemic and develop public health policies to support key goals. He asked USAID if fledgling CDC offices could share their space, which was, in Kampala, a large compound behind high walls that had once belonged to the British High Commission. Frequently, the answer was no.[6]

The answer came from the country mission directors, but it echoed sentiments from on high. Andrew Natsios, Bush's USAID administrator, didn't think much of the new country-based CDC offices, which had, he told me, "gutted" some countries' ministries of health by hiring away their best and brightest staff members.[7] He meant people like Ugandan physician Dr. Donna Kabatesi, one of the CDC's first hires in Uganda. She quickly encountered the challenge of explaining to her former health ministry colleagues what the CDC was and how it differed from USAID—which had long been the sole face of American development aid in the country.[8]

The agencies disagreed about how to do the work and about what work to do. Natsios's infamous soundbite about Africans lacking watches reflected real doubts on the part of his staff in the field.[9]

In 2000, Dr. Sten Vermund, then at University of Alabama at Birmingham and now dean of the School of Public Health at Yale, started a Lusaka-based project to provide the antiretroviral nevirapine to Zambian women with HIV to prevent transmission to their newborns, who also received a single dose after delivery. The program, which received initial funding from the LIFE initiative, was supposed to work closely with USAID and to expand its approach to the Northern Province, where USAID was working with mothers but focusing solely on nutritional support. (US agencies often worked in specific provinces or districts, carving out territory in a way that minimized conflict but also meant Americans in country didn't have to harmonize their approaches.)

USAID's resistance was fierce. The program, which focused on nutritional counseling, was "actually very militant about not taking up nevirapine," Vermund said, still frustrated years later. "In fact, they made a lot of trouble for us that we wanted to bring in nevirapine. We wanted to work with the government showing that this [nevirapine-based treatment for mothers and babies] was really very straightforward and very feasible. And AID was quite hostile to us at that time. They thought it was premature, they were worried that nevirapine might have some unanticipated side effects in pregnant women."[10]

One CDC doctor described it to me like this. "For CDC, they're like, 'Okay, well, we are the smart doctor people, we understand health care and health service delivery; on the other hand USAID, you don't know this stuff. So we're smart and you're stupid.' And on the other side, USAID was like, 'Okay, we've been doing development forever.' So both thought they were smarter than the other, in different ways."

PEPFAR's structure was designed to level the playing field for all of the US agencies working on HIV. But level ground takes many forms, including gladiatorial arenas. Putting PEPFAR in the State Department allowed CDC and the far smaller Department of

Defense program to compete for resources in countries where US-AID had spent decades developing its programs.

Deborah Birx had seen the opportunity and leapt into the interagency fray less than a week after the State of the Union, when she'd driven to the townhouse that housed the Office of National AIDS Policy to explain to its head, Dr. Joe O'Neill, that her parent agency, the Department of Defense, needed to get money from whatever the president's new program turned out to be. She remembered O'Neill's assistant popping her head into the office. He had to leave; he was late for another meeting. She didn't move. She had printed the slides out, hundreds of them, and she just kept going. "Poor Joe," she grinned when she told me this story years later.[11]

The Department of Defense didn't traditionally do development work, though it would, as the wars in Iraq and Afghanistan unfolded, become increasingly entangled in funding and managing projects designed to win hearts and minds. But the military had always had an HIV program. Enlisted Americans deployed and at home got the virus and required care. The troops would need an eventual vaccine. On that basis, Birx had, as head of the Walter Reed Army Institute of Research, led vaccine trials and preparatory work, including the formation of "cohorts," large groups of people followed over time to study rates of HIV, a baseline measurement needed to determine whether a trial had reduced infection rates at all.

Prior to PEPFAR and the Global Fund, research groups working on HIV in African countries that did not have free AIDS drugs faced a conundrum. If a study participant got HIV, it was ethically questionable not to offer treatment. But the offer of treatment might be an undue inducement to participate—even for HIV-negative people who feared acquiring the virus. This too raised ethical issues. At IAVI, I wrote about this issue and listened to scientists wring their hands over the conundrum. One afternoon, I called Birx to interview her about the topic, and she'd cheerily informed me that she was going to solve the problem for the military trials by providing treatment to everyone in the community where the trial was going to happen.

Participants wouldn't be induced to enroll because everyone who got HIV would have access to antiretrovirals.

Birx and her colleagues, including Kenyan physician Dr. Fred Sawe, set up an antiretroviral program in Kericho, Kenya, at a hospital adjacent to a tea plantation. She told me she decided to work in Kericho after visiting several other hospitals and clinics. At every stop, she asked how the staff diagnosed malaria. If the answer was "when a person has a fever," she moved on. In Kericho, she said, she'd been led to a lab where a tech had a microscope and slides whose edges had grown rounded from use and washing. Every malaria case was diagnosed on smear. Many illnesses caused fever. If there wasn't a lab confirming the diagnosis, meds got misused; diagnoses got missed. Laboratory diagnosis mattered for HIV too. In hard-hit African countries, many people who'd lost a spouse to AIDS assumed that they were HIV positive too; often they were not. A dead partner had been used as a proxy for diagnosis. Birx wasn't building an antiretroviral treatment (ART) program on such a flimsy foundation. In February 2003, she'd walked O'Neill through the results of her thoroughness: a testing and treatment program in a rural area, out ahead of this new program. Birx thought she could use the Kericho model to scale up treatment quickly, and she knew that moving with speed was a matter of life and death for millions of people in the countries PEPFAR proposed working in.

"You're not going to leave until I agree?" she remembered him saying. She wasn't. So he did. "Poor Joe," she sighed happily.[12]

Birx had gotten what she wanted, which was money. For USAID and CDC, there was more at stake: leadership over all, or part, of the program. Both agencies were deeply aggrieved that they had not been put in charge—which was precisely the reason they had been left out of the planning process. After hearing about the president's proposal, the head of the CDC's HIV program reportedly called the initiative "half-baked."[13] Reflecting back sixteen years later, Natsios said, "The decision . . . to have CDC play an equal role with AID in this, in the same countries, in my view, remains one of the major management problems that we still face."[14]

It wasn't that Natsios thought USAID could do everything. There were "things AID didn't have competency in," he explained. "So for example, we don't run, we don't want to run, we don't know how to run blood banks or laboratories, we don't run laboratories. So the CDC does that.... There are a whole bunch of things that CDC could have done in all of these countries, and then the stuff that we know how to do, we should have done." To Natsios and other USAID devotees, though, the agency should have overseen and coordinated the entire effort, using the systems for making and managing grants in country that had been decades in the making.

The CDC lacked that history but had competency in building a public health response in the field. Given that antiretroviral treatment was the major focus of the new program, it hardly made sense for the agency with the most expertise to be managed by the agency with the least competence and conviction that the drugs should be provided in the first place. "AID did not want to admit in any way that we did not have the capacity to manage treatment," Michele Moloney-Kitts, a nurse midwife turned USAID health expert who worked at PEPFAR headquarters in its earliest days, told me. "Basically, AID came into this with the feeling that we are the absolute, really best development agency on the planet. We're the most well funded. This is completely and one hundred percent our mandate by every way that you can figure. CDC, on the other hand, clearly had capacity in treatment that AID didn't necessarily have right on tap."[15]

Putting PEPFAR in the State Department with an ambassador-level head who had a direct line to the White House and a budget of unprecedented size contained, but did not resolve, the conflict. The sheer amount of money brought people to the table, but it didn't make them behave. USAID would never get over the fact that it had not been selected to house the new initiative, according to people from every US agency involved in PEPFAR. At several points, in the years after PEPFAR's launch, it would act with a level of aggrieved maneuvering that impacted PEPFAR's performance and decisions about ambitious, urgent pandemic-fighting initiatives. (The agency would achieve notable success with the president's Malaria Initiative, another Bush project launched in 2005.)

Many, including Dr. Mark Dybul, could only describe the interagency tensions in terms of violence and gore. Regarding the agencies' competition for resources from the very first months of the program, he'd later say, "It was just an absolute blood-on-the-floor nightmare."[16] Dybul experienced the nightmare firsthand. After the State of the Union, he'd worked alongside Joe O'Neill to get the new initiative up and running, borrowing space first from the townhouse occupied by O'Neill's Office of National AIDS Policy before moving to a State Department suite that still bore the name of its prior occupants: "Bush-Cheney Transition Office."[17]

In the Transition Office, O'Neill and Dybul assembled a team of support staff seconded from the major agencies, each represented by a high-ranking staffer, a "principal." Officially known as the deputy principals, or DPs, this group, who did much of the day-to-day work, quickly and cheekily dubbed themselves the "Unprincipals."[18] It fit with their mission, which was to set aside agency identities and core beliefs in the service of the nascent effort. When Moloney-Kitts was detailed from USAID to work in the DC office, her USAID colleagues told her she was "going over to the dark side." Other "Unprincipals," including Dr. R. J. Simonds, who supported Bill Steiger at HHS, and Connie Carrino, who supported USAID, likewise set aside their agencies' core tenets in order to figure out how to actually get the work done.

Dybul had one eye on the Millennium Challenge Corporation, by then a year old and still lacking the legislation needed to authorize its structure, budget, and activities. He knew that congressional confidence waned with delays, and he wanted the AIDS program—which had its law and mandate—to move as quickly as possible. He, O'Neill, and the Unprincipals devised a plan in which a first tranche of money would go out through "Track 1" grants to groups that could quickly scale up services in several countries; a second, larger "Track 2" budget line would finance country-level plans developed by the agencies, with the oversight of the ambassador. (In the first year,

Track 1.5 grants funded country-level work that was ready to take off at an accelerated pace.)

Track 1 was the first and only time that PEPFAR would assign roles, or "lanes," to the agencies receiving money. In recognition of the medical expertise housed at CDC, the group decided that HHS would manage the treatment grant, and USAID would take on prevention, which was, at that point, largely aimed at changing people's behavior and raising AIDS awareness—the "ABC" approach that was popular and unproven and required no clinical expertise to implement. Dybul was adamant that this division of labor must end with the Track 1 request for proposals. He said that when USAID leadership came and presented what he considered a "stupid" proposal to give all of the treatment work to CDC and leave all of prevention with USAID, he shot it down. He figured if the roles got broken apart, the tensions would become so great, both in DC and at the country level, that the damage would be irreparable. "I said, 'Once you do that we will never get the agencies together,'" he recalled.[19]

Moving the money fast was one way of proving PEPFAR worked; showing what it had paid for was another. Under the leadership of Kathy Marconi, a no-nonsense native New Yorker who'd developed the evaluation and reporting system for America's domestic AIDS program, and Ryan White, the deputy principals and their bosses hashed out a core set of things that the new program would measure and report on—"indicators" that would prove that the money wasn't just flowing; it was also saving lives.

Even this task involved navigating interagency tensions. When she'd asked about the information the agency currently collected on its work in the field, USAID offered a handful of "process" indicators—development of a plan, implementation of an education campaign, and so on. Few, if any, tied back to impact on HIV. CDC came with hundreds of epidemiological data points that it either had or wanted to gather. Marconi, who'd moved from her home in Arlington, Virginia, to a foldout couch in her daughter's DC flat, used her training in social psychology to find a middle ground and settle on twenty-odd core indicators for the program.[20]

If the staff in the Transition Office were moving as fast as they could, it still wasn't fast enough for AIDS activists who remained deeply concerned that the administration didn't intend to spend as much as had been authorized in the law. (All funds authorized in legislation still need to be appropriated in a separate legislative process.) A five-year, $15 billion program might be expected to spend $3 billion each year. But the White House's own leadership argued otherwise. On July 17, White House AIDS czar Joe O'Neill sent a letter to Senate Majority Leader Bill Frist stating that it was "inappropriate" to increase investments in the Global Fund and that appropriators should heed the president's ceiling for AIDS funds for both the Fund and the new bilateral PEPFAR, writing, "The Administration strongly opposes any efforts to increase funding beyond the $2 billion requested in the President's FY2004 budget."[21] "It is by careful design that the President's FY2004 budget request is for $2 billion. This request was based on the sound judgment that funds in excess of this amount could not be spent effectively in this first year." Birx told me the same thing, but from the outside looking in, it looked like lowballing and posturing, an extension of the approach the United States had taken with the still-beleaguered Global Fund.

July had been a bad month from beginning to end. On July 2 the White House had announced that Randall Tobias, a former Eli Lilly executive, would be the first US global AIDS ambassador to head the program.[22] By putting a drug company profiteer in charge, Bush seemed to be twisting the dagger, delivering the coup de grâce in his seizure of the global AIDS agenda from the transnational coalition of activists, many queer, Black, brown, pro-sex, and anticapitalist, who had brought the drug prices down over the vigorous resistance of people just like Tobias.

Tobias had doughy features, a little mouth, and a corporate comb over. He was a rich white man out of central casting who'd published a folksy, human-touch management manual, *Put the Moose on the Table*, that turned his ascent through corporate America into life lessons long on personal gumption and character.[23]

Easy to caricature, he was hard to pin down. When his first wife committed suicide in 1994, he talked about how Prozac, Eli Lilly's blockbuster drug, hadn't helped her.[24] Tobias had initially turned down the position when it appeared to be an interagency coordinating role. The offer had come as the United States was preparing to invade Iraq under the leadership of General Tommy Franks. "And I remember saying in some fashion very respectfully that if having a coordinator was such a good idea, why didn't we have General Franks as the coordinator of military forces?" He'd taken the position the second time he was asked—and it had the chain of command he recommended. "Randy will report to Colin Powell but will have a pretty direct line to me." Tobias recalled the president saying words to that effect to the assembled heads of the US agencies charged with implementing PEPFAR on the day of Tobias's appointment.[25] Behind the closed doors of the Transition Office, though, Tobias quickly earned the trust and admiration of the staff working on start-up. He proved adept at heading off long-term USAID contractors who assumed they would get first pass at large portions of the new funding, and he didn't hesitate to use his direct line to the White House to clarify whether the president wanted him to award funding to an established grantee or whether he wanted the initiative to focus on its "2-7-10" goals for treatment, prevention, and care.

"I've worked for tons of people, and tons of people worked for me," Moloney-Kitts told me. "And I absolutely loved working for Randy Tobias." She'd arrived at OGAC's first official office while the furniture was being bought and Tobias was demanding to know why Black-Berrys weren't allowed in the US government. "You can't emphasize enough in this story how really powerful leaders can change everything. We were going to fundamentally change the way we do business to be more efficient, deliver a service, and to achieve a result. Tobias was able to carry that in a way that I could not have imagined somebody coming from more inside the beltway being able to do."

Activists weren't interested in management savvy, though, and heard, in Tobias's repetition of doubts about condoms, a man who'd been handed a script and agreed to perform. August 2003 at least brought a glimmer of good news. On August 8, after five months of ongoing protest within South Africa—and solidarity actions in Washington, DC, London, and Amsterdam—the Treatment Action Campaign's (TAC) civil disobedience campaign focused on propelling the government to launch a national ART program paid off. That day, TAC announced the suspension of its civil disobedience campaign and reconsideration of its pending litigation after the South African government instructed the Ministry of Health to develop a plan for a public-sector antiretroviral treatment program. It was a victory too belated to be sweet. "We welcome the Cabinet's bold step today," the TAC statement wrote. "But we also remember the anguish, pain and unnecessary loss of lives over the last four years."[26]

If the South African government had conceded, the US continued to be an obstacle to meeting the transnational movement's demands. In October, the US delegation to the Global Fund unsuccessfully urged the body to delay launching the next funding round. Pro-Fund activists had to thread the needle on the new mechanism's performance to date: the amount of antiretroviral funding had dropped from one year to the next as countries submitted, and the Fund's Technical Review Panel approved, less ambitious policies.[27] Paul Davis thought that donor pressure on countries to keep their proposals small was "shitty, sneaky" maneuvering—he'd soon step back from activism focused on the Fund that he'd helped to conceive. Asia Russell would, in turn, take on leadership of Fund-focused activism, mastering and shaping its arcana and emerging as an indefatigable tactician.

At the year-end World AIDS Day protest, President Bush became "President Pinocchio," an effigy of a long-nosed liar who'd failed to heed the message on the banner: "Voters want AIDS Action, Not Weapons of Mass Deception." At that moment, the unproven plan looked shady and ego driven, even though the Fund had not yet proven itself a contender. "US jealousy and competition of [*sic*] [Global Fund to Fight AIDS, Tuberculosis and Malaria] led it to promise 93% of its resources to its own unproven, inoperational, and policy-flawed (abstinence-only) unilateral initiative," Health GAP, ACT UP, Housing Works, and other activist groups wrote in their 2003 "Year in Review."[28]

By the time the protests happened, the PEPFAR start-up team had completed a marathon two-week session at the State Plaza Hotel, working alongside country-based staffers flown in to hammer out a country operational planning approach for use across the program and to nail down the language for the Track 1 request for proposals. The request was launched on December 1, with a deadline of New Year's Eve that would see researchers like Phyllis Kanki, a Harvard-based veterinarian, printing documents at a Boston Kinko's in the hours before the ball dropped, and clinicians like Harvard doctor Rick Marlink, who'd helped launch a Botswana treatment program, temporarily commandeering a desk in the offices of the Elizabeth Glaser Pediatric AIDS Foundation to help hammer out their proposal.[29]

The pace did not abate in the first weeks of 2004. An initial tranche of the $2.4 billion budget was released on January 23, and exactly a month later, $350 million of those funds had moved out of OGAC and into the field to the Track 1 and 1.5 partners. That month also brought the passage of legislation creating the Millennium Challenge Account—the development innovation that Bush had proposed two years prior—a reminder of just how easily major presidential initiatives could bog down.[30]

During that same period, Cissy mastered the New York trains enough to make trips up to another Bronx clinic by herself. When I was able, I'd go with her, sometimes sitting with her in the office of a doctor who looked at her with an adoration and gratitude I recognized. Even when she was in extremis, Cissy seemed to be taking care of the people who were, ostensibly, providing assistance. The Bronx doctor managed to persuade a drug company to donate a year's supply of the medication Cissy required, and could not get in Kampala, for her ailment. Cissy made people want to show her their best selves, their most treasured things. He was seeing her for free, and when he learned she was a woman of faith, he'd invited her to see the Chagall windows in a Westchester church. One evening when she seemed somewhat more comfortable walking, I took her to see the blue whale hanging from the ceiling of the hall of marine mammals at the Museum of Natural History. When she was finally well enough to return home in February, I was relieved at her return to health but deeply sad to see her go.

— —

A MONTH AFTER CISSY went home, a fellow Ugandan named John Robert Engole swallowed the first PEPFAR-purchased antiretroviral pill on a leafy hill in Mbuya, not far from her home. Fourteen months after the US president had proposed that America pay for antiretrovirals for Africa, the program was underway.[31] The country's Global Fund grant, made a year earlier, had paid for little save offices in a swanky blue-glass-walled office building in downtown Kampala.

If PEPFAR and the Global Fund were judged on speed alone, then PEPFAR had won, at least in Uganda. When Engole took his pill, somewhere between 10,000 and 15,000 Ugandans had antiretroviral treatment. Six months later, there would be upward of 24,000—almost all supported directly by the Ugandan PEPFAR program, which would report 33,000, or 122 percent achievement of its Year 1 goal, in PEPFAR's first report to Congress, and 67,500, 113 percent of the target for the entire five years, in the second annual report, delivered in early 2006.[32]

But PEPFAR did not have a monopoly on speed. Malawi, landlocked and lake-bound like Uganda, but even more impoverished, didn't make PEPFAR's list of "focus countries" in 2004 and so launched its treatment program with a single funding source: the Global Fund. In 2004, before the program began, the country had nine sites serving 3,000 clients. The clinics were primarily in the public sector, and the care they provided was not standardized or guided by national government documents.

By the end of 2005, the country had sixty sites and 37,840 individuals in treatment—a more than one-hundred-fold increase in twelve months. The government had directed the rollout process, issuing guidance, setting accreditation standards, and advancing an "equity-based" approach that aimed for uniformity of services and nation-wide geographic coverage. The architects of the program recognized that they had less money than countries with grants from both PEP-FAR and the Global Fund, but they also felt they had more control.[33] The single funding source "allowed the country to build and sustain a cohesive national programme with a uniform direction for scale-up and no competing interests," they'd later write.

Malawi was proof positive that a PEPFAR program wasn't required for a fast, ambitious scale-up project with attention paid to training and quality. Uganda suggested that in some places the opposite was the case. Uganda had booked its Global Fund grant a full year prior to the president's State of the Union and hadn't spent a shilling on treatment by the time Engole swallowed his pill.[34] This wasn't for lack of local expertise. For a small nation, it had an enormous concentration of HIV-focused clinicians and researchers who, in turn, had a vast network of non-Ugandan partners and collaborators.

PEPFAR was also a key ally in South Africa, home to the largest HIV-positive population in sub-Saharan Africa. When Bush pledged his AIDS funding, Thabo Mbeki and Manto Tshabalala-Msimang still held the country in a lethal grip of AIDS denialism. The Pretoria-based PEPFAR team—led by USAID staffers—began what South African HIV clinician Dr. Francois Venter thought of as a "covert undercover operation." Every single resuscitation that Venter performed in the final year of his medical training had been on his knees on the floor. The hospital he'd worked at was, like virtually every other health facility, overwhelmed with people dying of AIDS—he reckoned it was at 300 percent capacity. Venter would never forget the people dying on the floor.[35]

Then the PEPFAR money had arrived. "PEPFAR played a very important role in getting ARVs out to the Western Cape and to ac-tivist doctors providing services in NGOs...before the government of South Africa was forced to do so by the courts of law," said Dr. Yogan Pillay, who joined the South African National Department of Health (NDOH) in 1996 and served as the coordinator of the AIDS response from 2008 to 2020.[36] "The brave people [at the US mission] in Pretoria assisted us to do whatever we could," said Venter, who ran the PEPFAR program at the Reproductive Health Institute at Witwatersrand University. The government was running a notoriously critical accreditation system, designed to find fault with clinics so that they could not provide antiretrovirals. Venter and his colleagues would go out in advance of the accreditation team and make sure the clinic—often a facility run by an activist doctor or nurse—was able to pass. PEPFAR paid for the health-care workers' training on how to administer ARVs and allowed this network of activist doctors and nurses to experiment with data-collection and patient-registration systems. Venter experienced those early years as ones of enormous flexibility and partnership. "If I had to guess, one million South Africans survived because of PEPFAR," Venter said. "It moved quickly, the funding was generous and it got shit done."

In the year prior to launching the ART plan, the national government blocked a Global Fund grant for KwaZulu-Natal, which had applied directly to the Fund and secured a one-year emergency grant for antiretrovirals. The government objected on the grounds that the grant hadn't been developed by a country coordinating mechanism (CCM)—though none existed—and dragged its heels on signing even when the Fund's executive director, Richard Feachem, flew into the country to work out the final details. At a news conference with Feachem, South African Anglican archbishop Njongonkulu Ndungane said, "I have no words to express my dismay. It seems that the health ministry or whoever is responsible for [the agreement is] fiddling while Rome is burning. People are dying."[37]

A neoliberal presumption that PEPFAR was the only way to bring AIDS drugs to Africa with speed was false; the antiglobalization, leftist assertion that all African countries would, if left to their own devices, take care of their most impoverished citizens also didn't hold up. The Western world had no monopoly on inequitable distributions of health and wealth across societies or on leaders who cared more for their militaries than their hospitals. White supremacy worked through Black and brown people too; it was the savage force, the strongest man.

In the context of an ongoing pandemic emergency, the American bilateral response saved lives quickly—and for the brave person whose life was spared, there was no question that the approach taken was the right one. "If you were somebody living with HIV and you didn't have access to ARVs except through NGO clinics set up by PEPFAR, you didn't care about PEPFAR. All you cared about was whether you could get ARVs," Pillay said. "It annoyed us [the South African NDOH] that this was a parallel system being put in place," he added, especially since the HIV clinic hadn't even treated tuberculosis, a common coinfection, in the early days.

It annoyed AIDS activists in the United States too. Matthew Kavanagh, the antiglobalization activist who'd viewed the Global Fund as a "postneoliberal dream," never stopped wondering about the counterfactual: What would have happened if the American investment had been in making the Global Fund work? If there had been $15 billion over five years that deployed Harvard-esque know-how to support countries to both build health systems and treat people at the same time? What if, he'd always wonder, all of the money and all of the energy that America put into PEPFAR had been put in the service of making the first new multilateral fund work?

I joined him in this enticing thought experiment in his office at Georgetown University fifteen years after PEPFAR launched. Kavanagh by that time had earned his PhD and knew so much about PEPFAR that activists encountering him for the first time sometimes thought he worked for the program. As we spoke, I thought of the pile of faxes in Jay Lefkowitz's correspondence file from PEPFAR authorization—how the Eagle Forum, Phyllis Schlafly, Representative Joe Pitts, Katy Talento, and just about every other conservative AIDS advocate thought that the Global Fund was a backdoor grant maker for abortionists and North Koreans. To imagine the sheer volume of US funding allocated to global AIDS going solely to the Global Fund was nearly impossible. Above and beyond its policies, the program itself reflected the nature of Talento's compromise: "Democrats pay for Republican policy change."

In many ways, PEPFAR was best suited for the countries where those enmeshed relationships had done the most damage—countries governed by leaders who knew there was little they could do to lose their donors' funding and their favor or whose raw experience with white supremacy and capitalism had warped their thinking about a virus and its remedies. Uganda was considered an island of political stability in the Great Lakes region, compared to the Democratic Republic of Congo, South Sudan, Burundi, and even Kenya, with its restive Islamic militant population. By the time PEPFAR arrived, President Yoweri Museveni had armed and instigated conflicts at the Rwandan and Congolese borders, committed human rights violations against his own and other countries' citizens, and flouted donor requests to consider a transfer of power. The funding had kept on flowing, with almost no conditions, as had the praise for an AIDS response that the funders were floating in its entirety. Museveni gave no sign of wanting to directly address his country's epidemic with a massive, government-led treatment program. There were historical antecedents, deep colonialist and neoliberal causes, but if you were a person living with HIV, you wanted the medications to treat the virus, not the interventions that would undo the twisted knots of colonialism's history and its present.[38]

PEPFAR was most palatable to those who could maintain a narrow focus on the AIDS epidemic as separate from geopolitics and history. If you saw the structures that caused the epidemic as part of the emergency, then PEPFAR's approach was harder to swallow. But the AIDS epidemic was indeed an emergency, and one that required a chronic medical intervention that had not been mounted before. PEPFAR was a uniquely well-funded and well-designed aid effort by American standards. This was true even though its diagnosis of the problem and its proposed solution reflected problems that the benefactors, and their ancestors, had caused and were invested in perpetuating. To say that it was the best possible effort that America could have put forward at that moment in time is not to say that it was the best possible solution to the problem. A capitalist, white supremacist America might never offer that sort of excellence. But to dismiss it for its limitations was to waste the evidence it offered for what the country could accomplish when it set out to fight a plague.

For the US Congress that had written the check for this new experiment in American altruism, the stock taking could not happen soon enough. In May 2004, not two months after the program had started spending money, PEPFAR head Randall Tobias was summoned to the Dirksen Senate Office Building to deliver a "progress report" to the Foreign Relations Committee. First, though, Lamar Alexander explained his hopes that the plague war reporting would take its lead from the Pentagon. "During the war with Iraq, winning the war, it was fairly easy to tell what progress we were making," he said (the hearing took place in the brief period where America could sustain the myth that it had won any war, that anything was over). "We had daily reports. Generals made the reports. They had clear benchmarks about their progress and we could see the progress."[39]

Tobias assured Alexander that his office would deliver the "report card" the senator repeatedly requested. "One of the things I learned in business school forty some years ago and has been confirmed repeatedly over time is that it's a good idea to start with the premise that if something can't be measured and isn't being measured, you need to question whether it's worth doing," Tobias said.

Tobias had a harder time addressing questions from Senator Russell Feingold about the program's legislated requirement that the funds pay solely for FDA-approved drugs, a stipulation that locked PEPFAR into buying expensive, brand-name drugs instead of cheaper generics. "I don't believe that the American taxpayers will tolerate decisions that favor saving fewer lives with patented pricey medications, if we can help more people with cheaper generic drug regimens," Feingold challenged.

Lulu Oguda, a Kenyan doctor who'd worked with Médecins Sans Frontières (MSF), backed up his concern with blunt testimony. "I have heard US government officials say that they will not tolerate a different standard for Africans. As an African doctor who has personally treated

hundreds of people with HIV/AIDS using these medicines and witnessed my patients' spectacular return from death's door, I find this
particularly appalling."

Oguda's testimony and Feingold's concern—which had been
piqued by a *Washington Post* article on America's outlier position on
generics—were testament to, and part of, an escalating campaign
that had been going on for months. It was, once again, an inside-
outside game. On March 29, Ellen 't Hoen, the director of policy for
MSF's Access to Medicines Campaign, had taken Mark Dybul to
task at a meeting that the United States had convened to discuss
fixed-dose combinations (FDCs)—simple, two-pill regimens made
only by generic manufacturers.[40]

The very fact that the United States wanted to talk about FDCs
instead of simply paying for them caused several groups, including
the European Medical Association, the equivalent of the FDA, to
boycott the meeting, insisting there wasn't anything to discuss at all.
While the United States contended that there were "issues" with
FDCs, much of the world countered that America's only issue was
that FDCs were solely made by generic manufacturers and sold for 40
to 50 percent less than the equivalent branded drugs. The World
Health Organization (WHO) had a "prequalification" process that
involved a rigorous review of bioequivalence data and manufacturing
plants. Drugs and other health commodities that passed through this
process landed on a list that many donors and governments shopped
from to supply their health programs. When Tobias parroted the official American stance that WHO wasn't a regulatory agency and that
only the United States' stringent FDA could do the job, Richard Hol-
brooke, then head of the Global Business Coalition on AIDS, said the
stance threatened much of the work that PEPFAR aimed to do.[41]

In his opening remarks, Dybul said that FDCs were conceptually
a good idea. FDCs weren't "conceptual," Ellen 't Hoen admonished.[42]
They existed, as did the principles for ensuring that they were safe. To
amplify the message, AIDS activists chained themselves to the headquarters of the pharmaceutical lobby on the day the meeting began.

At the Senate hearing, Tobias repeated the standard explanations about "principles" and "quality concerns" to little persuasive effect. Behind the scenes, though, his team had taken note of the protests, the bad press, and, perhaps, the evidence. Five weeks later, Tommy Thompson would announce a new "fast-track" approval process purpose-built to get fixed-dose combinations approved for PEPFAR purchase. It wasn't the fix activists wanted—the WHO process was adequate, they said, and the "fast track" would only slow things down. But if they hadn't gotten their precise ask, they'd proven that they could change the program.[43]

"The pressure that [the activists] deployed was obvious and palpable, and it absolutely drove an internal interagency process that resulted in the rapid-approval process for drugs that was totally unique," Tobias's chief of staff, Nazanin Ash, told me.[44] "There [were] a million things to do when you were deploying PEPFAR, and that activism really put it on the priority list and . . . created space for innovative solutions to be found in a much faster time frame."

The activists' analysis of the problem, marshaling of evidence, and partnership with doctors and clients using generics to fight HIV had changed the program. It was a moral victory, and one that would save lives and make PEPFAR more efficient with its available funds. Within four years, upward of 90 percent of the program's drugs were generics. It was indicative of the work that activists would take on, having realized that PEPFAR was not merely an empty promise and was perhaps the only way that the United States would ever spend as much money as they thought it should.

"Movements go in cycles, and politics goes in cycles. There are opportunities, and then everything after the opportunities is about keeping things moving in the right direction until there's another opportunity," Matthew Kavanagh said to me. There had been an opportunity with the Global Fund and the antiglobalization movement to do something wholly different—to rewrite the script. With that window closed, Kavanagh and his activist peers kept things moving— which meant keeping an eye on PEPFAR.

It had taken me years to ask activists about their initial opposition to PEPFAR—fifteen years later, it still felt somehow treasonous. One afternoon, I choked out the question to Sharonann Lynch: "Do you remember hating PEPFAR?" "I don't think we understood fully what we had," she said. "I think we were a bit churlish about it all, to tell you the truth."[45] She said it with such ease that I almost wished I'd asked years earlier, when I'd nursed private doubts about activists' assertions that PEPFAR was an empty promise. Though if I had, I might not have moved to Uganda to see for myself. Instead, in late 2004, I sublet my railroad flat and said good-bye to Liam Flaherty, the kind, singularly unflappable Brooklyn Irishman who'd quoted Naipaul to me at my friend's wedding. Over a slow-moving, months-long courtship, I'd been unable to scare him off with either tears, tipsy outbursts, or warnings that I was moving to Uganda. He had simply asked if I planned to come back, and because I was, by that time, in love with him, I said I would.

Then I left.

In October 2004, I moved into a flat on the Makerere University campus, pasted a postcard of Halley's Comet on the light switch above my stuccoed bedroom wall, and invited Cissy over for dinner. She came smiling, smooth-skinned, plump in a flowing chiffon blouse. She walked easily up the hill and into my red-floored flat, with its embassy hand-me-down furniture, and told me that the whole time she'd stayed with me, during all those months in which she'd entertained me by singing along to the theme song of *The Nanny* and dubbing the nearby Hoyt-Schermerhorn subway station *sukuma wiki*, the Swahili phrase for collards, which means, literally, "stretch the week," she'd been convinced she was going to die in my apartment. She said that she had slept every night for nearly two months worried about how in the world I would pay to ship her body home. She told me this, looked at my face, then burst out laughing at my shock and chagrin over what I hadn't seen.

CHAPTER 7

SMALL HEAVENS

K AMPALA, LIKE THE COUNTRY for which it is the major metrop-
olis, appears to be easy to know. It ranges over seven hills, several topped with landmarks that also tell the country's history:
Mulago Hospital, Makerere University, the Baháʼí Temple—one of
seven in the world. The largest palace of the king of Buganda sits on
top of Mengo Hill behind a round brick fence, close to the Anglican
cathedral that has adorned Namirembe Hill since the early twentieth
century, turning its red-brick face in the direction of the royal dwelling of the British-favored clan. In the oldest parts of town, like
Mengo and Old Kampala, dun-colored two-storied buildings with
overhanging balconies shading the sidewalk bore the year of construction and the occasional Hindu symbol for om in the crenella-
tion at the top of the facade. One can drive through the streets and,
by learning the landmarks, have the illusion of also learning history.

The city that I arrived in on October 24, 2004, was also easy to
traverse on foot. When I walked down from the Makerere University
campus to Bombo Road and thence to Mulago Hospital, I threaded
down a narrow pedestrian street of three-walled shops that stretched
up from Wandegeya Market. Nail salons, clothing stores, purveyors
of all things plastic—from baskets, to sandals, to the basins that students needed to do their laundry—sold their wares out of tiny,

ordered spaces. Alleys behind these stores led to more and smaller businesses, like Professor Ki Kati—whose name meant "What now?"—who had a phone-booth-sized wooden stall in a charcoal-brazier-studded courtyard used by a local restaurant, in which he hand-cranked a well-oiled contraption that emitted a metallic scream as it copied my keys.

When expats said, as they often did, "Kampala is a village," they were referring to the grazing animals and the maize that grew in plots next to office blocks. They meant, too, that for all its sprawl, it had a sense of intimacy and safety. One could move from the alley into the rear courtyard without crossing an invisible border demarcating here from there—poverty from wealth, public from private, safe from unsafe. White Westerners like me felt secure going almost anywhere. In Nairobi, whose verdant streets had a darker, evergreen hue, the shift from an NGO office adjacent to the Kabira slum, where the packed dirt was shot through with plastic bags, was so extreme that it was like jumping off a cliff; in Nairobi, carjackings were common, and the far superior sidewalks around the downtown hotels were often deemed unsafe for morning jogs.

Kampala hid modern conveniences like treasures amid its dirt roads and sprawling outdoor markets. There was, for a time, a pay phone in the post office on Kampala Road, across from the creamy white facade of the Barclays bank, that was unlabeled and, when the receiver was lifted, immediately connected to an international line from which you could use your calling card. The phone was singular, like many of the city's amenities at the start of the twenty-first century: the lone expat sports bar, Just Kicking, and the man in the parking lot outside with a basketful of DVDs of movies that had not yet been released overseas. You could set the metal receiver in its cradle and, in less than an hour, be at the side of Lake Victoria, where the noise of frogs and birds at the start of the day was a cacophony that made me think, time and again—and despite a sharp-tongued postcolonialist critique of my own musings—of Eden.

I woke to those noises most weekends, when I traveled out to my expat friends' lake houses: Mark Breda's in Munyoyno and Leslie

Nielsen's fairy house on stilts in Bunga, both technically suburbs of Kampala, where houses with coveted "mature" gardens of tall trees and thick, flowering bushes turned their faces toward the lake. Leslie was the nurse I'd met in Harlem who called me on September 11; she'd connected me to Mark, and together they'd welcomed me into the expat world, where weekends found public health–focused Americans and Brits congregating in houses thick with sun-bleached photographs from Zanzibar and Lamu and squat carved stools. I'd gorge myself on their duty-free wine and pasta with sun-dried tomatoes and sausages from the butcher beside the embassy.

Our expat delight in the long afternoons on Mark's giant wooden couch was, in part, a function of contrast. During the week, when we dispatched to our offices and inquiries, we entered a world that was equally navigable, though not always or even often physically lovely. From the top of Makerere Hill I could see Mulago Hill and its esteemed hospital, and I could see, too, the slum in the bowl in between, which flooded when the rains came and would, from time to time, be wracked with cholera outbreaks, even though the Ministry of Health was minutes away.

Many of my friends worked in offices at Mulago Hospital, in the jumble of many buildings housing Ugandan collaborations with international groups that studded Mulago Hospital's campus. There was the little white building with the outside staircase that housed the Case Western Reserve University project, where many of my expat friends worked on tuberculosis and other diseases with Dr. Roy Mugwera and Dr. Harriet Mayanja. Steps away sat the headquarters of the Makerere University–Johns Hopkins University project led by Dr. Frances Mmiro and Dr. Phillippa Musoke. Down at the bottom of the hill, in a 1960s-era building with a facade not unlike a Miami Beach motel, the Institute of Public Health housed Dr. David Serwadda, Dr. Nelson Sewankambo, and Dr. Fred Wabwire-Mangen, the trio of researchers who'd established the Rakai Health Sciences Program (RHSP) in the southern district where some of the earliest Ugandan cases were identified.

I could walk to these offices and, with enough advance planning, get an appointment to speak with these and other members of the

Ugandan brain trust of eminent scientists who'd worked on the front lines of HIV for years. From there, I could secure invitations to visit their clinics—my sole plan for the year had been to sit in different ART clinics to watch what happened. I could often even arrange a ride with a Kampala-based team member who was hitting the road to visit one of the sites of the new program.

I could do all of this and then walk from Mulago Hospital up Kira Road to Kisementi, the three-sided parking lot named for its crumbling cement, and sit at the Crocodile Café and get a chapati swaddled in cream sauce, wrapped around the filling of my choice, and a cappuccino with a crumbling butter cookie on the side, as I'd done on my first visit in 2000, when a tousled expat had sat down at my table and sighed, "I could spend a whole year here looking at clouds."

People who came to Uganda routinely fell in love, and the country's history—including its AIDS response—was inextricably linked with how strategically it managed this ardent affection. Winston Churchill had declared the country "the Pearl of Africa." His fore-bearer Gerald Portal's description of crossing into the "delightful, rich, and shady" Usoga region after a long march from the Kenyan coast evokes the instant when the Wizard of Oz switches from black and white to technicolor: "Our march the previous day had been, as usual, over monotonous, burnt, and barren plains . . . but now without any gradation or preparation, we suddenly passed into a land of fine trees, of endless banana gardens, of cool shade, and intelligent-looking, chocolate-coloured people." He goes on, "Now, indeed, we were in a land of plenty."[1]

Portal's brother would succumb to malaria during their stay in Kampala, and Portal himself perished soon after returning to Great Britain. Yet the attachment to the place and, in particular, the Ba-ganda people, whom the British would favor above all other tribes, persisted for the next sixty-nine years, as the East India Company staked its claim to a country it would never fully colonize but consid-ered a protectorate, a distinction that reflected the country's remote, landlocked location, which made full-scale plunder and occupation something of an inconvenience.

That distinction between protectorate and colony made a profound impression on the great Kenyan author Ngũgĩ wa Thiong'o, who in 1959 left his native country to attend Uganda's Makerere University. Gazing out the window on the westward train ride, he marked the shift from the grids of Kenyan colonizers' farms on stolen land to Uganda's verdant landscape of household farms, which seemed, like the vibrant Black-dominated streets of Kampala, unclaimed and untamed. He found the same energy and freedom in the campus's explosive intellectual scene, which was replete with playwrights, journalists, and theorists of Black African independence. It was also a place of contested narratives. Thiong'o wrote a play that portrayed a British army officer in an unfavorable light. It won an award, but the university declined to stage it. So he wrote another play and, with a multiracial cast of whites, Indians, and Africans, staged the first full-scale production by a Black African playwright in the country's history. Makerere University was "a place where the impossible seemed possible. Makerere was then a place of dreams," Thiong'o later wrote.[2]

To live in a city of hills is to live with long views. While Thiong'o pursued his undergraduate degree and worked on his first novel, he watched Black Africans assuming control of governments in protectorates and colonies taking care to preserve the colonizers' rules and definitions of order, lest the transitions be perceived as disorganized or chaotic. "Yes, we lived in paradise, but it was a paradise built on the uneven colonial structures we had sworn to maintain." He'd mark this as a time of cataclysmic change in which the gaze of white supremacy weighed heavy and mere perseverance felt Herculean. "Colonialism could not have been expected to nurture and encourage its opposite and survive. The class and ethnic divides could not be overcome by perpetuating the same vision" that had created them in the first place. Looking back decades later, Thiong'o rued the moment of checked ambitions. "The divisions could have been meaningfully encountered only by a bigger vision, certainly one different from the one that created and nurtured them. Thereby hangs a tale whose implications we could not and did not see at the time."[3]

— —

AFTER UGANDA GAINED ITS independence, a steady stream of well-intentioned whites arrived with offers of assistance. Americans, Canadians, Danes, Swedes, and Dutch roved Kampala and the lakeside capital, Entebbe, in such profusion that one Canadian volunteer engineer lamented, in 1972, that the sheer number of expats in Entebbe made it hard to meet the locals. Not that the expats were a boring crowd. This particular expat attended BYOBB (booze and bedding) bashes with Viking themes, promising "raping and pillaging." He would host his own house-warming party with two other expats after they'd located a cottage and left their three-month "imprisonment" in the lavish confines of the Lake Victoria Hotel.[4]

"It was sort of the smallest, most beautiful place you ever saw in your life," American diplomat Horace G. Dawson mused. "It was a paradise."[5] "It didn't have the colonial hang-ups," said Michael Pistor, a public affairs assistant who'd done a tour of duty in the 1960s.[6]

In the 1960s USAID missions pursued the serious business of securing alliances with newly independent African states with a steady stream of cultural imports. Louis Armstrong came to perform; American Golden Glove boxers flew in to face off with Ugandan pugilists. When the embassy staff aired kinescopes of the Nixon-Kennedy debates in its "dingy" library and auditorium, Ugandans lined up around the block to get in. They located and paid for an enormous lift van with special ice-making equipment to heave its way down Kampala streets. An indoor arena was flooded, and gasps went up all around when the first skaters glided out for "Holidays on Ice."[7]

Langston Hughes was flown in for a 1962 literary conference sponsored by the Congress of Cultural Freedom, an organization funded by the CIA. Participants used the occasion to meet needs that they—not the funder—defined. Thiong'o thrust the handwritten pages of a manuscript into the hands of Chinua Achebe. When

Hughes asked him for a tour of the city, he planned a day visiting the heights of the seven hills, then set that aside and followed the poet into the thick of Wandegeya Market, where he sipped *waragi,* the local gin, and roamed the outdoor market "absorbing the atmosphere of harmony in dissonance," that intoxicating mixture of gritty reality and dreams.

"Thank God I had no money and no influence because if I had, I would have used my own money to bet, or the United States' money to lavish on Uganda, because this was the country that was going to lead Africa," said Pistor.

Some forty years later, Jono Mermin, the first head of the US Centers for Disease Control and Prevention (CDC) program in Uganda felt much the same way. "Uganda portends the future of the epidemic," he said in a talk I attended shortly after I arrived in late 2004. A small man, he radiated enthusiasm, bouncing on the balls of his feet and moving in front of the projector beam so that his shadow flew up the wall behind him.

I'd come to the talk to introduce myself to Mermin, who I knew I had to meet to understand what America planned to do in Uganda. Mermin and his wife, social scientist Rebecca Bunnell, had teamed up with Ugandan collaborators to start the research endeavor known as the Home-Based AIDS Care project (HBAC). HBAC was "implementation science"—public-health speak for testing an approach to delivering service—and not an effort intended to be replicated on a national scale. Still, the project's motorcycle-riding home visitors had captivated Dr. Mark Dybul and persuaded him that large-scale antiretroviral treatment in rural, impoverished settings was possible.

As a research project, HBAC served a vanishingly small percentage of people in need of treatment for HIV—just 1,000 people in total. Designed to generate the scientific evidence to guide policies and programs across sub-Saharan Africa, it started from the premise that it wasn't clear exactly what African ART programs needed to look like to reach everyone, including the poorest of the poor. There was, within that question, the possibility that wholly new approaches might emerge. When I heard about it, I was as taken as Dybul. It sounded Utopian—a time-bound manifestation of the more equitable world that people fighting for AIDS drugs envisioned.

I wanted to meet Mermin to secure an invitation to HBAC. My sole plan for the year was to sit in clinics—to visit them regularly, watching what happened to the people who worked there and the people who came to receive the medications. I did not know what I'd see, but for the first time in my life, I did not have a predefined assignment for the story, which I described to Mermin and everyone else I approached that year as a book about what happened when AIDS drugs came to Uganda.

A New York City native, Mermin had trained at Harvard and earned his MD from Stanford University. Rebecca Bunnell, who hailed from upstate New York, was a Harvard-trained epidemiologist. Both were graduates of the CDC's Epidemiological Investigation Service training program, which turned out the epidemic-eradicating disease detectives widely considered to be the best in the world. In 1998, Mermin and Bunnell had each separately been offered jobs in Uganda. Bunnell had lived in country for four years, some years prior, working first for Médecins Sans Frontières and then becoming the first American on the staff of The AIDS Support Organisation (TASO), one of the earliest community-based groups in the country and the region. Her work had centered in the postwar devastation of the Luweero District where Milly Katana grew up.[8]

Prior to taking the Uganda post, Mermin had not worked overseas for more than a few months at a time. He was a self-described "global novice." But he'd never let his age or level of experience serve as a deterrent. Before graduating from medical school, he and his classmate Dr. Reuben Granich wrote a book about preventing and treating HIV in resource-poor settings that would be published in thirty-five languages;[9] the pair also fired off an opinionated letter to a medical journal about the fine points of testing strategies in Africa.[10]

"How old are you?" Dr. Kevin De Cock, the epidemiologist and physician then leading the CDC's division on HIV/AIDS prevention, asked Mermin when he flew to Atlanta in 2001 to interview for the job heading the Uganda program. When his deputy told him this question was illegal, De Cock moved on. Why, he asked, did Mermin want to go and start a CDC program someplace with so much existing strength—Dr. Peter Mugyenyi's Joint Clinical Research Center (JCRC) was there, along with the Rakai Health Sciences Program. Bunnell had done her dissertation work in that region. Biting back amusement—*You guys offered* me *the job*, he thought—he explained that he wanted to go to Uganda because it was at the cutting edge, ready to pave the way for a better future. "Uganda has an extraordinary set of human and scientific infrastructures," he recalled explaining. "So it will be setting the example for the next stage of HIV prevention [and treatment] in Africa."

Bunnell took the position she'd been offered leading HIV programs for USAID. After learning that they would not be able to live together in US government housing unless they arrived as a married couple, they'd exchanged rings and embarked—with their five-month-old daughter—for a country that was seen, once again, as a harbinger of the future and a crucible of dreams.

When they arrived, TASO—the organization Bunnell had worked for years prior—was waiting. The group had been founded by Noerine Kaleeba in 1987 after her husband died of AIDS. Bunnell had worked with Kaleeba in TASO's earliest days, when it, like the National Guidance and Empowerment Network, had focused on building community among people living with HIV. The group had an anthem, "Today It's Me, Tomorrow It's You," support groups for people living with HIV, and song-and-dance troupes who sang the anthem with a step-together-step, chest-thumping choreography that was church choir by way of the Supremes. While it lacked a substantial staff of doctors or pharmacists—or any experience providing medications—it was a vibrant group with a vast membership of people committed to supporting each other in any way they could. Kaleeba had also developed an agreement with the Ugandan Ministry of Health that allowed TASO chapters offering social support to be colocated at government hospitals and health facilities.

Both Mermin and Bunnell knew they needed to figure out how to provide antiretrovirals to people in the rural, impoverished communities where TASO members lived. To them, the members and the group's resilient structure mattered more than its medical know-how. Dr. Alex Coutinho agreed. A charismatic Ugandan physician, Coutinho earned his master's in public health studying the potential economic impact of HIV in Swaziland, then moved back to Uganda after Mermin and Bunnell arrived. Kaleeba had moved on to working with the UN some years earlier, and Coutinho became the head of TASO. To Coutinho, the deficits were an asset. "We could start afresh," he thought. "We don't have to learn all the complicated stuff; we can learn the future."[11]

Raised by a single mother, Coutinho learned early on to assume outsize responsibilities as a matter of necessity. His mother told him to attend mass before school in the morning; when he did, he often found himself the only celebrant besides the priest, who sometimes invited him up to the pulpit to read alongside him.[12] Mermin, too, had acquired some of his precocity out of necessity. His own father had died when he was four. As their mother worked to juggle child-rearing and her own work, she also conveyed the immense importance of academics to Mermin, his twin brother, and sister. Years later, he'd bond over this with Coutinho. "I had worked hard academically my whole life...to have skills that could help the world around me be just a bit better than if I hadn't existed," he told me. "Alex's drive seemed to be woven from similar fabric."[13]

One day, I climbed up the stairs to the TASO executive suite to visit Coutinho. On the wall behind him hung pictures of Kaleeba, along with images of Coutinho with actress Emma Thompson and the country's current UNAIDS representative, Dr. Ruben del Prado. "Providing ARVs is like building a house," he said. Prevention was the foundation—"unless we turn off the tap [of new infections] now, we are not going to be able to sustain [ART] delivery." Care and support for people living with HIV were the walls. TASO had built the foundation and erected the walls in the previous years; that was why it was ready to take on ART.

By that time, Coutinho, Mermin, and Bunnell had built on the previous agreement between the Ministry of Health and TASO, bringing them on board as an investigator in the HBAC study. Coutinho told me that they'd also persuaded the Ministry of Health to support TASO as an AIDS treatment provider, overcoming concerns that building the antiretroviral program through nongovernmental organizations like TASO would lead to the creation of a parallel health-care system. The CDC worked closely with government, funding a "cooperative agreement" that paid for laboratory and surveillance work and helped support policy development. But when it came to combatting the epidemic, the disease detectives wanted to build on the strongest foundation possible—programs that had core components of care and prevention already in place. "I have yet to see a house that starts with a roof," Coutinho said.

Mermin had been friendly the first day I'd met him and told me I was welcome in Tororo any time. But both he and Bunnell, like every American I encountered at the end of the program's first full year of operation, were fiendishly busy. In 2000, on my first trip to Uganda, I'd traveled down to the Rakai Health Sciences Program. At that time, it had been a research-focused endeavor, and one of its lead scientists, Dr. David Serwadda, had told me that he wasn't sure there was a place for antiretrovirals in a health-care system that failed to deliver basic, simpler remedies like antimalarials. Once PEPFAR was launched, though, Serwadda and his collaborators had come around, teaming up with the CDC to launch a treatment program that, like HBAC, sought to bring high-tech care closer to communities. In November 2004 I secured an invitation to visit its headquarters in Kalisizo—close to Cissy's home village—and made my way south, taking Masaka Road, which dropped south off the outskirts of Kampala by the lush green of Busega swamp and a store painted with an advertisement for shoe polish in which a white woman's hands gripped a black loafer. "Don't just shine, super shine my shoes."

Kalisizo was laid out on a simple grid, two main streets bisected by two others, wide and dusty as the thoroughfares in the Westerns my father had watched when I was growing up. The morning after I'd arrived, I walked out of the main building and into the dusty intersection, then climbed into a pickup truck loaded with metal foot lockers, nurses, and counselors who rotated through the district bringing the drugs close to the rural, impoverished population.

We drove to Kasasa, to a building classified as a Health Center III, pulling up on a flat-packed dirt parking area in front of two buildings set back from the road. One, small and covered in dingy cream-colored paint, was the government clinic, staffed by a nurse named Mary, who, when I asked her about her drug supplies, picked the bottles off her small dispensing table and rattled them like castanets so I could hear the thin click of a handful of pills inside. It was November 17; she'd last received drugs in September. She had the broad-spectrum antibiotic metronidazole and, for antimalarials, the colonial remedy of quinine, plus ten tablets of Fansidar—the preferred first-line treatment. It was enough to treat perhaps ten adults. She had a smattering of mebendazole for treating parasites and worms. She told me she lacked salbutamol, which helped with breathing, at least one malaria drug, and anything for the sexually transmitted infections that troubled so many of her clients. Of the thirty-odd a month who came to test for HIV, she reckoned fifteen were positive. She had not had condoms since July.

The RHSP staff took over the other building, which might otherwise have been used as an inpatient ward. It was a large, dusky square room whose only source of light came from the door and the square windows looking out on the bright green field and brush beyond. The room itself was empty save for what seemed like an enormous number of bed frames, all without mattresses, all made of varnished blonde wood. They stood at the odd and random angles of infrequent use. When the sun went behind a cloud, the room felt submerged, the pale wood seeming to gleam like bones. The RHSP team supplied the rest of the contents: medications for malaria and sexually transmitted diseases, antiretrovirals (ARVs), antifungals, medical charts in primary colors, a box filled to the brim with powder-coated latex gloves.

Next door, Mary had told me she had ten pairs of gloves and half a roll of cotton gauze and that five women had delivered at the hospital that day. On the RHSP side, I watched a nurse reach for a pair from the overstuffed box the team had brought. When several others popped out and then drifted like poppy petals to the floor, she scooped them up and shoved them into the trash.

The staff worked with a practiced efficiency—many of them played netball and football together on the Rakai project's teams, and they moved around the clinic with an athletic economy of motion. The physicians that day were Dr. Joseph Kagaayi, fresh from medical school, and Dr. Porto Kamya, who'd come out of retirement to help start the Rakai antiretroviral treatment (ART) program. Kagaayi, like many young doctors, had encountered a job market filled with demand for HIV physicians. Kamya had lived through the plague years when death was so pervasive that, for a time, the government tried to ban journalists from visiting the district.[14]

Kagaayi seemed to revel in the medical problems presented by the clients—many of whom had been sick with HIV for a long time. He thought aloud about getting testosterone for one patient who had lost his appetite and grinned at another woman who'd come back for her refill. He'd had to spend an hour with her to persuade her to take the drugs because another man in her village had started the drugs, then died. He held the pills in his hand—little plastic bags marked with suns and moons—and they inclined their heads toward the drugs she'd decided weren't poison after all. *Sawa z'emisana, sawa z'ekiro,* in the morning, at night; he pressed them with one finger, and she reached out and did the same. Their murmuring over those little tablets seemed a prayer, the medicines a Eucharist.

The first PEPFAR-funded AIDS-treatment program that I saw in action, RHSP was, in many ways, the best and worst of PEPFAR in one—a project literally running in parallel with a government clinic struggling to meet basic needs that had, within months of the money arriving, figured out a way to bring state-of-the-art care to the rural poor. But PEPFAR wasn't only paying for programs that broke molds and made temporary worlds, voluptuous with supplies and care. It was also paying to scale up treatment in the spoke-and-hub programs that had inspired its architects—including those run by Dr. Peter

Mugyenyi. When I went to see him, I found out how PEPFAR looked to the man who'd helped prove that it was possible.

— —

"THE PEPFAR PEOPLE FORGET that it is an emergency fund, and emergency is self-explanatory. It was put there precisely for the purpose of putting a stop to the carnage," Peter Mugyenyi, the director of the Joint Clinical Research Center, said to me when I went to find him—he'd moved out of the Rubaga building and into a smaller, more modern suite of offices nearby. That day, in early 2005, he was visibly frustrated, his leather office chair squeaking as he sat forward, then back, vibrating with emotion. JCRC was USAID's sole grantee, or "implementing partner," for providing antiretrovirals. Mugyenyi had initially balked at taking American money—he was suspicious of donors and their "godlike" approach to management, loathe to have external partners telling him what to do. But he'd been won over by Rob Cunnane and Amy Cunningham, the agency's local mission director and HIV advisor, respectively. Cunningham, a former French horn player who'd done a stint as a journalist in the navy, approached the collaboration with deference and patience. She'd book four hours each week for their meetings. She loved listening to him—it was like learning "from Gandhi." At opportune moments, she'd raise a reporting or financial requirement from USAID. "You basically want to clear the way for a visionary," Cunningham said. "I saw this as my job: clear the way, keep him safe."[15]

By both their accounts, Cunningham and Mugyenyi established a deep, trusting relationship. But that day it was clear to me that Cunningham, a mother of five, couldn't buffer the doctor from all of the US government requirements. He thought that PEPFAR was dictating, with too much precision, what the Ugandan programs could do. "At the end of the day, the donors will come to JCRC and say 'Mugyenyi, according to your protocol you are supposed to do ABCD, did you do ABCD? Show us.' Now if I was supposed to do ABCD and I did E, there is a technical term. They call it, 'non-compliance.'"[16]

USAID had been thinking about working with JCRC for several years prior—ever since Cunnane's boss asked him to develop a paper explaining how the agency would do antiretroviral treatment if it ever had to. JCRC had been the only option, as far as Cunnane was concerned. A Peace Corps alum who wore a suit like he'd rather be sailing, Cunnane believed in USAID, even though when he'd joined, in 1992, the agency was "on the verge of going out of business."[17]

To believe in USAID was to believe in "sustainability"—a grail-like quality of foreign aid and development assistance that describes conditions in which the services will continue on if the donor ceases to pay for them. "Leading up to PEPFAR, my strategy had us supporting the government ART rollout through third-party support," Cunnane told me. "And the only third party that was palatable was JCRC." Supporting government ART rollout meant using government facilities and hewing to government norms—staffing models that paid for nurses and doctors but not necessarily peer counselors like TASO members who helped new clients by sharing their own experiences. The drugs wouldn't follow the people to their homes, only to the nearest government health facility. "The linchpin would be Ministry of Health hospitals," Cunnane said.

The CDC's approach sought evidence to guide decisions about where the programs lived and how they ran. Mermin, Bunnell, and their Ugandan collaborators looked closely at cost-effectiveness and had designed the HBAC study in part to determine whether clients who received home visits could be well managed without the expensive viral-load and CD4-cell-count tests used in more resource-rich settings. But the primary focus was on defining the set of services that treated people, including those who, like most of the residents of Tororo, lived on less than twenty-five cents per day. JCRC's USAID-funded program provided free drugs for some clients—widows, pregnant women, and orphans—while asking others who were able to continue purchasing their medication. Its state-of-the-art laboratories would initially charge fees for running CD4 cell counts—including billing TASO programs, so that one American project ended up paying another one. Collecting fees for specific services was one way to build in a level of sustainability, according to USAID.

In Mugyenyi's office, a Macmillan map of Uganda hung on the wall, with pushpins marking the sites of JCRC centers. As we spoke, my eyes drifted to a yellow pushpin. I knew the clinic it marked very well. I'd found it by tagging along with a fellow Fulbright grant recipient who was conducting fieldwork many hours away from the capital city. We'd stayed in a simple, welcoming guest house, with a communal dining table that groaned with rich soups and handmade bread. I was looking for clinics to visit outside Kampala for the course of the year and knew I'd be happy to return here. When I asked the proprietor if there was an antiretroviral program in town, he'd directed me to what turned out to be one of the JCRC's Regional Centers of Excellence.

The hospital sat close to the main road of a town nestled in rolling hills that billowed, like a landlocked ocean, toward larger swells in the distance. It was a landscape of surpassing beauty. The dirt road from the guesthouse where I stayed to the hospital dipped between flowering bushes, and on sunny days when the sky was bright blue and the clouds white, I would stand on that road and think that the palate of green, white, and blue had the purity of earth seen from afar.

I made that walk for the first time on December 2, 2004, poking my head into a cramped room with gingham curtains at the end of a 1952 building with a long, covered verandah that served as the hospital's private ward. JCRC had borrowed the rooms from the hospital while it constructed a new building. Even though there was hardly room for two in the dispensary, the nurses seemed happy enough to have company that day. They offered me a stool beside a table packed with pills, ledgers, and files, more of which slopped out of cardboard boxes, one of which, labeled "Jambo Wine," rested by my feet. The taller of the two, whom I will call Sister Natalya, had a compact Afro and a lanky basketball player's frame. She sat folded into her chair like a carpenter's ruler, pursed her lips, looked at me, and sighed. "It's by God's mercy we survive."

The JCRC site was a world apart from the brisk-paced, all-inclusive mobile clinic model I'd seen in Rakai. Some of this was by design. In order to be sustainable, the clinic relied on government staff, with a limited number—Sister Natalya and one of the doctors—receiving compensation from JCRC for their duties related to the ART program. The clinic offered drugs for free to eligible groups, initially using funds from PEPFAR, the World Bank, and later, the Global Fund. The strategy of offering subsidized drugs to some, while maintaining paying clients, was a "cost-sharing" approach that prioritized revenue streams as well as public health services. This strategy, grounded in ideas about sustainability, stood apart from the CDC's model.

All of those categories of clients had specific days when they were supposed to appear at the clinic, but as I saw on that visit in December 2004, and in the visits I made nearly every month for the next ten months, few days went precisely as planned. Clients came when they had money or a free ride into town, not on their assigned days. The doctors came when they were not called away to the inpatient wards or working in private clinics in town—"freelancing," as one of them called it—for extra income.

Sister Natalya sat in a straight-backed chair that she tried to make more comfortable by padding it with sweaters and tried to deal with it all. She faced a desk and a bank teller's barred window with a semi-circular portion cut out of the bottom, its jagged edges padded with electrical tape. All day long, clients bent their heads down to the opening and spoke to her through that window. The room was so small that she could get almost everything she needed without rising from her chair. Office supplies sat in a safe beneath the desk, the antiretrovirals in a tall, locking double-doored metal cabinet jammed so close to the client services window that, when Sister Natalya wanted privacy, she swung open one of the long narrow doors to block the opening. She balanced her tea mug on a folded towel on the thick inner rim of the safe below her desk; every other surface was occupied. Files sat in cardboard boxes on the floor; there were antibiotics, antimalarials, and antifungals on a small wooden table alongside the plastic pill-counting aide—a gridded platform with a chute down the side—that Sister Natalya addressed by the brand name written across the top. "Come here, Daktarin."

The space evoked *Alice in Wonderland*, when she has drunk from a bottle and finds herself so large that her crooked neck jams up against the roof of the room. It was not just Sister Natalya's long, elegant frame or the configuration of chairs, desks, and boxes that prevented movement but the feeling that the work of managing the clinic was larger than what this structure could contain.

On the first day I visited, Sister Natalya tallied the clinic's clients for me. The JCRC clinic had started in 2003, providing drugs for clients who could pay. In December 2004, of the 611 who'd enrolled, just over half were on antiretrovirals; the others were eligible, meaning that their CD4 cell counts had fallen to 250 or below, but there weren't enough free drugs to start them. She showed me how the World Bank, PEPFAR, the Global Fund, and the JCRC's paying client pool each had a pharmacy ledger—a giant hard-backed book more than two feet long when opened flat. Patients had an assigned number based on which program they belonged to. When they moved from one drug source to another, their number also changed, scratched out in sharpie, a new one written by hand.

That day, another nurse poked her head around the door frame. Did the nurses have the stethoscope? There was one that moved around the clinic. They didn't have it. A sheet of flip-chart paper on the wall said that fifty clients had defaulted—had never come back at all. They made up about 15 percent of the total number of clients on antiretrovirals, and the clinic had no way of finding them. The hospital had a pair of vehicles—one for immunizations, the other for an ambulance—but even if they were on-site, they seldom had fuel, and if Sister Natalya went out in the vehicle looking for clients, there would be no one in the pharmacy to dispense the ARVs. At that point in the AIDS epidemic, a 10 percent loss to follow-up was considered acceptable.

When she was not worrying about lost clients, she and the doctor were juggling the slots between those who could pay and those who were running out of funds, those who'd been able to pay for a CD4 cell count at a hospital up the road—the JCRC machine was broken—and those who did not have the lab result used to determine eligibility for antiretrovirals. This woman came from the family of a local leader; she could pay. That person was "badly off," health-wise, even if he hadn't had a CD4 cell count; they'd use a complete blood count as a rough proxy. One day a bespectacled man rested his chin on his hands at the window opening and said Sister Natalya was the reason he was alive.

He handed his patient record book through the window to make his point. Flipping the pages, I saw a note from Sister Natalya urging the doctor to switch him from paying to a free slot. But on another day, when the doctor had disappeared for hours and the clinic's work ground to a halt, a different man in a sharp-brimmed fedora did a pitch-perfect imitation of Sister Natalya and her chin-up, arms-akimbo announcement that they'd all just have to wait. She'd smiled but looked like she might cry. When she said to me—as she often did—"It's by God's mercy we survive," she meant the clinic staff, not the clients.

Many hours from Kampala, the clinic had a close connection to JCRC and its charismatic leader. On one of my visits, in mid-2005, I settled onto the stool beside the gingham-curtained window in the pharmacy, and Sister Natalya told me that Mugyenyi had arrived by car earlier that week to check on the progress of the new clinic building. He'd been so frustrated by the progress that he nearly drove off to find the carpenter himself. "He was hot," she laughed. A man came to the window on another day—a schoolteacher who'd been badly off when he first arrived. Now he had a pedal bike and could work again. She wanted to take a picture to send it back to Dr. Mugyenyi himself. He'd be so pleased. The RHSP team swarmed into a building and then piled out, creating and dismantling a world once a day. The JCRC did indeed seem like it had always been there in the hospital. I knew which program I'd want to be seen by; I also knew which one seemed more likely to last.

━━ ━━

OUTSIDE KAMPALA, I OBSERVED clinics, many of which were supported by American money. In the city, I studied the Americans themselves. Mermin had a knack for making everything he said sound like a secret he'd saved just for you. Bunnell, a light brunette with a flushed, tensile strength, also spoke with an urgent intensity. But she was less conspiratorial, more gripped with unvarnished concern. When we spoke, it was usually in the backseat of her CDC vehicle, while she was riding from one meeting to another, her thoughts and worries about progress tumbling out with the rapid cadence of preoccupied thought. "We have a huge missed opportunity with prevention," she said to me one day in May 2005. She told me that if she "had a magic wand," she would ensure that every ART program had family-member testing. As it stood, an individual who received a diagnosis would be urged to return with a partner or children, but this wasn't a requirement, and programs working to start treatment programs did not always have the resources to seek out the contacts of people testing positive in a way that respected confidentiality. Bunnell was worried, too, about the women with HIV whose fertility was coming back when they started antiretrovirals. (Many women with HIV were so ill by the time they started treatment that their periods had ceased.) HBAC hadn't emphasized family planning, she said one day, and forty-three HBAC clients had become pregnant. Now they were "trying to catch up." "Most of them didn't want another pregnancy," she said.[18]

The USAID team was more formal, in its members' attire and in their conversations with me. Cunnane was seldom out of his suit; Cunningham, who wore her Crystal Gayle–length hair in a bun, glowed but seldom sweated. She seemed to exist in a different clime from the equatorial dry season that made me sweat and huff.

The two agencies' approaches and aesthetics mapped to their organizational philosophies. While USAID frequently awarded its contracts to American groups, which then built programs "on the ground," it seemed to aspire to a version of development in which America was nowhere to be seen—its projects were sustainable and locally owned. It favored backstage work that took place in offices and boardrooms. CDC's avatar is a detective, working the streets, knocking on doors, conducting "shoe-leather" epidemiology. To work for that agency was to show the effort, down to the holes in the soles of your shoes.

Mermin and Bunnell invited me to their home and served me tofu in T-shirts and bare feet. They told me how they'd done an economic analysis and concluded that the vast majority of people they hoped to reach with antiretrovirals had twenty-five cents of expendable income. They wanted to build the programs for *those* people. "That's what you do for public health: you work for the people who are least well off," Mermin said. They wanted, too, to build a program that included research—asking questions whose answers could inform policy. Before HBAC, they'd conducted a study in Tororo that showed that a single daily dose of a cheap antibiotic called cotrimoxazole reduced mortality in people living with HIV by 70 percent. When parents lived, their kids did too—an HIV-negative child whose parent died of HIV was twice as likely to die within a year as a comparable child whose parent survived.[19] The World Health Organization had taken those data and issued a guidance; now Uganda and many other countries had policies supporting national cotrimoxazole provision. You planned the research whose results would help you make a better program. It was, Mermin said, a "public health continuum from applied research to policy change to program scale up." You figured out what would work best for the least fortunate, then figured out what it would cost.

Cunningham and I ate hamburgers at Steers in Garden City mall. She was warm but viewed me with more formality, a distant friendliness, and a conviction that the agency knew what would work for the long term. When I asked Cunningham about the basic care package that the CDC team had tested and evaluated and was now seeking to scale up, beyond Tororo, she sniffed.[20] You couldn't put together kits forever. A better approach was to find a local source to make each component and sell them for a modest price. That way, it would be sustainable.

All of the Americans made some effort to conceal their frustrations with the divergent approaches, but the tensions were palpable—and common knowledge. "Did anyone tell you about the roses?" the

Peace Corps director asked me one night at a party at the ambassador's residence. At one of the many PEPFAR team meetings where the agencies were supposed to share and harmonize their plans, an issue had come up about how to do something, who would get the money. Someone had gotten up and left the room—she could not remember or would not say. The person had come back with a bunch of flowers—likely the tight-budded roses that were being factory-farmed in wetlands-consuming swathes by a local magnate named Sudhir—flung them on the table, and cried, "This is for all the people who have died since we started the meeting."[21]

Such interagency sparring was the norm across PEPFAR countries, and Uganda's team fared better than most by many accounts, thanks in no small part to Ambassador Jimmy Kolker. A career diplomat, Kolker had come to Uganda after a tour of duty as American ambassador to Burkina Faso, where he'd been impressed by the CDC's assistance with a meningitis outbreak. He'd come to Uganda with twenty-eight years of experience—including fifteen in Africa—and a hunger for a budget of his own. America's operating principle that aid was independent of America's interests meant that the State Department didn't have its own foreign aid funds, though it did approve USAID's annual budget and plan—a chafing level of oversight, from the development agency's perspective.

Under the PEPFAR structure, ambassadors were charged with coordinating the country plan. In Kolker's case, this meant arbitrating proposals about who would do what and partner with whom. He took to it with alacrity and a curiosity about what each agency could produce. In theory, he could have steered the country team toward a more streamlined ART program—perhaps putting CDC or USAID squarely in the lead. Instead, he took what he'd describe as a "Solomonic decision" to let each agency pursue its vision. "I decided to let one hundred flowers bloom."

In Washington, DC, the Office of the Global AIDS Coordinator refused to assign fixed roles or budget lines vis-à-vis provision of treatment, prevention, or orphan programs to USAID, the CDC, the Department of Defense, or the Peace Corps. This effectively kicked the issues down to the American team working in a given country; in many places, turf wars and personality conflicts between agency teams hampered work and led to conflicts that became the stuff of gossip and legend. High-drama meetings at the embassy notwithstanding, the Uganda program in its early years created space for the agencies to pursue their visions.

America also did not export its politicized agency dynamics to virgin territory. Mugyenyi, Coutinho, and Serwadda were all scrupulously respectful of each other in interviews and public conversations, all the while ensuring that each of their institutions secured PEPFAR funding. If this was out of ambition, it also reflected the long years spent tending to an untreated plague. They had not been idle during those killing years; they had been imagining the future and what they would do when the resources arrived. Strikingly, none of them appeared to have imagined a world in which their own government took the helm of the treatment program and brought a national Ugandan effort to scale.

I'd been warned about waning political leadership on AIDS in Uganda before. "Don't go to Uganda," Dr. Deborah Birx had told me a month or so before I'd packed my bags and left New York City. The Fulbright was in place; the flat on Makerere Campus was waiting for me. "If you want to see something work, go to Rwanda or Botswana," she'd said. "Not Uganda." I'd told her that I was going. I'd even ventured timorously that I thought perhaps she was wrong. She did not bother to repeat herself, saving her energy for other arguments that she actually needed to win. But as I began to apprehend the full cacophony of the Ugandan AIDS treatment program, her words came back to me. To be sure, the interagency infighting made for good gossip and addictive people watching, but it was like that in many countries, as I learned when I began to ask around. (This fighting, which sapped the energy of ambassadors, local collaborators, and foreign service nationals was one of the great, unquantified sources of waste in the entire program, even as the enforced presence of agencies with different capabilities was a major strength.) But a dearth of government leadership was of great concern.

From my base in Uganda, I collected stories about ART scale-up in other countries in the region and realized things were going differently. In Tanzania, the government put a policy in place that limited PEPFAR spending on more expensive brand-name drugs; in Rwanda and Botswana, the national government asserted control and ownership over the design and management of the program. Malawi was not working with PEPFAR at all but was instead pursuing rapid scale-up through its Global Fund grant. In each case, the government was taking a far more active role than it did in Uganda—the country that had once been the standard-bearer for an effective AIDS response in the region.

In April 2005, I asked Alex Coutinho if he could help me understand what I was seeing. He chose his words carefully. (He once told me that he thought in paragraphs, knowing what he would say many sentences beyond his current utterance.) It wasn't clear, he said, that presidential interest in antiretrovirals was there. "The degree of passion is not as much [for treatment] as for prevention," he said. "I believe President Museveni has not been fully-briefed on the intricacies of what it takes to roll out antiretrovirals."[22]

The intricacies were, in fact, phenomenal. The pills in their plastic sun and moon sachets had to be procured, shipped in, cleared through customs, stored, logged, and dispatched out to clinics across the country. Each HIV-related test—whether it was a diagnostic, a CD4 cell count, or a DNA PCR test used to confirm whether an infant had been born with HIV—required laboratory supplies and machinery. A lab required reagents, electricity, air-conditioning, gloves, sharps containers, and syringes. It required a way to log whose samples had come in, what results had been found. A printer to generate the information, a record system to receive the results so that the doctor had them the next time the patient walked in. No other disease affecting 6 to 10 percent of the adult population in Uganda— or any other country—had ever received such attention.

Some, like malaria, which was readily treatable, did not require it. Others, like tuberculosis, had national programs and protocols that had, years prior, deteriorated into a state of mediocrity. Each decision, from which forms to use to order drugs to what salaries to pay lab technicians, had implications for the nation's health system and for its clients. Dr. Christian Pitter, the CDC antiretroviral advisor, spent hours with TASO colleagues in rooms whose walls were thick with flip-chart paper. He'd sit on the edge of his bed one night with his head in his hands and wonder if this was even possible before leaning on the logic he'd come up with during his darkest days after emigrating to the United States from Jamaica. If you leave, you won't see what happens next, he told himself. He locked eyes with his Ugandan collaborators, including Dr. Bernard Etukoit, a towering physician who ran the TASO ART program. "We have to get this right," he said. "The world is watching."[23]

The Ugandan government didn't always seem to be. A few weeks after arriving in the country, I'd gone to see its head, Dr. David Kihumuro Apuuli, then the head of the Uganda AIDS Commission (UAC), whom I'd met on my first trip to the country in 2000, along with his deputy, Professor John Rwomushana, a stylish, bearded man given to cravats and spats, who'd leaned across the table and cried, "We're building the boat as we sail it," before cutting the interview short because he had other work to do. The country had thrummed with a domestic urgency. I had imagined that the arrival of the new AIDS drugs would activate new levels of excitement, urgency, and drive.

But when I'd gone to Apuuli's office in the year that PEPFAR arrived, I hadn't found that sense of urgency at all. There was a Shakespeare play in the inbox on his desk, one of the pocket-sized versions I'd studied in high school. He said he'd loved the theater when he was a younger man. We'd sat down, at first, in adjoining armchairs, which I recall as being upholstered in the red velour of a honeymoon suite. But then he'd moved us both so that we sat beside one another on the couch. He'd clasped my hands in his and turned toward me.

Now situated where he wanted to be, Apuuli began to speak—about not the future but the past. He told me how Yoweri Museveni had understood the great threat that AIDS posed to the country and done what no other leader had been able to do. The couch was low and soft, and he told the story, which he knew I knew, while my hands grew wet and warm.

"In Africa we use the drums," he said. "Africa"—the term that outsiders used, but also the term that the president used when he talked to the rest of the world. Dr. Apuuli served at the pleasure of the president; his job was to embody the national response, which was, like much else in Uganda, inseparable from the president himself.

That day, Apuuli told me the names of each of his siblings who had died and the years they had passed away. His face was sweet then, and sad, his eyes in the middle distance. There was an air of nostalgia about it all that was so discomfiting, I thought I had done something wrong. Perhaps I had not asked the right questions. It must have been my fault, I thought when I left, that the head of the UAC wanted to reminisce about the drug-less past at the moment when the drugs had arrived to save other people's siblings.

When I went to a meeting of the Uganda AIDS Commission's Partnership Committee, which was supposed to coordinate the national response, I began to see that the mixture of intimacy and degradation, bonhomie and inertia-inducing nostalgia wasn't personal but, instead, something of an official stance.

At that meeting, Amy Cunningham, the USAID technical advisor, urged the UAC to release the results of a mapping it had done to see where HIV resources were needed in the country. "We're crying out for it," she said when called on. She started all of her remarks, "Thank you, Mister Chair." But there was a problem, the Ugandans explained. The Ministry of Health was also doing a mapping. No one could say what it was for, and the ministry, which was widely known to be in competition with the UAC, had not attended the meeting. Perhaps it was the survey that the Global Fund office was undertaking, someone ventured. No one could clarify, and so the matter got tabled for a future meeting.

Afterward, I'd gone to lunch with Cunningham. A big red stone sat at her collar bone, a wrap top ruched around her yogi's torso. She told me that the US government had tried for months to no avail to get the Ugandan government to convene a single committee to

oversee all of the AIDS treatment programs. She'd sought to reconvene the "ARV implementation committee" created as a requirement
for the World Bank AIDS treatment grant, but that had disinte-
grated. There was a high-level committee overseeing PEPFAR work,
but it wasn't the same group that was overseeing the Global Fund
grant. They'd gotten permission to work on their own, but they
hadn't been embraced by the government.

In Rwanda, Uganda's neighbor to the west, President Paul Ka-
game and Agnes Binagwaho, director of the country's AIDS program, insisted that all of the funding for pharmaceuticals go into a
common drug-procurement fund. It might be donor money, but it
was Rwanda's program, they emphasized at every turn. To the east, in
Tanzania, the government had told PEPFAR not to buy any drugs at
all, as long as choice was restricted to high-priced branded drugs. It
would buy generics with money from the Global Fund, and PEPFAR
money could "wrap around" and support other things.

"He wasn't interested [in AIDS] anymore," Ambassador Kolker
would tell me of Museveni. In the meetings Kolker had with the
government as PEPFAR rolled out, the recurring topics were Museveni's plan to seek reelection, the passage of the African Growth and
Opportunity Act, and continued reinvestment in his country.[24]
Kolker urged President George W. Bush to use a head-of-state
meeting to persuade Museveni to step down at the end of his next
term. Didn't he want to spend more time on his ranch? Bush had
asked, one cattleman to another. Museveni had fixed him with an icy
stare.[25]

Kolker told me that in mid-2005, when Randall Tobias made his
first trip to Uganda as head of the Office of the US Global AIDS
Coordinator, he'd asked Museveni—who'd run so late for their meeting that his aides were worried Tobias would miss his plane—what
was uppermost in his mind. Museveni had replied with one of his
jazzman's riffs: twenty minutes on three or four topics, none of which
had anything to do with health care or AIDS. "Did he know who he
was talking to?" Tobias had wondered aloud to Kolker. The answer
was yes, of course he did.

PEPFAR had been maligned for investing in "parallel" health-care structures, for funding clinics and supply-chain systems separate from governmental facilities. These approaches didn't build the government's ability to take over in the future; they were redundant and often chaotic—without a national vision for a basic clinic structure, ART programs could be anything and everything. But at the end of the day with the Rakai Health Sciences Program in Kasasa, I'd asked the doctors if they thought that the government should be providing the treatment. They'd shaken their heads. Dr. Kagaayi, the younger one, wondered aloud how they would be able to manage. He was flush with mastery of the complexity of it all. Dr. Kamya seemed resigned. "They can't provide anti-malarials, so how could they do this?"

One afternoon, I'd left the JCRC clinic and walked about a kilometer out of town, past the roundabout with its Barclay's bank and the internet café with its monitors under fingerprint-smeared glass, and up the hill to the district health office headquarters that was, under the decentralized health system, supposed to oversee spending and performance of funds sent down from the central government. As the evening fell, I sat opposite a doctor and public health expert—he had his master's thesis in public health bound and sitting on his desk—who was charged with coordinating the district-wide response. I did not ask him why the clinic down the hill seemed ancient and fatigued, even though it was brand-new, but he'd given me an answer anyway.

"It's been a decade since the World Bank slammed this hiring restriction," he said. He searched for the phrase "structural adjustment." "That's it," he said. "They called it structural adjustment but that became so unpopular they named it the Poverty Eradication Action Plan [PEAP]. The principles remain the same."

The PEAP was the basis for the poverty reduction strategy that had so impressed the World Bank, Bono, Jamie Drummond, and the advocacy group they'd founded called the ONE Campaign. The local expert was having none of it. The regional referral hospital relied on central government funds for its staffing. The government had been subjected to the hiring restrictions; the Fort Portal hospital had spent "one whole decade of being starved of staff."

The district health expert explained to me that the situation in the district where we were speaking was particularly bad because, for the past decade, a European development agency had made a long-term investment in its health system. The government had funneled its resources elsewhere. In that respect, the end of the European funding was a good thing. "This could turn out to be a small heaven," he said of the donor project. "There could be a large heaven coming next." He didn't want any more donor funding. The large heaven he envisioned depended on it. He thought that the government could provide antiretroviral drugs with a "home-grown approach" structured by the Ministry of Health. He wanted to see routine testing for people who came in sick and a system where people who tested positive were immediately enrolled in clinical care. The PEAP had been one of Museveni's signature interventions in the development space, an embrace of the World Bank's principles that had earned it debt relief and donor praise. The government had acceded to the conditionalities that were structural adjustment by another name. But he felt that problem lay with aid in general, that without it the country would figure out what it needed to do.

If aid stopped flowing, he and many other critics of foreign donors argued, countries would take on the task of providing basic services. He voiced a common critique of aid that flowed regardless of outcome and government accountability. The most compelling arguments paired this assessment with prescriptions for what else needed to change: trade agreements, tax avoidance by multinational corporations, wealth and resource extraction by Western nations far in excess of what they gave in return. A true heaven was a place where funders gave less and took less and countries took on the lion's share of responsibility.

Of all the small heavens in Uganda in that first year that AIDS treatment began, none was more notorious or fantastical than the motorcycle-based HBAC program out in Tororo. I began visiting Rakai and the JCRC clinic in November 2004. Five months later, in April 2005, I finally hitched a ride in a CDC car out to Tororo and stood in the gasoline-scented air of the spotless garage, filled with the blue-and-white Suzukis and their bug-eyed rearview mirrors that roared out each day to test the idea that the only way to end a plague was to do whatever was required to treat the poorest of the poor. The bikes were part of a research study, not a permanent part of the landscape, but they represented Mermin, Bunnell, and Coutinho's shared conviction that you used the money you had to make the future, not preserve the status quo.

On that first visit, I met grinning women research team members whose jobs on those bikes was itself a manifestation of a feminist future. I met a woman with HIV who'd trained in aromatherapy for the clients, and I listened to the research team as they debated what to do about clients with HIV who'd returned to health and so were not at home when they went to find them. I hadn't been invited onto a bike, though, and so two months later, I returned, climbing onto the back of one of the blue-and-white Suzukis, riding behind a tall, bespectacled research counselor named James Mugeni, who drove with me to the home of a woman who had, of late, refused to take her medication. He sat with her while she held her head in her hands as chickens crowed and children's faces crowded the windows. He'd brought everything she and those children and her aging father needed—bed nets, clean water, simple antibiotics. He'd brought, too, a sense of companionship that was nearly holy. He sat and let that silence fill with a patience and warmth, something that felt akin to love. I'd still been glowing quietly as we'd bumped along the dirt track away from the house. The engine purring, and not roaring as it did when it opened up to full throttle, Mugeni had half turned his head over his shoulder and said, as though reading my thoughts, "This can never last."

CHAPTER 8

THE MEANING OF LIFE

Tororo is a town of monuments. A flat-topped, vine-strewn, blackened hunk of carbonatite called, simply, Tororo Rock dominates the horizon. A geologic Eiffel Tower, it is visible from most vantage points, astonishing every time. The Rock has its own Facebook page and, at its base, a ramshackle hut where a man in flip-flops waits each day to guide people who want to make the climb. Looking out from the top, to the east and west, ash-gray pits gouge the green patchwork of cultivated land and lower, flat-topped formations that hunker by the Rock like giant ottomans. The pits, thick with cables and machinery, are the town's cement quarries, established by the British after completion of a geologic survey that defined the composition of Tororo Rock and guided the colonizers toward the resources they wanted to extract: calcium carbonate in the east, copper and cobalt in the West.[1]

The British wanted other resources, and from the top of the Rock, one can see what is left of them. A tidy square of green studded with white is the commonwealth cemetery, the final resting place for the members of the East African Labour Corps, men conscripted to carry the belongings of British colonialists seeking to defend their colonized territories from other Europeans. It is the site of the graves of Private Jeremiah Oloo Osiro, a member of the East African Corps of

Signals who had been trained on radio, flag semaphore, and the code of lamps flashing in the dark, before perishing on May 14, 1946, and Erifaze Kidza, a member of the African Pioneer Corps, a quasi-independent African brigade formed after East African leaders convinced the colonialists to allow them to create a force of their subjects.[2] Kidza died almost as soon as the corps was established in 1941. There are whites there too: men and women and children. They lie, set apart, in a row nestled against the manicured box hedges that provide the burial ground's only shade.

Three kilometers west, the clocktower in the center of the green quadrangle of the Tororo Girls Secondary School is another monument to cement, the West, and human potential. When the US Agency for International Development erected the school in 1963, the British sniffed and scoffed at the extravagance.[3] America's first major educational project in the newly independent country had multistoried buildings accented with sherbet-colored fiberglass panels and sans serif metal letters screwed to the doors. Such details added to the glamor and drove up the price, purchased as they had to be, per congressional orders, from America. The girls who climbed to the second-story of their dorms would lean out and shout that they were in America, so rare was it to see the world from such a height. In the center, the clocktower, a brutalist phallus, was the center of their new world. But the Americans had also bought the rebar from their own country, or perhaps it had been the cement. The building had, within a year of its completion, begun to crumble as the rain seeped in and caused a reaction between cement and metal alloy. The Americans were unmoved by reports of early crumbling.[4] The problem was not theirs to fix. Some parts of their structure were remarkably strong. When I walked onto the quadrangle in 2018, the colored panels were still there; the original buildings remained. The clocktower was surrounded with scaffolding though, the rebar showing through like bone in a deep wound.

James Mugeni was a hometown Tororo boy, born in January 1964, less than two years after the town celebrated the country's Independence Day with a red, gold, and yellow arch across Bazaar Street and another on the main road, decorated with lions, African silhouettes, and the word "Uhuru," meaning freedom.[5] Eight years after his birth, men, women, and children from Uganda's sizeable Asian population took the east-bound road toward the Kenyan border, after Idi Amin ordered their expulsion.[6] He'd grown up under the regimes of Amin and Milton Obote. Little had been stable; much had been lost. When he said that the Home-Based AIDS Care (HBAC) project couldn't last, it was not an opinion but a fact. It had never been any other way.

"Who would pay for the motorcycles and the gas?" Mugeni asked, a magician shucking off his coat backstage. Moments prior, in a round house with chalk drawings on the side, he had sat in silence with the woman, Agnes, and then spoken with her father about whether she would ever take medications again. She had been treated once before for depression. This itself was extraordinary. In a place where aspirin was a treasure and every day a matter of survival, diagnosis and treatment of mental health issues was nearly unheard of. "Leave me to God," she'd whispered through the palms she kept over her face. "I'm here as a friend," Mugeni replied, then sat a while longer.

Mugeni carried his shoulders light and square, like the javelin thrower he'd once been. He was proud of his job and happy he had it. When he said it couldn't last, it wasn't because he wanted it to come to an end. He, like many other Ugandans I'd met, could and did tell me to the shilling what he made as a staff member of a US-funded project and about the pittance that government health workers made by comparison. He was coaching a track team of his own; he'd become a prominent man in town. But this kind of program would never blend into the environment. So many people needed treatment, and yet he had just spent half a day with a woman who had been offered everything and decided she didn't want it.

If Mugeni doubted HBAC would endure, he knew the problems it sought to address would. PEPFAR was just over a year old, and the Global Fund, while older, had not yet begun providing treatment in Uganda. Yet both initiatives, like the AIDS response they sought to support, were already confronting a fundamental challenge with the task of saving lives. Even with a sizeable influx of funding, it was a task that required choices: Did mental health matter, or hunger, or domestic violence, or lack of education? How much time and energy did one devote to someone who had antiretrovirals (ARVs) and didn't want to take them when there was surely someone who did? Antiretrovirals prevented illness and staved off death. They left survivors who faced other challenges and needed many other things. The questions came in many forms, but each grappled with what it meant to save a life. To address that, one had to define what life was as well. Was it merely the removal of the fear of imminent death—or was it something else?

Mugeni and I rode on his motorbike to see Agnes in May 2005. A month earlier, he'd escorted me and a visiting anthropologist in a car to meet a woman named Rose. She too lived in a round-walled house with a metal roof near a father who loved her very much. Like Agnes, Rose sat on the floor, resting on one hip with her knees tucked beside her. Rose also brought her hand to her mouth. But she'd smiled behind her hand, then burst out laughing as she relayed—and James translated—her story. Rose had been widowed while pregnant; she'd been filled with despair until her father welcomed her home. She'd found strength from talking about her HIV status and joined TASO, then eventually HBAC. She'd decided that she wanted the cow that had been marital property, even though she had no claim to it under Ugandan law. She'd gone to her late husband's family and demanded it back. "Have some food," her father-in-law had replied. Rose had refused several times, like Persephone in Hades. But her father-in-law persisted. Finally, she'd reached toward the communal pot. As soon as she did, he'd slapped her hand. "See, you want our food which tastes so sweet," he'd jeered. "Come back and stay with us. Don't come to take what isn't yours."

Rose had turned to a local women's organization for legal support; she'd gotten local government involved. Eventually she'd got the cow back. She crowed with laughter. But then, James turned to me to translate, she'd told them to keep it. She wanted to prove it was hers, but she didn't actually want it. Like Agnes, she had refused something that could sustain her. But in Rose's case, pride, not hopelessness, was involved.

Two women who looked to have much in common contained wholly different worlds. In most cases, the health system did not concern itself with such things. An immunization program could do its work without curiosity about whether the woman with the card in her hand, the baby on her hip, was an Agnes or a Rose. A contraceptive program that administered Depo-Provera, the three-month injectable birth control shot, did not need to know what the woman felt or wanted from her time on earth for the jab to do its work. Once administered, it could not be undone.

But AIDS treatment, which had to be taken every day as scheduled for as long as a person lived, demanded a reckoning with biography. No plague war in the world had been waged against a virus that required lifelong medication. Therefore no plague war had ever depended, for its success, on calibrating a level of curiosity about people's lives. As the free AIDS drugs programs rolled out across Africa, this calibration often looked dismally reductive. "The politics of compassion produce a stepped-down notion of humanity," Ippolytos Kalofonos wrote in an anthropological study of people living with HIV and their support groups in Mozambique after the advent of free ARVs. He called this notion of humanity "bare life," defined by "suffering bodies and biological life devoid of social and political context."[7]

Kalofonos titled his study "All I Eat Is ARVs," a quote from one of the Mozambican informants who explained how the programs that supplied the drugs had not brought food support or addressed the underlying conditions of poverty to which many people living with HIV (PLHIV) returned when antiretrovirals restored to them a modicum of life.

Everyone knew that poor people with HIV needed to eat—more so when they got the medications. That basic fact had been used to confound the demand for AIDS drugs for Africa. But PEPFAR and the Global Fund were not built to address all the symptoms of poverty, just the infectious ones. One evening, I sat on a couch at Ambassador Jimmy Kolker's residence and asked PEPFAR head Randall Tobias about PEPFAR's focus. He held his hands apart, palms facing each other, at about the width of a bread box. There was food—he marched his hands together—and education and other illnesses. He moved his palms toward each other with each word. When he was done, there was a bread slice worth of space between his hands. PEP-FAR was going to pay for what was contained there: medications, testing, programs to persuade people not to have sex, or to only have sex with one person, and programs for orphans and vulnerable children (OVC)—an area beset with definitional challenges, since all children were, in some way, vulnerable. He'd brokered deals with USAID and food donation programs; he knew the whole bread box mattered. But he couldn't lead a program that tried to take all of that on.

Tobias thought that the bread box, or the universe, of explanations for why people got HIV and died of AIDS could not be addressed by a single aid program. Many African activists felt that a single virus also could not be understood except in the context of that universe. These activists had preceded PEPFAR and the Global Fund and persisted in their work after it. For all the support groups like the ones that Kalofonos visited, where the sense of purpose was altered and often defined by the new resources, there were networks intent on setting the definitions. Prudence Mabele's Positive Women's Network emphasized psychosocial support, counseling, and food packets. Her organizational budget included funeral policies for members so that if they died, their burial costs would be covered. "She didn't want to do service provision," South African HIV activist Yvette Raphael said. "She wanted to go and bury a woman who couldn't be buried. She wanted to go and be able to take [someone's] son to school."[8]

In Rwanda, women who had acquired HIV during the genocide wanted their AIDS treatment programs to acknowledge history too. An estimated 250,000 women had been raped during the genocide in 1994; a decade on, the perpetrators, some of whom had been jailed, were more likely to be receiving HIV treatment than the women they had infected. The women wanted treatment, but they needed a program that addressed their trauma first.[9] A woman who had gotten HIV from a *génocidaire* rapist did not want to go to a clinic where she might see him, where he might look at her with a glint of satisfaction in his eye as if to say, "I know you have it too." Even if you did not see your rapist, the pill itself was a reminder of the virus and the event through which you had acquired it. Anne-christine d'Adesky, the activist-journalist who'd founded *HIV Plus,* had heard these and other explanations when, in 2004, she began talking to Rwandan women's groups. She'd been curious about how antiretrovirals would impact women's bodies, and the Rwandan women had explained that this question couldn't even be posed until there was trauma counseling and support for them to explore their bodies' other wounds. Working with feminist HIV researchers in the United States, d'Adesky had secured a small grant from the voluble, passionate UN global AIDS ambassador, Stephen Lewis, and then persuaded Dr. Agnes Binagwaho, the coordinator of Rwanda's centralized HIV response, to let their small NGO, called WE-ACTx, partner with the government.[10]

In Uganda, in the years before PEPFAR and the Global Fund arrived, members of the National Guidance and Empowerment Network gathered resources and donations to support a handful of their members. Lillian Mworeko never forgot one meeting. We "had medicine for only seven people...and everybody wanted to be on treatment, but at that moment we were like, 'No, you know what, it can only be these people.'" Everyone concurred on the same names.

Mworeko herself had been able to start ART after her supervisor at an AIDS organization wrote a budget line for her treatment into a grant from the British government, arguing that if his staffer wasn't alive, they couldn't deliver the project. She recalled the decision about the seven slots being unanimous and easy. "I don't remember anybody complaining." She told me this story beneath the shade of a drooping tree on the lawn of her home in a village outside Kampala. The house was filled with children, relatives, and an orderly hum. It was the sort of "normal" life that had seemed out of reach when she was first diagnosed. But there was something about the caring that suffused those days that stayed with her. "Where did that moment go?" she asked.[11]

In the pretreatment era, many other groups offered similar spaces of refuge and solidarity. In Zimbabwe, Gays and Lesbians of Zimbabwe (GALZ) had, by 2004, evolved from a social club for urban elites into a multifaceted, community-led human rights and health-education advocacy organization. GALZ was the first LGBT group in Zimbabwe to launch an HIV-awareness campaign, and it did so with an emphasis on the ways homophobia and transphobia embedded in communities and often enshrined in laws were themselves a public health threat.[12] Martha Tholanah, a family therapist by training, launched health programs at both GALZ and the Zimbabwean Network of Women Living with HIV after receiving her own HIV diagnosis. For Tholanah, work with GALZ was an extension of her own "long journey to accept myself as a woman living with HIV." She wanted everyone to arrive at a place of "self-love."[13]

Kenyan Dorothy Onyango had, in 1994, founded Women Fighting AIDS in Kenya for similar reasons. She'd waited five years to disclose her own status and then realized that survival for herself and other women depended on creating spaces to tell their stories of resilience and, often, rejection by their family members.[14]

In Zambia, Felix Mwanza had been an IT manager and a blazingly talented footballer before his diagnosis with HIV. He'd grown up in Copperbelt Province, in a mining company home whose verdant flower beds were the envy of the neighborhood. His father, a middle manager in the mines, had tended them. On his diagnosis, Mwanza had a CD4 cell count in the single digits; he soon learned that it was remarkable that he'd been able to get a CD4 cell count at all. There were only three machines to measure immune health in the entire country. He'd "dance on the head" of the minister of health to get them to expand the coverage of services, working alongside fellow activists like Winstone Zulu, Paul Kasonkomona, Eunice Sinyemu, and Kuyima Banda. In 2003, Mwanza took over the leadership of Zambia's Treatment Advocacy and Literacy Campaign, a group inspired by South Africa's Treatment Action Campaign. He ran the organization out of his car for the first few months, pulling together a strategic plan that set out roles for people living with HIV as monitors and providers of services—not just recipients of care. They would count the CD4 cell-count machines, monitor the drugs on the shelves, and demand that the lived experience of navigating stigma, side effects, and adherence be valued as expertise. PLHIV were uniquely suited to help newly diagnosed individuals absorb their diagnosis.[15]

These networks and groups organized by and for people and women living with HIV existed in every country PEPFAR planned to work in and in every country in the world with an HIV epidemic. They'd begun in private homes and the backs of cars, and by 2004 many had grown, becoming well established, with national chapters, somewhat steady funding, and a broad portfolio of issues addressed, including property and inheritance rights, housing and food insecurity, rape, gender-based violence, homophobia, and police harassment of sex workers and emigrants. These groups provided places for people to gather and utter truths that they were unable to voice anywhere else and to talk about their fears, hopes, and defiance.

All of the things on this long and varied list were the stuff of healing. No other disease in the history of the African subcontinent, let alone the world, had prompted such a comprehensive, clarion definition of health—one that encompassed human rights, housing, social support, and a life free of stigma, sexual violence, and shame. In the absence of the medications, these groups had sought to provide almost everything else. They also served as the basis for the powerful activist organizing that led to the advent of the medications. (Many of these groups belonged to the Pan-African Treatment Access Movement, which Milly Katana and Zackie Achmat launched in late 2002, with the goal of bringing all of the access-focused work in sub-Saharan Africa under a single umbrella coalition.)[16] But when the pills arrived, physicians rewrote the definition of health. Much of the preceding work either did not fit within the clinic walls or did not fit within PEPFAR's scope at all.[17]

This was not because it was impossible. WE-ACTx and Reach Out Mbuya were both small, community-derived projects that had been designed by and for people who also needed antiretrovirals.[18] These community-embedded HIV programs operated with endorsement and support from governments and funding institutions. But if they showed what was possible, they were the exception, not the rule. Regardless of the source of funding, the vast majority of the AIDS treatment programs that rolled out across sub-Saharan Africa did not seek to put the pills in the context of clients' other needs.

For some AIDS activists, this was the safest approach. In South Africa, AIDS doctor Francois Venter had designed "lean-and-mean" clinics and approached design with a "Protestant work ethic." Always worried that the funding would diminish or disappear, he wanted to build programs that delivered quality at the lowest possible cost. "Please God, don't hire anyone you can't afford to fire," he'd tell his team.[19] In 2005, New York–based AIDS activist and public health expert Rachel Cohen moved to Lesotho to lead a Médecins Sans Frontières collaboration with the Basotho government focused on expanding antiretrovirals in a rural area using nurse-initiated care. Her partner, Sharonann Lynch, one of the original Health GAP staff members, traveled with her and helped train the nurses and peer educators. She, too, grew worried about programs that created "bullshit health cadres" and added bells and whistles that would never be absorbed into the broader health-care system. "Innovation before consolidation," became Lynch's mantra, by which she meant defining a robust, lean program that could be folded into the broader health-care system.[20]

The tension between lean, mean biomedical programs and holistic health need not have been as great as it was. Simply asking people what their priorities were, what else they needed, and where they'd like to have those needs met could and did yield community-based and -led programs that complemented clinical services. But exploring such an integrated approach wasn't a priority for PEPFAR, and it wasn't a requirement for countries submitting grants to the Global Fund. In this way, for all of their innovation, both funding streams replicated patterns of decades of aid that did not begin with questions about what people needed most and how they wanted to be helped.

In Tororo, at the HBAC program, counselors like Mugeni paid exquisite attention to their clients, asking all manner of questions about their health and well-being. But Mugeni also knew that such attention was fleeting. What had once been USAID's flagship school for girls was now less well kept than a British graveyard. The soldiers' lives had been undervalued; the girls' lives had, for a time, been considered treasures. Mugeni might have been paid handsomely to ask the questions of the clients, but it was not worth it to him to conceal the truth. He wasn't sure the answers would change anything.

— —

IN TORORO AND RAKAI, the clinics traveled to the clients. I could see what happened when people arrived at the clinic, but it was hard to follow them out the door and into their lives. One morning, I picked my way down Wandegeya Hill, shook my head at the minibus taxi drivers who saw me and shouted, "*Mzungu*, come and we go," and picked my steps across the slick of soap and water by the sponge-and-bucket car wash. There was the man selling suits who wore all of his wares on his shoulders, and there, in a Doppler whine, was Shania Twain singing "Ain't No Particular Way"—the anthem of obsessive devotion that was ubiquitous as a soundtrack in the city that year. I climbed up Mulago Hill and greeted the buxom parking guard who always clasped her hands, bowed her head, and said, "*Nee how*," to a doctor and expat acquaintance, Jeanne, who was Korean, not Chinese.

I walked through the clinic's double doors and turned right, away from the waiting area, with its shelves of donated books and a video tape of Olympic track-and-field events playing on repeat on the television bolted to the wall. I passed the phlebotomy clinic with its incessant wails of needle-stuck pain on my left and the *Mwanamujimu* nutrition room to the right, from which vats of fortified porridge emerged in a cloud of thick, wholesome steam every day. I said hello to each nurse I passed, pausing to hold her hand and exchanging the Lugandan greeting, which ended with *gyebaleko*, "thank you for your work." "Mmmm," one said in reply. Then returned the appreciation. Thank you for your work.

At last, I knocked on the door to Cissy's small office and entered to find a thin man with a baby in his lap sitting in a chair pressed against the wall. The man, whom I will call Taata, sat loose, his arms down by his sides rather than holding the boy.[21] He did not look neglectful, just relaxed, like a parent who had held a few kids in his time. The boy was nearly inert, awake but hardly stirring. Taata didn't speak any English, so Cissy talked about him in the third person. "It's unusual for a father to be bringing in a baby like this," she said. "I like this man."

Taata had large, almond-shaped eyes with luxuriant lashes. He had a high forehead, an elegantly pointed chin, and, he would say, a "long nose." That day, a faint shadow of a beard traced the contour of his jawline. His mouth was expressive, his expression gentle. I asked Cissy to explain who I was and was not. I was a writer, not a doctor. Whether he talked to me or not wouldn't affect his care here in the least, Cissy communicated to him on my behalf.

That's fine, Taata said. He might have been thinking about how his father had been friends with a white priest. In the years to come, he'd tell me about that man many times. The priest visited and ate with them, and sometimes his father went to eat with him. When his father died, the priest had brought a lantern and put it in his father's grave, a sign of immense respect for the late Ugandan man. "It was as though he was a president," he remembered.[22]

We agreed that I would come to their next appointment. I would, in the meantime, find a translator. Then we would go together back to Taata's home. The boy, Apollo, had crust around his nose and yellow-orange hair in patches on his scalp. "What's his prognosis?" I asked Cissy after they had left. She pursed her lips and shook her head at me. I was not sure whether she was being discreet or superstitious or merely conveying that the answer was utterly obvious. She wouldn't say anything out loud.

I feared that Apollo would not be at the next appointment. He was, but Taata was not. That day, instead, the boy had been brought by his mother, whom I will call Maama Apollo. She was taut with energy. She moved with a bouncing stride, and her arms flew to the four corners of the room when she spoke, daring the listener to underestimate her. If she didn't like a response, she dimmed her gaze and looked past you, as though you did not exist at all. But before she was Apollo's mother, Taata's second wife had a different family. She'd given birth to her first child when she was sixteen, back in her home village, which was, like Taata's home place, close to the Uganda-Rwanda border, the most verdant and dramatic of all of Uganda's landscapes, with towering trees whose branches touched across the gravel roads and mountains that soared toward the high, wide sky. She'd had two more children with that same man, but it was never easy between them. She was jealous, suspicious of him. They argued frequently and often so ferociously that she'd leave him and go home to her parents' place for the night. He'd come to get her the next day, and things would be all right for a time, but then it would start again.

Eventually, Maama Apollo had discovered him having an affair with a friend of hers in a shop he kept in town. She'd refused to keep his transgressions to herself, reporting him to the local leader, then deciding that she'd better leave for good. A local women's group paid for two bus tickets to send Maama Apollo and her youngest daughter, Olivia, to her aunt's place in the town where Taata had grown up, after his father, a cattleman with a long stride who'd walked the family across the country, had decided to settle down.

Taata's father raised fifteen children. It was at the funeral of his last daughter, the last surviving child besides Taata in fact, that Taata met Maama Apollo, who was working as a maid. He saw that she was nice to his children and especially kind to his littlest girl, Stella, who'd been so young when her mother died that she had been sure, when they'd come carrying her body down the hill, that she was drunk, not dead, and so had danced at the songs they sang at the funeral. Taata decided to marry Maama Apollo even though, as he said, he'd "given up on such things."

He was more than twice Maama Apollo's age. When I met them, he was fifty-five to her twenty-seven. Slender even at his strongest, Taata was a slight, friendly, gentle man, unlike Maama Apollo's first man, who'd been tall and strong. But Maama Apollo liked how Taata, who had only stopped carrying his long, rancher's staff when he'd completed training as a chef and gotten a good job, sent meat home in a car. She did not know how to read or write, and he was a professional with steady work and a solid, if basic, home. She had seen no need to tell her first husband that she was leaving, and he'd complained to the local council that she had disappeared. They'd told him where she'd gone. That's fine, he said. She'll be back. I'll bewitch her so she returns. When that story reached her, though, she was even more determined to stay.

Maama Apollo moved in with Taata, in the little brick house in the venerable slum within walking distance of Mulago that he'd lived in since the 1970s, long enough to know the neighbors, to remember the army man who had kidnapped the woman who brewed *marua* across the courtyard, violated her and extorted money, then brought her back. He remembered how that man had been killed when political power had changed hands, how the trees had been cut down, how the woman, the *marua* brewer, had stuck around and was still a friend.

Maama Apollo entered Taata's life and two-room home with just one of her children, Olivia, who had round eyes, her mother's crackling mischievous energy, and shining deep brown skin. Olivia's stepsisters were Catherine, Stella, and the oldest girl, Peace, who was in secondary school and spoke some English. She slipped into the house quietly, one day carrying a handful of straight nails she'd collected from the building site, sometimes scooping up her young half brother. Usually, though, she sat behind the curtain separating the living and sleeping areas while her siblings clasped my hands, pulled at the hairs in my moles, and crawled into my lap.

The first day we met, Maama Apollo stopped by the close-quartered rooms in the brick house, then led me to another dwelling nearby. It was larger and better ventilated, with a corrugated metal roof, a charcoal brazier by the side wall, and at the foot of the mattress, a mosquito net hanging above it, a box of the brassieres that she walked around the city selling every day. A tarpaulin covered the dirt floor; a cloth tucked under a piece of the floor caught the leaks when it rained.

Apollo's twin sister had died in March 2005, about two months before I met them. Both Taata and Maama Apollo had been tested for HIV after the girl sickened. In their family, as in many others, a baby's failure to thrive was the first warning sign that the virus had entered the home. Maama Apollo had gotten her home after the HIV diagnosis—it was paid for by a charitable group that sought to support women living with the virus.

I wasn't surprised to hear that she'd received help so rapidly. The slum the family lived in was easy to access from more comfortable places in Kampala. I could walk to it from my flat on Makerere Campus. This proximity was one of the reasons Cissy had introduced me to Taata in the first place. Yet it was still a desperately poor area without plumbing, sanitation, or reliable electricity. Neither the national government nor the city had made any inroads into improving living conditions in the slum; instead, a steady stream of relief projects offered different services to different types of people, streams of charitable compassion as thin and meandering as the brown tributaries that flowed down the slum's chipped, makeshift drains. After Maama Apollo's diagnosis, a charity group for single women found her and paid the rent for her new home, as well as school fees for the girls. If some of the neighbors claimed she'd gotten these things by saying that Taata was her brother rather than her husband, Maama Apollo didn't care.

When I'd first met Taata, I had said, in both English and Luganda, that I was not a doctor and that I had nothing to offer by way of assistance. I had asked Cissy to translate for me too. As I became a regular visitor at Taata's house, it became clear that this made me the exception, not the rule, among the white people who came walking down the hill from the main road, past the dry goods shops with bags of beans and rice and the women selling jars of minnow-sized silver fish and larger, sepia-colored smoked fish on worn wooden boards.

Many people came to help out in the slums; many came to Taata's home. Sometimes when I came for my weekly visit, there would be a new plastic kitchen shelf, a bag of maize, a sack of beans sitting by the window. Uniforms for one child, school fees for another. Sometimes there were visitors who did not help but pretended otherwise. One day I arrived to find his niece in tears because a set of charitable volunteers had come and fussed over Taata, then asked him to pose for pictures and give testimony that they had been helping him all along when they had given him nothing before that day.

Taata, too, had been put out by being asked to perform his poverty. It had not been so long ago that he'd been the generous one. Thirty cats used to come around when he cooked to get their rewards. Now there was just the one, with a feathery orange tail, who glided between our legs over the pebble-pocked film of contact paper spread on the floor. His father had recently died, Taata said one day, looking at that cat with affection. But this one still visited.

On another visit, Taata told me that he'd heard the news on the radio that the Ugandan Global Fund grant had been suspended after an independent audit uncovered evidence of massive corruption.[23] He thought the free AIDS drug programs were going to go away. I explained to him that the Global Fund wasn't all of the AIDS money; there was also American money, I said, which was not going anywhere. He ducked his chin toward his chest while I spoke. His head looked large and heavy for his body, which was so thin that his clavicles had the definition of flying buttresses on a cathedral. His rosary hung down on his smooth, hairless chest. He smiled when I was finished talking and my translator was done simplifying whatever it was I'd tried to say. He understood that there was new money, but he didn't think it was here to stay.

His doubt about the new AIDS money was one of the reasons that Taata hadn't joined Maama Apollo at TASO up the hill or at the pediatric clinic's family center, which sought to simplify appointments, pharmacy visits, and labs by seeing everyone with HIV at the same time. Taata preferred to go to a nearby Catholic clinic about ten minutes from where we sat. He liked knowing people and being known; he liked people who had been around for as long as he had. He liked his faith.

A better, easier clinic for AIDS medications was too much of an unknown. It might not endure; it might not get to know him or care for him the way that the Catholic clinic had. When we met, he'd recently been discharged from the hospital where he was treated for terrible gastric distress—"I feel like my heart is hanging down in my chest," he said. On the day he came home, the head of the clinic had come down the hill and walked with Taata four times around his small house. When he was done encircling his home with a man from the clinic who knew how to find it, he'd felt almost well again.

——— ———

FROM APRIL 2005 UNTIL I returned to the United States in November of that year, I went to visit Taata and Maama Apollo every week that I was in Kampala. One week out of the month, I returned to the USAID-funded Joint Clinical Research Center (JCRC) clinic, which expected its clients to get everything but medication elsewhere in the community. I began visiting in late 2004, returning monthly for the next fifteen months. Over the course of that first year, the clinic did not have a dedicated, paid counselor on its staff or a standard offering of pep talks and health advice, as many programs had. Clients came with their HIV-positive diagnosis on a slip of paper. The person who provided the slip likely had been a counselor who'd dispensed messages about "living positively," local support groups, and the promise of medications.

The mere fact that a person turned up with her diagnosis suggested either that the counselor had done something right or that the person had enormous reserves of self-assurance and self-preservation. There was space for no more than eight people in the narrow hallway inside the clinic building. Everyone else who came sat on the verandah in full view of the busy road steps below. To bring your test slip and sit there was to announce your status to the entire community. People who did so had already decided that life mattered more than stigma or shame.

Clients on the verandah weren't asked about their lives or their decisions; if they had been asked, they might not have answered, since the silence that settled in that space was thick and attentive. The wait was long, and there was little to pass the time. If anyone struck up a conversation, everyone would listen.

The silence was only reliably broken on Wednesdays, when the clinic saw its pediatric clients. On those days, there was some chatter.

The children who came with their guardians were generally silent, sitting still and docile. Many wore their best clothes, the girls in party dresses stacked with stiff plastic crinolines going gray at the hem, the boys in school uniforms. Those children said little. The noise came from the boys who brought themselves alone.

They arrived with their black plastic bags, *caveras*, in which they carried their pill bottles and patient record books, the soft-covered, side-stapled school examination booklets that every client possessed. These boys sat on the wall and kicked their heels. When Sister Natalya told them to go and get a relative to escort them, they shook their heads and refused, sometimes gesturing across the road that ran between the hospital and the market, insisting that an auntie or mother or guardian was just there, working, as if that were close enough.

The boys also noticed me. "Of Simon of Mulindwa," one of them announced to me one day. He had a wizened face and the herky-jerky walk of a stiff old man.[24] Though he looked about ten, he was in fact sixteen. HIV stunts growth, especially when it is untreated and undiagnosed. A widespread belief that children with HIV didn't live past the age of five meant many children didn't get tested in the era before antiretrovirals, even when they were regularly sick, even when, as was the case with Simon, both parents had died.

"Of Emily," I replied. I'd been sitting on the wide cement ledge of the clinic's verandah, my steno notebook open on my lap, a fancy Teva flip-flop hanging off my callused heel. Simon reached over and took my pad and pen. He drew a Ugandan flag and the country's national bird, a crested crane. We named the presidents in our respective countries. I asked him if he liked to play sports, and he said that he did, especially football, but that he did not play often because he was weak. We spoke haltingly, trading more words and phrases than sentences. He looked at me forthrightly, as though he was accustomed to people being interested in him. He showed his age most clearly when he smiled. Bright and private at the same time, his was an adolescent grin that only half sought to conceal amusement at the adult sitting opposite.

"Of stomach of paining of food," he said. He did not want a banana from my bag. After I tried all of the foods I knew from my Luganda lessons, he had agreed that we should get some pork, and so we had climbed down the steps of the verandah, followed the dirt path to the main road, and threaded around the perimeter of the market edge, where one vendor's giant pile of black men's shoes on a plastic tarp always made me think of a display I'd seen in Auschwitz. We then headed back into the market to a pork joint where the man hacked flesh from bone with a cleaver before your eyes. We'd waited in the company of a woman with a fur stole and a man with glassy eyes and a juice glass of clear, astringent-smelling alcohol. "Are you doing some kind of excavation?" the man asked. He told me that he'd been to Geneva. "Just because you have heard of a place, doesn't mean you have been there," the proprietor chided. Simon and I ate in companionable silence, then asked for the leftovers to be packed up for him to take away. "Stubborn," he said to me when we stood outside and tilted his head apologetically toward the interior, where the customers sat drinking. "Alcohol," I said, and he smiled, as though reassured that I understood whom we'd encountered.

Then he stopped smiling, shifted the bag of leftovers and the bag of medications and records into one hand, held out the other, and asked me for my pen. I'd refused. I had just one with me, I was always losing and misplacing pens, and I was going back to the clinic, which did not have a single thing to spare. I felt, too, that I had been generous enough. He didn't wait to hear the explanation, though. While I was still shaking my head, Simon turned on his heel and walked away with a wave, explaining that a reverend from a local church was waiting to give him a ride home.

I'd come to know that reverend in time. He had noticed Simon, a boy who greeted him from the side of the road when he went out for his evening walks. He'd been poorly off but still friendly, and the reverend had taken an interest in him. For Simon, securing what governments and funders called "social support" was a personal project that involved being affable and focused on basic needs at the same time. Over the years I knew him, I'd watch the work Simon had made seem so easy and natural that day take its toll.

In theory, he shouldn't have been working that hard at all. One afternoon, shortly after I'd met Simon for the first time, I'd walked up the dirt road that ran past the guesthouse I stayed in and ascended toward the ridge where the military barracks lay. I knocked on the door of a building that bore the insignia UPHOLD, the acronym for Uganda Program for Human and Holistic Development. It was a multi-million-dollar PEPFAR project that had received an infusion of "Track 1.5" funds—money to help preexisting projects pivot quickly to meet PEPFAR's new goals. Its stated goal "to increase the utilization, quality, support and sustainability of services in education, health and HIV/AIDS through an integrated approach" was standard USAID-ese. I took it to mean that the project would provide the wraparound support that the JCRC clinic did not offer and asked the woman behind the desk how they were coordinating with that USAID-funded venture.[25]

She shook her head. They weren't. This was, she said apologetically, a regional headquarters. UPHOLD was not working in the town at all. They were providing palliative care, though, for people dying of AIDS in their homes. They had a program to help train local community members to provide support for those afflicted individuals who—she did not say this—had not made it to the clinic and never would.

UPHOLD had many missions: education, sexual and reproductive health, teacher training. But 10 percent of PEPFAR funds were earmarked specifically for orphans and vulnerable children like Simon. Those programs were not required to nest within AIDS treatment clinics, however, or even to link up with them. The money for OVC programming went through one set of partners, money for antiretrovirals through another. The government ministries were also divided—health sat apart from the Ministry of Gender, Labor, and Social Development and the Ministry of Education, both of which did work that touched on the things a child like Simon might need. Funding for orphan care often also came with a script that swapped development lingo for local vocabulary. At one training to "sensitize" community leaders in a town near the JCRC clinic, I watched a local woman with HIV copy from a sheaf of pages. "Psychosocial Support. Define Psycho. Define Social. Define Support," she wrote on a flip chart. The entire meeting was conducted in such jargon, as though simple words and local ideas were inadequate.

The next time I'd seen Simon, Helen, a volunteer at the clinic, told me that he'd been there since the night before. He'd arrived alone and refused to leave. He'd had no blanket and no mattress, and he wouldn't go home. The private ward nurses initially refused to let him stay, but Helen had intervened, and they'd relented. She smacked the top of her closed fist with her hand. That's what she thought of their lack of compassion. She was also living with HIV and had explained to me that she was sorry to be "on the drugs of India"—that generics, while free, had given her side effects she hadn't had when she was buying branded medications from the cash-and-carry window. I often felt guiltily impatient with Helen, who used the JCRC computer with its rare internet connection to search for online visa applications and to browse websites selling shoes, but that day I was glad she'd been able to help Simon find a place to stay for the night. It hadn't been her job, but she'd done it anyway.

I asked Simon what was wrong. "Feet of fire," he replied. "Feet of fire." He lifted up the back of the red sweater he was wearing and showed me the skin on his back. A white hoarfrost of rash crept up from his waistband and covered his skin. Perhaps he had a fungal infection; perhaps his feet were tingling from the neuropathy caused by both HIV and some of the medications that treated it.

He'd gone in to see the doctor and then come out again and sat on the floor of the verandah trying to push the smaller of his bottles into the mouth of a larger one. A pair of women had arrived, one in a Christmas sweater and another carrying a clutch purse with a pair of crossed knobs as the clasp. As they'd stood over him, arguing, the woman with the clutch purse snapped the clasp open and shut. Helen explained that they were his cousins and that Simon wanted money to take a *boda boda* motorcycle home. They didn't want to give it to him. After a while, one looked up and said, "Why don't you get money from your *mzungu*?" "That's not my job," I said to Helen. "What will happen when I'm not here." They left, then, picking their way down the cement path.

I opened my steno notebook to a blank page. "Do you want to draw?" I asked Simon. He didn't. I drew a house, a quick cube with a triangle on top. He reached over for my paper and pen and bent low. I thought he was tracing the shape to see how I'd created the illusion of three dimensions, but he was, I saw, going over the corners to connect the lines that I'd sketched so that the house was sealed up all the way around. He drew a boom box radio next, a pair of dark whorled shapes inside an oblong. "For listening to the news of the world," he explained. He added "Mother Maria," a woman snaking an arm up to steady a pile of wood on her head.

"Draw yourself," I suggested to him. He placed a small, owlish shape, whose limbs were hardly discernible, at the bottom of the page. Unlike Maria, his own figure did not have a means to move.

His cousins returned while we drew, and Clutch Purse dropped a grimy folded shilling note into his lap.

"What is Simon thinking about?" I pointed at the drawing.

"He's thinking about going home."

— —

STORIES OF DEVELOPMENT BOONDOGGLES and anecdotes of the aid beneficiaries they fail are easy to find, dangerous to extrapolate from—as is any evidence that hovers, as scientists like to say, around the threshold of an "*n* of 1." But the aggregate picture of the world created by the free AIDS drug programs bore out what I saw when I kicked my heels on the wall with Simon or sat on the chair facing the door in Taata's home. The pills had arrived in conditions of poverty, trauma, and daily struggle that a virus-focused effort could not afford to ignore or seek to abate. As money went from social support groups to medicalized services, the meaning of living with HIV and, therefore, the purpose and identity of the groups that had been formed to support "living positively" also changed—and not always for the better.

THE MEANING OF LIFE

Kalofonos, the anthropologist, found that the PLHIV organizations split into different groups, each competing for coveted food vouchers. The notion of "therapeutic citizenship," advanced by another anthropologist, Vinh-Kim Nguyen, described the set of rights and responsibilities that PLHIV had defined in the context of demanding access to the drugs.[26] Yvette Raphael took the medications to support children left behind; Cissy took them to take care of her own children and those at the clinic; others took them so they could testify to their benefits to people who thought the medications were poison. In the era before treatment access, therapeutic citizenship meant residing in a specific world where the pills were scarce and their meaning clear. When pills became relatively abundant, the meaning shifted, and the borders of that terrain dissolved, leaving the real world, with all its miseries, and the question of whether AIDS programs should seek to address some or all of those miseries or whether the broader arena of development could or should do that work.

The chair I occupied in Taata's house was one of just two, low and splintery, and only occasionally cushioned with a scrap of yellowed salvaged foam. I got the seat with the most fresh air, which meant, too, that I got wallops of sewage when the wind blew past the pit latrine or the gutters where it ran, thick and brown, when it rained. I'd breathe through my mouth while I handled the client record book and bottles of medication that Taata sometimes handed me, taking the pills out of their *cavera* and the record book out of the brown pleather purse that held important documents and hung on a nail pounded into the brick wall above my head.

Taata understood that I was interested in his family because they had HIV. To him, this meant that I wanted, or needed, to see their records. I was glad he was taking the medications. I was glad, too, that Taata, through gentle ministrations, had been able to persuade Apollo to swallow his liquid formulations. As the months went by, his hair darkened again; the crust at the corner of his lips went away. He began to grow. Eventually, when Peace called out to him in her husky voice, he would sometimes hold the edge of the rickety wooden chair, bob his knees, and dance.

But they never had enough to eat. In the front room they had, in addition to the purse, a charcoal brazier, a metal pot with a thin, flat lid, and a knife whose blade wobbled in the wooden handle. I'd know them for two years before I saw the fire lit while I was there. They had soap sometimes, because I'd join Maama Apollo while she bent double from her waist and slapped soapy clothes in and out of basins. But sometimes they did not, and when that happened, the girls whose school fees were paid got sent home because their uniforms were dirty. There was a communal tap to draw water from, but it was not filtered or reliably clean. In the AIDS activist movement, antiretrovirals were what Sharonann Lynch called "the crowbar in the crack," prizing open the portal to a world filled with more equity and justice. In Taata's home, they assumed their actual size: small enough that if one rolled off the palm and into a corner of the room, it would be difficult to find at all.

When I asked Randall Tobias why PEPFAR was a slice-sized program, he explained that other resources were filling the gaps. Both the Millennium Challenge Corporation (MCC) and USAID were supposed to be part of America's new compact for development, one that would, through an insistence on good governance, prioritizing the people, and delivering impact, put an end to the patchwork of charity in Taata's slum and to Simon's rural *Lord of the Flies* existence. George W. Bush had, after launching PEPFAR and the MCC, poured money into overseas development aid, doubling investments and promoting the performance-based approach advocated by Gary Edson.

But by the time Tobias and I met in 2005, it was clear that the wholesale overhaul of American humanitarianism hadn't gone as planned. Unlike PEPFAR, the MCC had been slow off the block. The US Treasury and members of Congress had deliberated for over a year about whether the new fund should be within or outside USAID; a free-standing bill setting up the new mechanism—as the US Leadership Act had for PEPFAR—had failed to pass, and the MCC had finally been legislated into existence in 2004 as a line buried in an omnibus appropriations bill.

After that, the initiative had tried and failed to make up for lost time. It had been fast to form a board and announce eligibility criteria but slow to get the "compacts" for countries signed and out the door. Many of the initial countries opted for big infrastructure projects instead of the health and education investments "in the people" that the compacts were supposed to prioritize, and in many instances the overall funding level was dwarfed by other, non-US funders. "Between the program's founding vision and its meager results thus far, there is a vast gap. The lack of progress could just be chalked up to the growing pains of a new program, but it is also possible that the program needs much more congressional guidance to keep it true to its potential," Representative Tom Lantos pointed out in a 2005 hearing, adding, "The MCC grants didn't have enough clout to effect lasting change."[27]

Over the years, the program would earn praise. In 2008, three former USAID administrators dubbed it "one of the United States' most innovative foreign aid programs; it is free of earmarks and promotes genuine partnership with recipient countries."[28] This partnership took the form of a rigorous planning process, including requirements for country-led analyses of the major obstacles to economic growth and of the anticipated economic rate of return for the project. With a few notable exceptions, the MCC refused to fund projects where the anticipated rate of return was less than the initial investment. The program could not spend $1 million on an agriculture project that would provide the farmers or farm owners with $600,000—or less. "These important innovations took the rudimentary accounting approach written into the legislation and created a comprehensive results-focused approach that would impose economic logic and quantitative rigor on every program, from inception to completion, across the institution's entire portfolio in a manner only occasionally seen in the practices of other foreign assistance agencies," one independent review concluded.[29]

In spite of the former administrators' praise, USAID only occasionally used the same standards for its projects. USAID also still made the lion's share of American development grants, meaning that eligible countries could pass up the chance to pitch projects to the MCC. "Countries just divide and conquer because they're getting a hundred million dollars a year for five years from the MCC but they have to jump through all these hoops for it. And over here they get a hundred million dollars from USAID with [fewer preconditions]," said Nazanin Ash, a veteran development expert who worked on PEPFAR in its earliest days and served as Randall Tobias's chief of staff at USAID.[30]

Bush's original vision had called for MCC to be funded at $5 billion per year; in its first decade, a skeptical Congress authorized $1 billion. Even at its full funding level, the initiative's budget would have been half the size of that of USAID and the State Department. It could not compete with other US agencies; in countries, its grants were often dwarfed by other public and private funding flows. "Programs of this size are unlikely to have any discernible effect on investment and growth at the macro level."[31]

Even underfunded, there was some evidence of a salutary "MCC effect" whereby governments adopted the policies and approaches that would earn them eligibility, tackling corruption or fiscal issues that rendered them ineligible.[32] An in-depth study found that empowered technical working groups established to work on MCC issues had a positive "disruptive" effect—forming nodes of influence and catalytic action that propelled government action.[33] But celebrating these accomplishments as the MCC's intent was to diminish the original ambition.

MCC had not been set up solely to change policies and shift attitudes, just as PEPFAR had not been devised as a source of inspiration for government-led action. Both had been designed to make things happen directly, not obliquely. They had also been designed to work in tandem with USAID. When he'd explained this to me, Bush's first-term advisor on economics and security, Gary Edson, held up three fingers flat, parallel to the table. MCC, USAID, and PEPFAR were to have been coequals, with heads who had the same level of seniority, each performing a specific function. USAID would help countries prepare for MCC eligibility; PEPFAR would tackle a modern plague with biomedical strategies, while the paired development efforts supported countries to build the health, education, and governance systems to heal the structural drivers of the intervention.

Such a proposition was ripe for critique. The MCC's primary strategy for economic growth was making countries more appealing for private-sector investment. Aid flowing from a country invested in reaping the profits of a capitalist extractive economy could not be expected to catalyze wholesale, pro-poor change in other economies. The MCC is "one small vehicle [in America's] pursuit of economic hegemony through the extension and ever-deepening penetration of neoliberal capitalism," wrote one British development expert.[34]

Such critiques left little room for inquiry about how America's other development investments might help address a plague that required more than medicine as its remedy. To ask if the United States was missing the chance to use its development aid to make its AIDS war more effective was to accept the premise of that aid in the first place. With PEPFAR, one could always point to the people taking the medications. The program might be neoliberal, but the patients didn't care. Development aid didn't offer a comparable loophole for countenancing America's bilateral version of compassion. AIDS activists reached a détente with PEPFAR, working to make it as good as it could be until the next moment for wholesale transformation arrived. They would tackle debt relief, trade policies, and the entrenched issues with intellectual property and access to essential medicines, but they would seldom, if ever, ask the United States to do more with its non-HIV-related aid.

Nor was it solely, or even primarily, activists' responsibility to ask this question. That task sat with the politicians in the White House and on Capitol Hill who agreed that AIDS was a global scourge and that the American aid architecture was in desperate need of an overhaul, yet seldom connected the issues, in part because they did not have to.

By the metrics PEPFAR laid out for itself, Bush's program was a resounding success. The president had never specified the quality of the lives he wanted his plague war to save, and the stories that the program offered of people lifted up off their deathbeds generally emphasized the fate from which they'd been spared, not the future to which they'd been delivered. PEPFAR kept Taata alive so that he could push pieces of a chapati bought with a one-hundred-shilling coin from inside his handkerchief into Apollo's mouth; it restored Simon's health so that his face could fall when I told him there was nothing else I was willing to give him.

——— ———

In April 2005, around the time that I met Taata and Maama Apollo, Health GAP issued a starkly worded report. "The Global Fund's granting and grant management system is experiencing a meltdown—millions of dollars sit in bank accounts in Geneva and in nations' capitals while thousands of people die needlessly," Health GAP's Brook Baker wrote. "The health management and health delivery system in most developing countries is broken. The GF thinks that by auditing a broken system, you can make it work."[35]

The issue, Health GAP and allies argued, was that money alone couldn't fix years of neglect and donor-driven destruction of primary health care. The secretariat needed to ensure that the entities receiving Global Fund money had help along the way so that services got delivered as quickly as possible, while systems got built for the long term. But the secretariat wasn't insisting on this, and so money either wasn't being turned into grants or grants were arriving, as they had in Uganda, and then sitting in bank accounts, paying for swank offices and sketchy NGOs with links to the president and his reelection campaign.

The Global Fund was, in other words, struggling to do the thing PEPFAR had been given license to avoid: support bottom-up, well-governed aid plans devised and owned by the people in the country. This required a focus on speed and long-term systems. It was a monumental task—which was, in part, why PEPFAR had decided to work through NGOs and faith-based hospitals that could begin providing treatment right away.

In theory, the MCC and USAID could have propelled work on the longer-term agendas. Arguably, a true commitment to addressing

AIDS in Africa would have resulted in a US strategy that encompassed all its foreign aid. But that was not to be. PEPFAR was Bush's favorite, precious as a firstborn son. The president championed his AIDS initiative at every turn, departing from the text of public remarks to quote the Book of Luke, asking for updates. He enthused over progress and supported Josh Bolten when, as the director of the Office of Management and Budget, he twice turned over hundreds of millions in reserve funding to cover gaps in costs.[36]

Meanwhile, the MCC dropped off the president's radar, and other efforts to revamp aid failed in their desired aims. When Bush and Condoleezza Rice tried to rationalize and elevate USAID's role by giving Tobias a "dual-hatted" role as head of USAID and director of a State Department–housed bureau of foreign aid, this effort failed too. USAID balked, and initial implementation, which cut USAID's budget even further, set off alarms that the reorganization was a poorly disguised hit on the beleaguered institution.[37] When Tobias left Washington, DC, in ignominy after his phone number was found in the contacts of a DC madam, some of the changes he'd been charged with putting in place remained, but much was as it had always been.

Amid a sea of aid innovations that aimed high and fell short, PEPFAR was the sole initiative of the Bush administration that delivered on its promise. As the president entered his second term, it was clear that PEPFAR had done more than skeptics had expected, if less than it might have done had it been situated amid a robust, complementary, American-funded development effort or an adequately supported, strategically structured Global Fund. It was five years old and far from finished with what it had set out to do. As Bush entered the final year of his presidency, with his other wars devolving into chaos and pointless carnage, he embarked on a project to ensure PEPFAR's long-term survival.

CHAPTER 9

WHERE THE BODIES ARE BURIED

I N MAY 2007, AS President George W. Bush's second and final term in office passed its midpoint, the impact, extent, form, and content of his military wars were known in rich detail. On May 30, the *New York Times*' front page carried an article detailing intelligence experts' grave fears that America's "enhanced interrogation" tactics—waterboarding, sleep deprivation, humiliation via nudity and simulated homosexual acts, intimidation with slavering dogs—were out of date and, more importantly, ineffective. There was no evidence, this particular article explained, that torture made people divulge the truth. It was a finer cut at the issue of American interrogation techniques, which had dominated the news cycle in prior months. Other experts, other stories took aim at issues of morality, American identity, and the administration's brutal manipulation of the language of international law. This article was primarily concerned with cause and effect. As a psychologist who consulted for the Defense Department said, "There's an assumption that often passes for common sense that the more pain imposed on someone, the more likely they are to comply."[1]

"My patience for this war, it's run out," a Bush supporter was quoted as saying in another article in the paper on that penultimate day of the month of May. "I think this is the most expensive, stupid-est thing ever done."[2] Other expensive, stupid things were soon to come to light. It had been just under two months since New Century, an American real estate venture specializing in subprime lending and securitization, filed for bankruptcy.[3] One of the dominoes that triggered the global economic crisis had already fallen.

Meanwhile, the treatment component of the president's AIDS war looked like a far wiser investment. In South Africa, PEPFAR support had helped the monthly initiation rate quadruple between 2005 and 2009. Now, there were 24,622 South Africans on antiretroviral treatment (ART) every thirty days.[4] In Uganda, PEPFAR supported two-thirds of all Ugandans on antiretrovirals and planned, in 2008, to double both the number of PEPFAR-supported ART clinics and the number of adults started on antiretrovirals each month.[5] These rapid jumps in speed and scale—a "hockey stick" shaped curve—were a sign that start-up was over. Systems built and staff trained, the program could shift to the massive task of bringing antiretrovirals to all who needed them. In some cases, growth had heightened concern about PEPFAR and its parallel system. One evaluation of the South African PEPFAR ART program offered an "unequivocal yes" to the question of whether the US funds had helped close the treatment gap but noted that health workers were also gravitating to higher-paying, better-supported PEPFAR positions that offered more hands-on training and management than many government posts. "While PEPFAR has undoubtedly supported its own program, there are repercussions in terms of the overall HRH [human resources for health] outlook."[6] Nevertheless, the numbers in 2007 showed initial victory in an effort that had not been guaranteed. With the World Health Organization (WHO) now recommending antiretrovirals for people with CD4 cell counts of 350, not 200, even more people with HIV were eligible for ART. The concept proven, the emergency unabated, it was time to pick up speed.

On May 30, 2007, it was a beautiful, sunny day in Washington, DC, when the president who'd authorized the enhanced interrogation stepped into the dappled shade of the Rose Garden to ask that

PEPFAR be continued and expanded. "This investment has yielded the best possible return: saved lives," he said. Just over one million people were now on antiretrovirals thanks to US government support.[7] "This is a promising start," he said. But it was time to plan for the next phase. "Without further action, the legislation that funded this emergency plan is set to expire in 2008."

Presidential press conferences to request reauthorization of a piece of legislation are few and far between. The event was a sign of how seriously Bush took the matter of his AIDS program and his legacy. So, too, was the amount of money he asked for: $30 billion for the next five years, a doubling of the $15 billion budget authorized in the law that created PEPFAR 1.0.[8] Much had been done; much more was needed. This was, for a change, a welcome truth.

UNAIDS estimated that in 2006 roughly three million people had died of AIDS, roughly 40 million people were living with HIV, and roughly 4.3 million had contracted the virus.[9] At the end of that year, roughly two million people in low- and middle-income countries had access to antiretrovirals—a 54 percent increase over the previous year's total. But access wasn't happening fast enough. In low- and middle-income countries, the lifesaving pills were reaching less than one-third of the people who qualified.[10] To meet its treatment targets, PEPFAR had, in every country it worked in, paid to train doctors, nurses, and pharmacists in delivering the drugs, which had specific dosing requirements, drug-drug interactions, and side effects. It had, with the largest contract in USAID's history, established the Supply Chain Management System (SCMS), which bulk-purchased and delivered the test kits, medications, laboratory reagents, and other commodities for PEPFAR-supported clinics.[11] The SCMS was yet another piece of parallel programming—a vast procurement operation that ran alongside governmental systems. Like the program it served, the SCMS was expensive, bilateral—and effective.[12] In places like Uganda, where corruption and inefficiency beset the National Medical Stores, the SCMS-supported procurement system was a stopgap for drug stockouts. PEPFAR Uganda supplied tuberculosis medications and sometimes antiretrovirals when the drugs that the government should have been supplying either didn't arrive or ran out.[13]

Parallel systems had other benefits that spilled over into the public sector too. Dr. Mark Dybul, who'd taken over from Randall Tobias as the new PEPFAR head, would tell Congress that in Rwanda, after seven PEPFAR-funded sites had been operating for just two months, the number of hospitalizations fell by 21 percent.[14] Freeing up beds that had once been occupied by people dying from AIDS didn't mean that the services necessarily got better, but it did mean that the hospitals weren't straining—and that the resources available could be spent on other things. (PEPFAR didn't invest in hospitals, and clinicians regularly bemoaned the fate of the clients who were "admitted." On my first visit to Rakai, I'd heard of one client who had been deafened as the result of an accidental overdose of quinine provided in a local hospital; another had been sent to the hospital for a lumbar puncture and been turned away.[15])

PEPFAR was excelling at both doing the work and reporting on it. It could say, with more specificity than any prior American foreign aid program, how much money it had given out and how much of that money had actually been spent. The latter information—expenditures—was not a required component of reporting on foreign aid. But Dybul, working alongside Tobias, had ensured that the program provided that information. By 2007, PEPFAR had obligated 97 percent of its allocated funds to specific agencies and the subgrantees known, in PEPFAR parlance, as implementing partners; more than two-thirds of that had been outlaid or spent.[16] PEPFAR was the first major US foreign aid effort to report on both in the aggregate and by individual country. It also tracked what got paid for, reporting biannually on performance against the key indicators that Kathy Marconi had hammered out with the US government agencies in the program's first year. Among these, the numbers of people tested for HIV and treated with antiretrovirals were quantitative measures of a service with a direct, satisfying impact. Treatment offered the romance of Camille rising off the couch, the awesome power of Lazarus rising from his deathbed. It was redemption and recovery, providing the sort of emotional satisfaction that prevention never could. If legislators focused on these resurrections and not the technical complexity of this work in their remarks from the floor, the program's sophistication was still palpable, tangible. The program was smart, perhaps even brilliant, as well as merciful.

Even so, the fact that the president would, in 2008, get what he requested that day in May 2007—and more—was quite extraordinary. American governmental attention spans for health emergencies are short, and sympathy for a given disease is often fleeting. In 2007, the American AIDS epidemic was no longer an emergency, even though, as a Centers for Disease Control and Prevention (CDC) research team, including Gregorio Millett, an openly gay, Black public health expert, would note, "Black MSM [men who have sex with men] are the only population in the U.S. with HIV prevalence and incidence rates that rival those in the developing world." They also noted that HIV risk was often a function of the state, not the individual. Mass incarceration, poverty, and inequitable access to quality health care all played a role, and there was a dearth of information about what community-led, culturally competent services might look like. "Failure to heed this call and to address the devastating HIV rates among [B]lack MSM will be our collective legacy and another sad chapter as we observe, once again, *And the Band Played On.*"[17]

This ongoing crisis hardly registered with the general public. Prior to the advent of antiretroviral therapy (ART), 44 percent of Americans surveyed said that HIV/AIDS was the most urgent problem facing the nation; by 2006, that number had dropped to 17 percent, even as rates of HIV in Black communities climbed and federal funding for HIV prevention plummeted—dropping 19 percent during the Bush administration. When surveyed, Black Americans were more likely to be concerned about both their communities and the country.[18]

The AIDS epidemic among Black Americans simply didn't prompt the same sympathy and call for mercy from the Bush White House as African epidemics of the same scale. Many lawmakers and activists sought redress for their communities; activist researchers like Greg Millett and Adaora Adimora produced a steady stream of research into the relationships, communities, and social factors that impacted HIV risk. Black-led organizations focusing on HIV had existed since the earliest days of the epidemic, often written out of the dominant ACT UP–focused narrative; many of these had endured but seen already scanty budgets further sliced when AIDS drugs arrived. As in Africa, community centers and clinics were placed in competition, when they should have been in partnership.[19]

The root cause of the epidemics within the United States and beyond its borders were, in many respects, the same: a white supremacist state whose wealth and privilege depended on and derived from economic and political practices that devalued the lives of nonwhites and actively sought to keep them from obtaining money, privilege, and power. To begin to address and acknowledge this in America was, in Bush's administration, untenable. In Africa, though, Bush entertained the fantasy that colonialism existed in the past and that PEPFAR was part of a movement toward equality. It was possible, then, to tell a story about the plague war that provided a satisfying narrative arc—possessed of a beginning, a middle, and an end. As the White House sought to secure his legacy, this is precisely what it did.

The storytelling began that day in May, with the trio standing behind the president in the Rose Garden. They could have been PEPFAR's magi, so closely did they hew to the archetypes of the heroes in the stories PEPFAR told about itself. There was Dr. Jean Pape, the Haitian doctor who'd been flown in to advise the Office of Management and Budget when PEPFAR was still the brainchild of a rump group of White House staffers; Bishop Paul of the Coptic Orthodox Church in Africa; and Kunene Tantoh, a South African woman living with HIV who ran a support group for fellow HIV-positive mothers: the compassionate doctor who'd made something out of nothing, the man of faith with a large cross swinging low by the waist of his belted robe, and the woman who'd saved the life of her child with American money. Kunene proved, the president said, that "people with HIV could lead productive lives."[20]

Kunene, Pape, and Bishop Paul also could have strolled out of the pages of any one of PEPFAR's annual reports to Congress, which had, for the past three years, been thick with images of children, women, doctors, and people of faith. The illustrations put a human face on the numbers that read like a venture capitalist's dream. According to the annual report issued a few months before the Rose Garden ceremony, PEPFAR was, by September 2006, adding approximately 50,000 people per month to its treatment rolls; the number of sites providing treatment had increased by 139 percent from FY2005 to FY2006, and each month an average of about ninety-three new ART sites came on line.[21] The United States had also put just over $1 billion into the Global Fund's coffers in 2006–2007, and that investment was also paying off.[22] In mid-2007, the Fund announced that, together with PEPFAR, it had doubled the number of people on treatment in the past year. Untangling who'd paid for what was tricky, but the Fund reported an even split—with PEPFAR and the Fund each supporting 1.1 million people on treatment.[23]

The law that created PEPFAR covered 2003 to 2008. Technically, PEPFAR didn't need a new law to continue. A line item in the foreign aid appropriations bill would have maintained the budget and allowed it to continue. But without legislation specifying structure, targets, and budget, Bush's legacy would not be secure. The plague war needed to be reauthorized with a new law, its purpose and strategy reviewed and retooled.

Over the course of four hearings in the House and two in the Senate, Congress sought to set the course for the program's second phase. In these open forums, the lawmakers took an even more active role in defining PEPFAR's purpose and strategy than they'd done in 2003, when the president's White House–based team supplied the details, targets, and structure for the new initiative. It was, in many ways, a transfer of ownership—for while the program would keep the word "president" in its acronym, Bush was in the last year of his presidency, and no one knew whether his successor would be a champion. Congressional support had always been important; now it was essential.

Statistics seldom warm hearts like stories do, and in the months after the president called for expanding his program, congressional staffers traveled to African countries receiving PEPFAR funds. In a village outside Gaborone in Botswana, Brian McKeon, an aide to Joe Biden, reviewed a patient ledger with a nurse who'd come out of retirement to help with her country's response. She showed him how she'd once put a red mark beside the names of clients who had died and exclaimed, "with great joy and pride," that the red marks had ceased.[24] McKeon carried the news back to Biden, then chair of the Senate Foreign Relations Committee (SFRC) and a candidate for the US presidency. "Over one million death sentences have been suspended," Biden said at an SFRC hearing on October 24, 2007.[25] If his language made discomfiting references to America's racially biased capital punishment system, it also signaled support for continuing the program that saved so many Black and brown bodies overseas.

Warning that the "relentless enemy" had not yet been vanquished, Biden said that the program now needed to begin to turn control over to countries, chiefly by removing the prior legislation's earmarks, which set percentages of funding for treatment, orphans, prevention, and—within prevention—abstinence-only education. Each country had its own epidemic and should set its own strategy; that strategy required an intensified emphasis on prevention, Biden said, citing the findings of an exhaustive independent assessment by the Institute of Medicine (IOM) that had been published a few months prior.

The assessment fulfilled a requirement written into law that created PEPFAR, and it was, on balance, profoundly positive. Dr. Jaime Sepúlveda, the Mexican physician and public health expert who led the process, wrote in his introduction, "Though the programs evaluated are still young, it was clear that millions of people are being served and life-saving medical care is being delivered on a large scale in some of the world's most challenging settings. I strongly believe that the American people, acting through PEPFAR, are to be complimented for supporting this remarkable humanitarian undertaking."[26]

The IOM report was positive but not uncritical. Like many other evaluations before and after, the 397-page assessment noted that PEPFAR programming for orphans and vulnerable children was vaguely defined and therefore difficult to evaluate in terms of actual impact on children's health and well-being. Giving a child a blanket or a set of pencils did not have the same reliable benefit as offering pills; you could count services offered without knowing if they'd changed anything at all. Primary prevention for HIV-negative people had the same problem. Condoms and abstinence-promoting comics were not proxies for numbers of infections averted.

The report reserved some of its strongest language for the earmarks in the original law. PEPFAR had

> made spending money in a particular way an end in itself, rather than a means to an end....Although they may have been helpful initially in ensuring a balance of attention to activities within the four categories of prevention, treatment, care, and orphans and vulnerable children, the Committee concludes that rigid congressional budget allocations among categories, and even more so within categories, have also limited PEPFAR's ability to tailor its activities in each country to the local epidemic and to coordinate with the level of activities in the countries' national plans.[27]

Earmarks had been essential to the program's initial bipartisan support. The treatment carve-out had satisfied the Left and Right alike; the apportioning of a strict percentage of prevention dollars for abstinence programs provided Christian conservatives with confidence that they'd limited funding for sexual and reproductive health programs favored by their ideological foes.

Five years on, though, the program had to meet other requirements, including positions about the ontology of aid. Humanitarian aid is assistance offered in response to an emergency. Both the aid and the emergency are expected to be finite. Humanitarian aid is, to aid professionals, a thing apart from "development aid," which is funding designed for the long haul. Helicopters to save people from disastrous floods are humanitarian aid; flood-tolerant rice is development aid.

Epidemics, which do not behave like crop cycles, bedevil these classifications. Some, like flu, do have a seasonality, but others arrive and persist in a state of emergency that does not abate but only appears to wane because of the human ability to accept once-unthinkable conditions as normal. "It is in our human nature to better respond to emergencies than to sustain efforts over time," the Institute of Medicine report warned.[28] When it came to a pandemic of a pathogen that did not immediately kill its human hosts, the challenge was to conceive of a *longue durée* emergency, to ensure that compassion did not fade before the epidemic had been brought "under control," a phrase that is itself subject to debate but often defined as the point at which the ratio of new infections to deaths is less than one. When more humans carrying the virus are leaving the world than entering it, then eventually the epidemic will wane.

The paradoxical solution to sustaining this support was to argue that the program was no longer going to act as though the epidemic was an emergency. A House report on proposed reauthorizing legislation read, "In the first five years of the U.S. response to the global HIV/AIDS pandemic, U.S. policy was driven by the urgency of an emergency response. Under this Act, the United States will develop and implement strategies to transition from the emergency phase to long-term sustainability that can be maintained by the host countries."[29] It was time for PEPFAR to ensure that countries had control over, and by extension took responsibility for, their AIDS fights. Under this logic, the earmarks had to go. This argument was far harder for conservatives to refute than the more compelling and urgent claim—amply borne out by evidence—that the prevention earmarks in particular had done far more harm than good.

——— ———

In April 2007, I returned to Taata and Maama Apollo's house for the first visit in more than a year. The house was cold, and Maama Apollo sat on the floor with her arms wrapped around her legs, staring into the middle distance. Taata looked as though he did not have the strength to hold up his head. He sat pinching the bridge of his nose, eyes cast down to the floor.

I was not surprised. Ten months prior, in June 2006, just before I'd left the country for an extended period, they'd lost a newborn baby girl. In 2006, Maama Apollo had been jubilant in her pregnancy, big and bouncing and filled with pride. Delivered at home, the baby had been like her mother: big and round and "brown," the Ugandan delineation for lighter skin. She had drunk some sugar water while Maama Apollo waited for her milk to come in, and then, before she'd been a full day on this earth, the girl had died.

When I returned in April 2007, it seemed to me as though mourning still stalked their home, as it stalked mine. In January 2007, my partner Liam's mother, Carolyn, died. I'd moved back to the States from Uganda at the end of my Fulbright just over a year prior, in November 2005. I had planned to remain based in New York, while returning to Uganda for several months at a time every year. I took a job at the AIDS Vaccine Advocacy Coalition (AVAC), a nonprofit focused on HIV-prevention research that made this possible. With relevant research underway in Uganda and better internet with every passing year, I could work for AVAC from Kampala for periods of time—while also continuing to research the book.

When we were together in the city, Liam plotted weekend adventures to far-flung neighborhoods, treating the city like a microcosm of the world. During the summers, when he wasn't teaching, he planned trips farther afield. In 2006, I traveled back to Uganda and planned to meet him in Madagascar when I was done. But Liam called one afternoon and explained, over the windy hum of our transatlantic line, that his mother's doctor didn't like something he'd seen on her X-ray.

Taata and Maama Apollo's baby died a day or so after that doctor's call, and I'd been somewhat distracted when I visited the small brick house to pay my condolences. Taata told me how he'd wrapped the baby's body in bedsheets and placed it in a suitcase, then taken it by public minibus taxi back to his home place, where his relatives had been amazed that such a large, strong child had been born to a man so frail. He'd been proud of that and of how he'd managed to give this baby a dignified burial in her home place.

I left promising to come back and sit with them again, but a few days later, the news from New York was worse. I left what I had intended to be a months-long stay in Uganda on five hours' notice. Liam and I got married while Carolyn was well enough to walk her son down the aisle. But her decline had been mercilessly fast. When she died in January 2007, grief suffused my new husband and the Brooklyn apartment he'd grown up in, which had become our first shared home.

In April 2007, when I returned to Taata and Maama Apollo's house, I set aside my role as observer. I had learned how to act quickly when a life appeared to be draining away before my eyes. I called Torkin Wakefield, an expat who'd started a highly successful income-generating project that taught women how to fashion beads and jewelry out of shellac and paper from posters and magazines. I implored her to take on a woman I knew. BeadforLife offered trainings for women by neighborhood so that they could, on "graduation," form local associations. They were about to start a group for women in Maama Apollo's slum, and Torkin agreed that she could join. At first, Maama Apollo demurred. Her buoyant energy concealed fears about her abilities. She could not read or write. She asked whether she could send a friend instead. "No," I said, "just you. You don't have to go, but I think perhaps you should." Eventually, she agreed.

— —

"SHE DID IT FOR chapatis," Taata said bitterly when I returned three months later, in July 2007. Peace stared at the ground. Moments earlier, it had been one of the best days I had ever spent in the small brick house. Peace had, for once, come out from behind the curtain. She stood in the small main room cutting up a red onion with the knife with the wobbly blade, dropping the pieces into the pot that sat on live coals, sizzling with oil. Potatoes and tomatoes sat in neat piles, ready to be turned into a savory sauce. Maama Apollo's voice ricocheted off the walls as it did when she was happy. She'd long since moved back in from the little house that the charity had paid for. Once the subsidized rent had stopped—as it almost always did— she'd come back to Taata's home. "We are like blood," Taata said of himself and Maama Apollo. "We are a family now."

Maama Apollo had completed the training. The house, hung with strips of beads, felt festive and bright. There was food in the baskets behind the curtain. Maama Apollo beamed, and Taata held his head up high. As for Peace, she never spoke all that much anyway. She was a young woman with a round, full body who seemed to want privacy in a house that offered none. I tried to give it to her in the ways I could. I did not ask her too many questions; I did not pry. But that day, because she was standing right beside me, the room so small that my knee grazed her shin, I'd asked why she was home and not at school.

"You tell her," Taata muttered with surprising bitterness. "You tell her." And she finally had. She was pregnant, and though she was not showing, she had stopped going to school. Her teachers mocked her, they said. When she nodded at her desk, her body feeling the exhaustion of first trimester gestation, they laughed at her. When other girls dozed off, the teachers asked if they wanted to end up just like her.

Peace's father said she had traded her body for food, but when she walked me and my translator up the hill after we left, she explained that it hadn't been quite that way. The boy, whose name was Adam, had shut the door one day when his mother wasn't around. She'd asked him about condoms, and he'd told her he did not have AIDS. She wasn't worried about AIDS, she'd replied, but she did not want a child. Now she had one on the way. She wanted an abortion and knew where to get one. Taata had told her that if she went looking for one, he'd throw her out of the house.

As we spoke, we walked up the hill past the women with their tables of fish, pyramids of tomatoes, and piles of small potatoes that many Ugandans called "Irish." We passed the tarps piled with knock-off Crocs and slip-on sandals like the bright orange ones Peace had on her own feet. She put her body between mine and the cars that came careening down the road and told me to keep my hand on my bag, just as Maama Apollo did when she accompanied me on the ascent from the slum up to the main road. I looked at her more fully than I had before. She wore a T-shirt with the insignia of her father's beloved Catholic clinic atop gray-washed capri jeans, and there was both light and resignation in her eyes. She liked this boy, Adam. Her eyes shone when she said his name. She just didn't like the pregnancy.

We passed the clinic as we talked, its yellow gate opening inward. It offered free care to any family member with the card that the clinic had issued to Taata. But other than the T-shirt, it had nothing to offer Peace. Earlier that year, it had begun receiving PEPFAR funding via Catholic Relief Services (CRS). The conscience clause written into the original PEPFAR law stipulated that faith-based groups did not have to provide any services or commodities that violated their faith or principles. No condoms, no sexual education, no pregnancy termination. In the proposed reauthorization, this provision was further strengthened. The clinics did not have to offer the services, and they could not be required to acknowledge that they existed, to provide referrals for requested care.

When the closest free clinic did not offer young women and men anything but abstinence-until-marriage education, pregnancies were inevitable. Pregnant women were at far higher risk of getting HIV than nonpregnant women; women with HIV who had unplanned pregnancies were more likely to struggle taking their antiretrovirals, leading to a higher viral load. This put their health at risk as well as that of their children.[30] Providing services to plan, prevent, and—when absolutely necessary—terminate their pregnancies was, without a doubt, HIV prevention. But when Ken Hackett of Catholic Relief Services appeared at a December 2007 Senate hearing on PEPFAR—Peace was, by then, large with child—he pleaded with Congress, "Do not require PEPFAR implementers to offer family planning and reproductive services." In his written remarks, he pushed further. It was not just that the services should not be required; they should not be recognized as something a woman with HIV would need. CRS was, the submitted testimony said, "very concerned about efforts to define 'comprehensive services' for HIV-positive women as necessarily including family planning and reproductive health services. CRS regrets these efforts and asks that such proposals be rejected." If he was ignored, he warned the committee, "millions of people" would lose their care.[31]

But the hearings also included people who were champions for Peace and other young women like her. In September 2007, Helene Gayle, the physician and public health luminary who'd left the Bill & Melinda Gates Foundation to lead the girl-focused NGO CARE International, appeared before the House Committee on Foreign Affairs to advocate for young women like Peace. "Addressing HIV and AIDS solely as a medical challenge is like treating the symptoms, but not really the cause of the disease," she said. For the women and girls who made up 60 percent of new HIV infections in Africa, more had to be done to keep them healthy.

Gayle said that this meant drawing from programs like those of CARE, which provided loans and vocational training, food aid, and support groups. She wanted women and adolescent girls who needed family planning to be able to get contraceptives. She drew a sharp distinction between these programs and the strategy that had been enshrined in the first legislation, the Uganda-derived Abstain, Be Faithful, Use Condoms (ABC) approach. "While we believe that the ABC strategy is critical and has to be a foundation, we feel that an ABC-plus strategy that really looks at some of these other issues that are critical for the vulnerability of women is essential."[32]

Chris Smith, the representative from New Jersey who had, five years prior, said, "Hell, I'd support 15 billion," wasted no time in getting to the heart of the matter. "That sounds reasonable on its face until you understand what they mean by reproductive health. To many of us, it simply means abortion." He wanted Gayle to clarify. "So how do you define reproductive health? Is it abortion?"

Gayle tried to answer, explaining comprehensive needs and how women who had one child born with HIV were likely to have another. Smith cut her off. "But do you define reproductive health as abortion?"[33]

In truth, it did not matter how Gayle answered. Smith believed, along with Representative Joe Pitts, the Republican Pro-Life Caucus, and many other conservative members of Congress, that reproductive health meant abortion, comprehensive women's health meant abortion, and sexual rights meant abortion. The conviction that all terms associated with women's health were code was so deep that it extended beyond the vocabulary of sexual and reproductive services. Researchers interviewing Hill staff about perceptions of coded speech reported, "House staff members were very surprised to discover that some offices believed that 'behavior change' meant masturbation training.... These examples are cited as a caution to anyone seeking to find common ground."[34]

Dr. Joia Mukherjee, a Partners in Health physician and Harvard professor who worked with Paul Farmer in Haiti, sat beside Helene Gayle that day in September. She began her remarks with a concise, powerful indictment of International Monetary Fund policies' impact on health systems before making her own plea for expanding PEPFAR's remit to include education and other so-called structural interventions. She said, "Something that we do in Partners in Health as risk prevention, is thinking about getting rid of school fees; is helping children to go to school. And is that an abstinence program? Well, in fact, it is. Because every study—again these are studies—... shows that the longer time girls are in school, the more likely they are to delay the onset of sexual intercourse."[35]

A debate over PEPFAR's ideological provisions was also brewing inside the White House. By 2007, many of the original West Wing staff who'd helped launch PEPFAR had moved on. Dybul found himself working with a far more conservative team that wanted the reauthorizing legislation to both preserve the abstinence-until-marriage funding earmark and ensure that family planning didn't get mentioned in the bill at all. At one particularly tough meeting, Dybul sat and listened to deputy staffers declare, "No, you can't mention family planning; no, you can't give on abstinence; no, you can't do any of this." Dybul said he refused to get on board, ultimately raising the issue with Condoleezza Rice and, eventually, the president, who supported Dybul's position that the bill move forward even if the abstinence earmark changed and family planning appeared in the text.[36]

Dybul, who'd once considered becoming a poet or a philosopher, was viewed by many legislators and their aides as a savvy, skillful political advocate for PEPFAR on Capitol Hill. While he pushed back against West Wing conservatives, he took care to keep those on the Hill comfortable with the program's direction.

Dybul wasn't by any means confident that reauthorization was a slam dunk, and so when he appeared before Congress in late 2007, he offered the assembled senators the commitments that could earn bipartisan support. He told them that PEPFAR 2.0 would have a broader development agenda, addressing far more than the virus that was its singular foe. It would hand ever more responsibility off to countries, and it would, as they'd asked, focus on prevention. The change would be one of intensity, not strategy, he explained, offering this reassuring assessment: "Our best hope for generalized epidemics, such as those in Africa, is what's called and was created by Africans as ABC—or Abstain, Be Faithful, and Correct and Consistent Use of Condoms."[37]

He would champion a reauthorization that upheld conservatives' core beliefs, while also taking care to demur on issues like the education investments that Mukherjee advocated, which might be considered mission creep. In the question-and-answer portion of the October 24 SFRC hearing, Democratic senators came armed with questions about the kinds of structural strategies that could help reduce girls' risk.[38]

How many PEPFAR countries had universal primary education? Biden asked. "I'd actually have to doublecheck. Most of them do actually have universally available primary education," Dybul said. Biden wanted to know whether, if money were no object, supporting elementary and secondary schools that treated boys and girls equally would help reduce their HIV risk. "Is that likely to have any positive impact on what we're talking about here?" the senator asked. "It's something we intend to look at," said the US Global AIDS ambassador. "I don't know. You could say that it would and it very well might, but we're not 100 percent certain."[39]

— —

PEPFAR THE POLITICAL BEAST was always different from PEPFAR the program "on the ground" in the countries where it operated. The past five years had seen both subversion and implementation of the program's strictures on women's sexual and reproductive health. On the one hand, nurse midwife Michele Moloney-Kitts, one of the early "Unprincipals" who'd remained on the PEPFAR team, and other US-based staff urged the country teams to consider ways to integrate contraceptive programming: USAID could buy the supplies; PEPFAR programs could pay for provider training, even if the program didn't deliver the services.[40] But over the same five-year period that PEPFAR funds had soared, USAID funding for family planning had flatlined.[41]

South African AIDS activist Yvette Raphael saw the ways that PEPFAR-funded programs negotiated the politics of family planning when, in 2007, she took a middle-management position at a PEPFAR-funded communications project run by Johns Hopkins University. In her job interview, she'd announced that she'd like to be running the organization, or an equivalent, within five years. When she got to her monitoring and evaluation qualifications—the skills she'd honed at the gun-collection program—the white man interviewing her told her to stop. She was hired.[42]

By this time, Raphael had been working with Americans for years on the "underground" system that shared donated medications, treatment literacy materials, and activist strategy. She'd imagined PEPFAR would be an extension of that work. "When I came into the system with the American people I was actually shocked that there were so many conditions for this funding," she said. "It took me a while to understand and accept it as aid."

She'd found a set of rules and regulations but also an organization that was willing to push the envelope—to a certain extent. In trainings she could provide information and address questions that fell in the realm of comprehensive sexuality education; she could also provide referrals to and information about abortion clinics if a young woman asked. "There were smart ways around it," she said. She took notice of her boss's posh home and ample household staff but concluded that, in spite of it all, he was "a good-hearted American white man doing stuff for South Africa." The contradictions and compromises made her squirm, but it also seemed like the best option for fulfilling the mission—shared with Prudence Mabele—of making adolescent and young women's lives better and safer. When she looked outside her organization, she saw "a denialist government and a denialist America." Denial referred not just to whether HIV caused AIDS but to the fact that sexual and reproductive health were inseparable from HIV programs. Inside the PEPFAR-funded NGO, things looked better, though by no means perfect. She could see her boss "pushing the envelope, you know, but not too much, not to the detriment of the funding to the organization."[43]

Back in Washington, DC, though, these nuances couldn't be allowed to filter into the reauthorization. Dybul believed a bill aiming to expand the program's investments in women's health would never get passed, and when a draft that sought just that emerged from the House drafting process—with Peter Yeo and Pearl-Alice Marsh again at the helm—he made sure the worrisome language got scrubbed out before it reached the conservative champions it needed.

Yeo and Marsh had worked on the bill despite, and because of, the loss of their revered leader, Representative Tom Lantos, who had succumbed to cancer in early 2008. Before it was over, the legislation would be named in honor of Lantos and Henry Hyde, his Republican counterpart, who'd died some months before. Once again, Marsh practiced her grassroots statecraft, opening up the process to the advocates and activists who had, in the past five years, come to accept PEPFAR as part of the AIDS funding architecture and, anticipating the reauthorization debate, had in early 2007 begun a campaign to secure the program's continuation with expanded funding.

━━ ━━

ON OCTOBER 24, 2007, when Joe Biden talked about how PEPFAR had offered stays of execution to people with AIDS, he also said that he thought the president's $30 billion funding ask should be treated as a floor, not a ceiling. Activists had let his campaign team know what would happen if he didn't. For months, Health GAP had been working tirelessly on a campaign called '08 Stop AIDS. The group and its network of allies, including college and medical students and church leaders, had "bird-dogged" the entire presidential campaign field, appearing at public events and demanding that the candidates pledge to give $50 billion to PEPFAR if elected.

By late October, Biden and fellow candidates Hillary Clinton and Barack Obama were the only holdouts. The trio were headed for a Halloween night debate at Philadelphia's Drexel University—ACT UP Philly's home turf. Activist Paul Davis and his comrades planned a Halloween-themed protest complete with wheelbarrows, torches, grim reaper costumes, and signs declaring that candidates who didn't sign the pledge wanted Africans to "dig more graves." A day or so before the debate, Davis decided that he favored "dread over surprise" and so called up the campaign staffs of Biden, Obama, and Clinton to warn them of what awaited them in Philadelphia if they did not sign on to the pledge. Clinton and Obama agreed; Biden held out—he still hadn't signed on October 27, when he convened the Senate committee.

Davis counted it as a partial win. He changed the messages on the signs and put the brakes on media outreach. With its fiery torches and flapping reapers, it was one of the most beautiful actions he'd ever tried to hide. After the debate, he and a couple of activist "good eggs" tracked Biden down at his after-party at a University of Pennsylvania bar and asked him once again if he'd sign on and announce it on his campaign website. Davis and others there that night say the candidate agreed.[44]

The $50 billion pledge was a high bar but not an outlandish request, since Congress had, year after year, appropriated more than the president had asked for—a total of $19 billion by 2007. Annualizing $30 billion over five years would bump the funding up a little bit—$50 billion could change the game. Repealing the abstinence earmark was another point of easy agreement for the liberal activist coalition. At a January 2007 meeting, as the bird-dogging efforts got underway, the Prevention Working Group of the Global AIDS Roundtable—the umbrella coalition for DC-focused work on AIDS—took stock of the program's prevention efforts. "We need to stop treating sex like a disease but as part of human development," declared Jodi Jacobson, leader of the sexual and reproductive rights advocacy group the Center for Health and Gender Equity. "Practicing safer sex means you aren't subject to GBV [gender-based violence] and you can choose when and with whom you have sex." An activist phoning in from AIDS Project Los Angeles pointed out that gay men and transgender people needed "sex positive" interventions that were "grounded in human rights." Daniel Raymond, a leading harm-reduction activist laid out the ways that the program could do more to address HIV in people who used drugs. Other than Ukraine and Vietnam, PEPFAR did not work in many of the countries where HIV infections acquired via drug use drove the epidemic. But HIV and the criminalization of drug use were issues in all countries, and PEPFAR had been unambitious with its harm-reduction programming. It need not have been. It was technically not bound by the domestic regulations that prohibited federal funding for syringe exchange and had leeway to pay for essential harm reduction activities even if it chose not to purchase syringes.[45]

The treatment activists thought big—and also pragmatically. When the drafting process began some months later, women's health advocates, including Heather Boonstra from the Guttmacher Institute and Jacobson and Serra Sippel with the Center for Health and Gender Equity, advanced a strong reproductive health agenda even as allies like Paul Davis and Paul Zeitz worried that this might jeopardize bipartisan support. They ignored these issues, asking for female condoms and a clear expansion of the program to cover sexual and reproductive health—which they took pains to define as exclusive of abortion. Marsh had, once again, taken the activists' suggested wording, making no promises about what would happen. "I'll put it in, you have to defend it," she liked to say.[46] She developed a draft that Sippel would call the "Dream Bill"—one that didn't go as far as Gayle might have liked in endorsing structural interventions like education and microfinance but at least mentioned "reproductive health," "family planning," and "contraception" as integral to a public health approach to fighting AIDS.[47]

When Dybul got wind of the draft, though, he had a deputy write a letter expressing the opposition of the Office of the US Global AIDS Coordinator. "We warned them—the Democrats threw reproductive health and family planning all through the document," Dybul later said. "We told them don't do that.... Have 'family planning' over here and 'reproductive health' in another paragraph. Don't put them together." To women's health advocates, the two phrases referred to distinct and complementary activities. To conservatives, the pairing was code for abortion.

Dybul's deputy put the warning in writing in a letter to the House Foreign Relations Committee. The Office of the Global AIDS Coordinator couldn't back that kind of language. "We are deeply concerned that the draft repeatedly invokes 'reproductive health' and 'family planning,' and requires linkages, referrals, reporting on training, support and direct funding for these activities." HIV-positive women with unplanned pregnancies were more likely to transmit HIV to their infants; pregnancy planning helped ensure women had children when they were able to access the health care they needed. Nevertheless, the letter objected to the notion that contraception could help reduce the risk of mother-to-child transmission, saying that it suggested that "it is necessary to prevent [babies] from being born" to reduce HIV risk, a suggestion that ran counter to PEPFAR's "life-saving principle."[48]

On Capitol Hill, work on consensus language for women's health hit a logjam. Seasoned staffers who'd worked on the issue before, including Lantos aide Peter Yeo, found the staff of Ileana Ros-Lehtinen, the ranking Republican, unwilling to strike a deal on compromise language that would allow the legislation to move into a committee hearing. Representative Howard Berman, the ranking House democrat, placed a call to the White House seeking a means to break the stalemate, Peter Yeo recalled. "The next meeting, Mark Dybul walks in, and we had a deal within half an hour." Dybul arrived on the eve of the House International Relations Committee meeting to mark up the bill. With no time to lose, he steered a revision that effectively killed the Dream Bill. Berman had given Yeo instructions on where to give and where to stand firm in order to move things forward. "I was willing to sacrifice a lot of the language we had included from the women and gender community in order to get a compromise bill that would be signed into law by the Bush administration."[49]

At the eleventh hour, the lawmakers removed almost all mention of reproductive health and family planning from the bill. The revised bill was not circulated to committee members in advance; the copies that arrived in their hands were still warm from the printer. Heather Boonstra was standing in line, waiting to get a seat in the hearing room, when she heard the news. "I lost my sense of purpose," she'd recall. "All that I had been working for melted away."[50]

Peter Yeo explained what had happened to Boonstra, Sippel, Jacobson, and other women's health advocates in an empty conference room adjacent to the hearing. Marsh thought he'd cried that day, which he would remember as the worst day of his professional life. But when Yeo had called his mother—"She'd be ashamed of you," the women had said—Reverend Eleanor Yeo told him she understood. She knew precisely how hard the American government would work to control women's reproductive lives.

The bill that came out of the Dybul-brokered deal making pleased Representative Chris Smith to no end. "I am glad that the whole focus of the bill, originally, which would have been toward enriching the abortion industry, has been done away with," he said, and with that the other House Republicans fell in line. Just before 12:15 p.m., the vote was called, and the ayes carried the day.[51]

The bill they'd voted for had also found a delicate way to deal with the matter of the earmarks. In lieu of a specific percentage of funds allocated to treatment, it provided a numerical target—an additional three million people were to be treated in the program's next five years. The prevention carve-out had also been dispensed with, replaced with the requirement that each country develop a strategy for preventing sexual transmission of the epidemic, and if that strategy allocated less than 50 percent of these funds for behavior-change programs (abstinence, delay of sexual debut, monogamy, fidelity, and partner reduction), the program would, within thirty days of issuance of the strategy, submit a "justification for this decision."

Countries could be trusted—but not too much. African nations that did not dedicate at least 50 percent of their prevention dollars to the A and B elements of the "African" ABC strategy still had to explain themselves to America. This was not ideal, but the Christian conservatives could live with it.

The same could not be said for the new approach to antiretroviral treatment, at least on the Senate side. There, Katy Talento was, once again, ready to fight tooth and nail for the program to put as much money as possible into treatment. For anyone who'd missed the first round of negotiations, she was there to remind them. "By [2008] everyone had left who had been there the first time around, and we were back to a bunch of Hill staffers who didn't know the issue, didn't know where the bodies were buried on these policies. They were being snookered into watering down these policies when blood had been spilled over [them]." She meant, in particular, the program's clarity on spending money on antiretrovirals above all. It was her job to explain, "Don't you dare water them down when [they are] the only reason why this program's different."[52]

Without the treatment earmark, Talento saw no safeguard against USAID coming in and spending money on billboards, conferences, condom airlifts, and other pointless, low-impact programming. The three-million-person treatment target didn't allay her fears. The program had put over a million and a half people on treatment in its first four years, according to the March 2008 report to Congress—and that had been starting from square one. In those first four years, the program had needed to create clinics, train staff, and alert people that the drugs had finally arrived. The program was on track to treat two million people by the end of 2008, which meant that in the next five years, for twice the budget, PEPFAR would put just one million people onto antiretroviral drugs.

Katy Talento's views hadn't changed, but her position had. In 2005, she joined Oklahoma Republican senator Tom Coburn's team as staff director on the Federal Management Subcommittee of the Senate Homeland Security Committee. When the bill left the House for the Senate, she launched a campaign to get a treatment "floor" or earmark put back in. She had, in Coburn, an ally who could make that happen. There were forty-eight Democratic senators in 2007, forty-seven in 2008. Two independent senators caucused with the Democrats, providing a wafer-thin majority. Of the many challenges this majority faced in passing legislation, none was as formidable as Dr. Coburn, an

OB-GYN who'd continued delivering babies for several years while serving in government. He'd earned and reveled in the title "Dr. No" for his frequent use of the Senate's hold procedure to block debate on bills he did not like, often because he said that they appeared to duplicate other programs or would waste taxpayers' money.

Talento was a perfect foil for Coburn. They were both commanding congressional strategists who burned with hatred of waste and suspicion of government spending and who blended science and faith in their bone-deep beliefs about the value of abstinence and fidelity. Coburn, an MD, would give slide talks on sexually transmitted infections (STIs), complete with images of suppurating ulcers, to his young staff to persuade them to avoid sex outside marriage. "The plow runs deep," he said about Talento. "She is well rooted in the principles of liberty."[53]

With Coburn at the helm and Talento at his side, the pair put a strategy in motion to get the bill they wanted. On March 12, 2008, before the House bill could reach the floor, Coburn introduced his own "message" bill, which proposed, among other things, a target of putting seven million people on antiretrovirals in the next five years.[54] Arizona Republican senator Jon Kyl cosponsored Coburn's bill and also introduced his own bill—Talento praised it as a "nastygram" intended to communicate that concerned senators were playing to win. Kyl's bill aimed to prohibit the extension of PEPFAR funds to new countries with higher incomes or nuclear programs. He also condemned the Senate's wishy-washiness on the issue of reproductive health. "It appears the Senate Committee bill would pander to the so-called 'family planning' agenda."[55]

There were now three bills—the "pandering" one that had passed through the House of Representatives after Dybul's eleventh-hour intervention, Coburn's message bill, and Kyl's nastygram—the latter two of which were intended to gum up the works with conditions that the Senate would need to debate before they could move on any legislation.

This wasn't what the White House wanted. Bush wanted to take PEPFAR 2.0 to the next Group of Eight summit. He also wanted to be able to tell the African heads of state, who had written a letter to him expressing concerns about continuity in their funding, that they need not worry. He wanted the law before it was too late to get that kind of money. In March 2008, as members of Congress invoked the nation's unstable footing in their opposition to the $50 billion price tag for PEPFAR 2.0, the Federal Reserve held its first emergency weekend meeting in thirty years to try to save investment bank Bear Stearns, which, if it collapsed, might imperil other overleveraged investment banks and thence the entire economy.[56]

Paul Davis, Paul Zeitz, and the American AIDS activists working on reauthorization shared the president's urgency. They'd secured candidates' pledges for the '08 Stop AIDS platform, which called for the $50 billion investment, with allocations for hiring and training 100,000 health-care workers and a bumped-up contribution to the Global Fund. Now they turned to the business of getting that content into the draft legislation and seeing the bill passed, then signed into law.

It was a different time for them too. The sense of emergency had abated for the American Left. When Bush cut his enormous check for fighting global AIDS, he'd turned the revolution into a work of mercy, and many potential allies dismissed the effort all together. AIDS activist and historian Sarah Schulman wrote, "Marketed as 'AIDS in Africa,' ongoing international AIDS has inspired a kind of insipid charity mentality in the citizen who expresses her opinions through the products she consumes." About PEPFAR, Schulman lamented, "The United States has responded with programs both government and corporate that fluctuate in level of support and fail to address underlying issues."[57] Many other left-leaning American activists shared the sense that the Bush program had to be bad news. If it was another morally corrupt, neoliberal capitalist venture, then it could be dismissed outright. Yet many American AIDS activists opted for the work of influencing the system. A blanket dismissal of both the aid program and the activist work to hold it to account threatened to obscure critical efforts to improve a system many still hoped to revolutionize.

The work of watchdogging a "win" like PEPFAR had far less moral clarity and sex appeal than mobilizations that called Bush a murderer and a liar and took him to task for his disastrous wars and conservative domestic agenda, which included assaults on comprehensive sex education, affordable prescription drugs, and much more. Diminished in size, the cadre of activists who'd come to terms with PEPFAR fought against the flagging energy. Good organizers build and ride momentum. In fallow times, great organizers become the momentum—carrying it with them in their bodies, sometimes all alone. As '08 Stop AIDS unfolded, Kaytee Ray-Riek, a Health GAP staffer in charge of grassroots organizing on the presidential campaign trail, drove hundreds of miles back and forth across Iowa, listening to Harry Potter audiobooks to pass the time. That season, Ray-Riek realized that if she wanted someone from a church group or an activist cell to ask a candidate a question, she had to be there herself, sitting beside them, feeling her own body fill with adrenalin as she waited for the person next to her to shoot a hand into the air.[58]

Davis, too, realized he needed to be in the room. In later years, he'd rattle off the names—and subsequent life histories—of all the "church ladies" and "white coats" (members of faith-based groups and medical student associations) he'd brought with him. But he himself had gone to almost every one of the hundreds of Hill meetings Health GAP arranged—always with an ask and an argument tailored to the audience, each with follow-up, and then more follow-up after that. Global justice organizer Matthew Kavanagh arrived periodically with reinforcements—busloads of students who'd sleep on church floors overnight, then get briefed on what they were asking for and why. Davis rarely complains about anything but evil Republican policies and makes almost everything sound like enormous fun. But when he remembered that work—the first time he'd tried to pass a bill—he couldn't muster the enthusiasm. It had been "just this enormous grind."[59]

As activists from the Left and Center went to one set of offices, Katy Talento and AIDS Healthcare Foundation (AHF) executive Michael Weinstein canvassed others, with Weinstein explaining that

AHF could provide drugs far more cheaply than the $1,000 per person per year figure PEPFAR supplied.[60] Talento and Weinstein had worked together during the drafting process of the 2003 legislation and shared a passion for seeing their arguments prevail. Weinstein kept a note from Talento reading *Aut inveniam viam aut faciam*—Latin for "I shall either find a way or make one"—in a frame on his desk.

With a presidential champion and little precedent for providing large-scale treatment in poor countries, PEPFAR began as a program for which money was no object. Five years on, under scrutiny from an empowered Congress, the cost of doing business mattered very much indeed. Remarkably enough, considering that the majority of American aid did not calculate return on investment or cost per intervention, PEPFAR had an answer, even if it was one that Talento and Weinstein didn't like.

The $1,000-per-person-per-year figure came from a wry, brainy, informal economist named John Blandford who'd been sent up to the Office of the US Global AIDS Coordinator by his boss, Deborah Birx—who'd moved from the Department of Defense to head the CDC's global AIDS work—to help Mark Dybul get the PEPFAR budget right. Blandford had collected numbers from actual programs in the field to get a handle on what people were spending—not just for the pills but for the "buffer stock," the total inventory required in national and regional warehouses and in clinics to keep shelves full at all times, as well as for salaries, equipment, furniture, and rent. Weinstein's costs were lower because they didn't account for these "fully-loaded" costs.[61]

The Institute of Medicine report had urged PEPFAR to be a "learning organization"—and it already was. Paying for an economist to collect data from forty-five sites across five countries in order to calculate the per-person cost for services was yet another step that no other American foreign aid initiative had taken. But as far as Talento, Coburn, and his allies—Sam Brownback, Jon Kyl, and Mike Enzi among them—were concerned, there were other lessons PEPFAR had to learn. On March 13, the Senate Foreign Relations Committee voted eighteen to three to order the Lantos-Hyde bill, in honor of two bygone champions, to the floor.[62] On March 31, as Coburn had done eighty-odd times in the past twelve months, he sent a letter to Mitch McConnell that placed a hold on the bill on the basis of "mission creep," "irresponsible spending," and "elimination of safeguards" that would require the money to be spent on treatment.[63]

The hold lasted exactly three months, from March 31 to July 1, 2008, as the White House sought in vain to persuade right-wing groups to support the legislation, and Kaytee Ray-Riek, gripped in a bear hug by John McCain in a meet-and-greet line on the campaign trail implored the candidate to get his colleagues to lift the hold.[64]

Once again, Dybul stepped in with a solution. He proposed that the earmark be replaced by a stipulation that "more than half" of PEPFAR funds go for "life-saving care," a bucket filled to the brim with services including antiretrovirals, testing, medical monitoring, food support, and more. The hodgepodge sounded like treatment to Talento and like everything under the sun to the Democrats and therefore made everyone happy. In addition, there would be a requirement that the target for treating people rose in proportion to the amount of money appropriated each year. If all $50 billion were to be appropriated, then the target would rise to five million additional people on antiretrovirals. Talento, who'd called their strategy "a game of chicken," looked at this offer and assumed they'd won.

On July 1, Coburn sent a letter lifting the hold, and the bill passed in the Senate on July 16, 2008. It included $50 billion, the treatment formula, and a $2 million earmark for health on Native American reservations inserted by Senator Kyl. It passed even after Kyl introduced an amendment that would have applied Kemp-Kasten language, forbidding the expenditure of funds on coercive abortion, to the bill, an action that could have been prevented had the floor manager from Biden's staff been paying closer attention. Putting Kemp-Kasten into the bill would, effectively, have meant that the Mexico City Policy was back in play. It was a near crisis—since even the Republicans had agreed not to seek MCP expansion. But overnight phone calls to the conservatives implored them to table the amendment, not to vote against it but simply not to consider it. And because this was a treatment bill, a bill of massive mercy with the hierarchy of priorities clear as the pyramid on the back of the one-dollar bill, they had agreed.

━━ ━━

ON JULY 2, 2008, two weeks before the bill passed and one day after Coburn sent the hold letter, Peace and I once again walked together up the hill. She'd given birth to a baby boy named Adam, after the father. Then she peered into my face and asked for advice. Something was wrong between her legs. She wore a maxi pad to catch the pus that was pouring out of her all the time. "Go get treated," I said, and pressed a folded-up bill into her hands. "Go see someone soon." I hoped I was not too late.

Several studies had been done to evaluate the HIV-prevention benefit of treating sexually transmitted infections. It made sense: a person with open sores in their genitals had more portals for the virus to enter—both physically, in the sense of breaks in the skin, and at a cellular level, since the immune cells that gathered around an ulcer or infection were the ones that the virus infected to survive.

One of those studies, conducted in Tanzania, had found that treating STIs reduced a person's risk of getting HIV.[65] Other studies seeking to duplicate that result had not found the same thing, and as part of the explanation, the vast mystery of the private parts of women's bodies had been invoked.[66] There was so much going on down there. Diagnosis and treatment of STIs had not made it into the ABC strategy and therefore not into PEPFAR—in its first incarnation or in the Lantos-Hyde bill that President Bush signed into law on July 30, 2008. That law, which represented the first and last time that substantive changes would be made to the legal framework of PEPFAR, did not in fact include or stipulate any HIV-prevention service that asked people how their bodies felt, whether something burned or itched or dripped, and then offered a remedy for those most private wounds.

As the senators had made clear before they passed the reauthorization, this program was a salve for America too. In 2003, Bush had not launched the AIDS war to improve the American brand. But in 2008, the senators were plain about how they needed it to burnish

America's image in the eyes of the world. "Our sustained commitment to the treatment, prevention, and care of HIV/AIDS globally through this law has helped us make great strides toward helping repair our Nation's image overseas so badly damaged by the war in Iraq," said Christopher Dodd. "So, I tell my colleagues, the eyes of the world are upon us. We must reauthorize this program and we cannot wait another day to do it."[67]

"I think this is our most successful foreign policy initiative in my lifetime—I was born after the Marshall Plan started or thereabouts," Coburn said. "This is the most effective thing we have done to build American prestige, esteem and respect and thankfulness in my lifetime."[68] Coburn's comparison of PEPFAR to the Marshall Plan was, in its framing, more apt than most, since the post–World War II effort had been a politically calculated intervention aimed at ensuring that countries ravaged by that conflict did not turn to Communist Russia for help, alliances, and aid. Economic restoration was important; so was how the recipient countries felt about and acted toward the United States as a result.

Moving forward, these champions would be essential.

"Come on, Bishop," President Bush had called to Kunene Tantoh's son, who sat in his blue wax cloth ensemble, clowning around with sunglasses, at that Rose Garden ceremony at the end of May 2007. There was no response. That wasn't the boy's name. "Come on, Baron." The little boy came trotting. When the president dropped into a crouch, grinning, arms wide, the child had leapt into Bush's arms. The president stood then, hoisting Baron onto his hip. He'd raised his hand and waved at the crowd, motioning to Baron to do the same. Bush was the program's first and only fully committed presidential champion. He was an imperfect progenitor and protector—he'd made countless errors far greater than forgetting a boy's name. But he'd provided PEPFAR with a mandate from the White House that it would never have again. Both America and the countries it served suffer as a result.

Baron didn't lift up his hand until his mother plucked at his sleeve. Finally, Baron followed the president's lead. He lifted his hand and waved. *Good-bye.*

CHAPTER 10

ARRESTED DEVELOPMENT

H OW QUICKLY THE WORLD changed. In the morning of Tuesday, November 4, 2008, President George W. Bush believed in boots-on-the-ground war and in PEPFAR as a mission of mercy that was "off to a good start" but nowhere near complete. For eight years, he'd been accompanied by the angel and her whirlwind, which had first appeared in a letter between slave owners at the dawn of the country's independence.

That night, when the votes had been tallied, a new president-elect walked out to greet the country with his Black skin and his Black family. His wife wore a red dress with a black cross over her chest. The red ate into the black, Dixie consumed by flames. On inauguration night in January 2009, though, she wore white, for she was the angel now. History and its lashes were at her back. Standing in lavender on a tiny dais, Beyoncé was the love child of Harriet Tubman and Botticelli's Venus. She stretched her arm out toward them and made a love song a redemption song. Dancing—foreheads touching—the Obamas made their love a redemption of all sundered families, of the nation's soul, its moral center. She thrust her arm up into the air. *At last.*

It was a time, if ever there was one, for thinking about the future. It was also a time for endings, America being enamored of the story-book form, the conclusion. The end of racism, of war—a hope so fervent that it permeated the globe, with the president of postracial America awarded the Nobel Peace Prize just eleven months after taking office.

The world could not be remade quickly enough. On November 8, 2008, just a day after the election, a pair of ethicists published an article, "US Health AID Beyond PEPFAR." In a handful of sentences, the pair put an expanding PEPFAR in the past. It had been a success, authors Dr. Ezekiel Emanuel and Dr. Colleen Denny wrote. It had benefited countries and boosted America's "moral legitimacy," and, yes, it had also recently been reauthorized for $50 billion. This portended a problem, they wrote:

> Doubling or tripling PEPFAR's funding is not the best use of international health funding. In focusing heavily on HIV/AIDS treatments, the United States misses huge opportunities. By extending funds to simple but more deadly diseases such as respiratory and diarrheal diseases, the US government could save more lives—especially young lives—at substantially lower cost.[1]

One day, PEPFAR had been a moral imperative. The next day, it was a program that could not ethically continue to expand, at least according to the principles the authors proposed: save the most lives, prioritize young lives, spend on the most cost-effective interventions possible, meaning the ones that did the most for the least amount of money. The authors themselves had developed these principles. There had never been an American ethical framework for global health, or any other, foreign aid.

"Zeke" Emanuel, the brother of Rahm, Barack Obama's irascible campaign manager and a future mayor of Chicago, was no stranger to developing ethical frameworks. Some years prior, he'd worked with a team of researchers and ethicists to devise both principles and benchmarks for assessing the ethics of conducting clinical trials in resource-poor settings. He'd done that at a time when US-funded research networks wanted to test HIV vaccines and other experimental HIV prevention tools on Africans and had been stymied by what to do when people in those trials acquired HIV.[2]

Dr. Deborah Birx had looked at the dilemma and decided the question was all wrong: it wasn't "How could you do trials where antiretroviral treatment (ART) wasn't available?" but "How could you make ART available to everyone where the trial was happening?" That was why she'd started the ART program in Kericho, Kenya. Birx liked to remake the world; Emanuel liked to provide principles for the world as it was. And that world, in late 2008, was in the midst of a massive recession, an economic slowdown that, he reckoned, meant there would be finite funds for global health and a need for an ethical framework to guide spending in a time of scarcity.

PEPFAR, he and Denny suggested, failed on most counts. It did not save as many lives as, say, a mass childhood immunization campaign. It did not prioritize children, for as much as the legislation and the annual reports spoke of orphans and vulnerable children and of preventing mother-to-child transmission, these areas lagged far behind in being able to show concrete results. It paid for antiretrovirals (ARVs), which were absolutely not the most cost-effective AIDS response. It was always cheaper to prevent an illness than to treat it.

Emanuel and Denny did not want to end PEPFAR; they just didn't want it to grow at the rate that it had been, even if that meant that America ceased to pay for more people to start ARVs. Those drugs were expensive, even with the price reductions and the shift toward generics—by the time they wrote their article more than three-quarters of all antiretrovirals purchased by the program came from generic manufacturers.

Emanuel wasn't the first or only person to take issue with PEPFAR's disease-specific, treatment-focused approach. But he would soon be in a unique position to make his case. By February 2009, Dr. Emanuel was a special advisor in the White House Office of Management and Budget (OMB). His remit in that position was twofold: guide Obama's health-care reform effort and overhaul American spending to align with the ethical principles he and Denny had designed.

Lin Liu, a budget examiner at OMB, had been waiting for a boss like Emanuel. Six or seven months prior, even before the election, she'd been looking at the different streams of money that the US government spent on health, and she'd been troubled by how disconnected they were—how PEPFAR dwarfed most other investments and didn't connect up with the maternal-child health account or the President's Malaria Initiative, which sat within USAID.[3]

It looked inefficient, suboptimal, and like PEPFAR was a giant disease-specific stovepipe that was spending too much money on one thing. She worked up a proposal for a way to streamline all of these budgets and, on Emanuel's first or second day on the job, presented her vision to him. He loved it. Pooling the money and streamlining the spending was the operational side of the ethics-driven global health investment portfolio he'd envisioned.

On May 29, 2009, President Obama announced the program that reflected this new vision. "In the 21st century, disease flows freely across borders and oceans, and, in recent days, the 2009 H1N1 virus has reminded us of the urgent need for action," he said. "We cannot wall ourselves off from the world and hope for the best, nor ignore the public health challenges beyond our borders. An outbreak in Indonesia can reach Indiana within days, and public health crises abroad can cause widespread suffering, conflict, and economic contraction. We simply cannot confront individual preventable diseases in isolation."[4]

The president asked for $8.6 billion in the coming year, as part of a $63 billion, six-year investment to "shape a new, comprehensive global health strategy," designed to expand on the previous administration's work, including PEPFAR. "As a US Senator, I joined a bipartisan majority in supporting the Bush Administration's effective President's Emergency Plan for AIDS Relief," Obama continued. "But I also recognize that we will not be successful in our efforts to end deaths from AIDS, malaria and tuberculosis unless we do more to improve health systems around the world, focus our efforts on child and maternal health, and ensure that best practices drive the funding for these programs."

The new program, called the Global Health Initiative (GHI), was as cool and cerebral as President Bush's hunger for mercy had been hot with emotion. It emerged in the context of an administration that would, in the president's words, be "guided by science." On taking office, the Obama administration abolished the Office of Health and Security that Dr. Kenneth Bernard had helped set up under the Bush administration, but when the novel H1N1 flu emerged, the White House reacted quickly with a proactive preparedness strategy that won kudos from many public health experts.[5]

In the speech launching the Global Health Initiative, Obama seemed to link the investment in other countries' basic health needs to America's own security against emergent infectious diseases. But as details about the program emerged, this connection disappeared. The White House fact sheet declared that GHI would contribute to national security as a "smart power" tool that stabilized poor countries' government institutions so that their societies didn't crumble—and create a vacuum for terrorists—when a pandemic emerged. Global health investments helped make good neighbors; they weren't viewed as essential to America's health at home.[6]

In other ways, the proposal was prescient. The AIDS activists all agreed that far more work needed to be done in other health arenas. But even though GHI purportedly sought to build on PEPFAR's success, it ignored its most important lessons: bring significant money to the table and put a single, White House–backed person in charge. PEPFAR soared in part because of its sheer largesse—the checks cut for countries were big enough to keep the interagency squabbling to a dull roar. But not only did GHI lack significant new funds; it also brought a budget cut for PEPFAR. The activists figured this out on May 30, the day after the GHI announcement, when the White House released its proposed budget for the coming fiscal year.

The Lantos-Hyde Act authorized $48 billion over five years; stretching that figure to GHI's six-year time frame would mean a $57.6 billion allocation for AIDS. But the budget sought just $51 billion for six years—an adjustment the activists deemed a $6 billion cut. Adding to the concern, in the full budget request, Obama sought just $366 million more for PEPFAR than it had received the previous year,[7] the smallest year-to-year increase in the program's history, and reduced the American contribution to the Global Fund. "President Obama is betraying the trust of millions of people around the world, many of whom will die as a result," said Paul Zeitz from the Global AIDS Alliance.[8]

Reflecting back on that time, Emanuel told me that he thought activists' outcry reflected "naivete on budgeting," saying, "Anyone who does budgets knows you cannot grow at the same rate. You are going to inevitably slow down your growth. And again, if you look historically at any new programs, NASA, EPA, NIH, they all go through the same process. It's inevitable. Plus we were in a major recession, facing huge budget deficits."[9]

The effect of having to relitigate the scope and ambitions of the AIDS war came as something of a shock to the activists for whom Obama's election was, in so many other ways, a longed-for reprieve. In 2009, Sharonann Lynch and Rachel Cohen were newly returned to the United States after three years in Lesotho. Lynch, now working for the Médecins Sans Frontières (MSF) access campaign, expected her job to entail a fight for continued and expanded spending on global AIDS. She knew that as the wards emptied of skeletal bodies and treatment clinics filled with people who needed medications every day for life, the romance of global AIDS would wear off, and the expensive, mundane realities would set in. She'd heard from MSF colleagues that health economists were beginning to say that "the global city" could not afford to carry the costs of medication for people living with HIV in low- and lower-middle-income countries and that critics thought the whole concept of stand-alone AIDS treatment programs was wrong. AIDS programs were vertical—shooting money into countries for a single disease—when real, lasting solutions needed to be horizontal.

Lynch knew the conceptual fight was coming, but she didn't anticipate that she'd have to fight for the importance of providing antiretroviral treatment to people living with HIV in what several activists described to me as table-thumping, combative meetings with Emanuel. "When we had a meeting with him, it's the only time I ever got a migraine in a meeting because he was so upsetting," she remembered. "He literally wagged his finger at Tido [von Schoen-Angerer], my ED [executive director], saying, 'Who are you going to save? Who are you going to save? A child who has diarrhea, or you want to put all the money in ARVs? Who? No, you have to pick. Who?' "[10]

—— ——

JOHN BLANDFORD, THE HEALTH economist Birx had seconded up to the Office of the US Global AIDS Coordinator (OGAC), was also taken by surprise by the new administration's stance on America's AIDS investments. In early 2009, his phone started ringing—a lot. As he recalled, Lin Liu was often on the other end. She and her OMB colleagues had reviewed and signed off on the PEPFAR budget submitted in late 2008. (Every year, PEPFAR turns its budget in to OMB, and every year OMB reviews it, paying close attention to the treatment budget.) In late 2008, the budget had sailed through, but when Blandford picked up the phone, Liu wanted him to run another scenario through his cost model. What would costs look like if America capped its investment in AIDS treatment, or if it added some people and then ceased expansion? Each model gave a different price tag for a different level of ambition. "We ran twenty-five or thirty scenarios in a two-week period," Blandford said. "The questions were becoming more and more systematic and inquisitive."[11]

By this time, Blandford's boss, Dr. Mark Dybul, had left the building. One day, Blandford had seen him, ashen but still amiable, coming through the door at OGAC headquarters. The next, he was gone. In the capital, rumors circulated that the women's groups had gone to the new secretary of state, Hillary Clinton, a staunch women's health advocate in her own right, raised concerns about Dybul's policies, and helped to secure his early ouster. After being appointed executive director of the Global Fund to Fight AIDS, Tuberculosis, and Malaria in 2012, Dybul would make investments in health and education for adolescent girls and young women a signature theme. But in 2009, women's groups did little to conceal their glee at the departure of a man who, they thought, had done "everything he could to work with the far right to tighten policies, deny women access to reproductive and sexual health care, and put in place guidance that further restricted women's choices," as Jodi Jacobson wrote in a blog post titled "Dybul Out: Thank You, Hillary!"[12]

But many of the core staff in the Office of the Global AIDS Coordinator remained. John Blandford worked closely with Dr. Charles Holmes, a dark-haired, amiable midwestern physician who'd helped write Malawi's first proposal to the Global Fund. Holmes had joined OGAC as the antiretroviral advisor in 2008. In that capacity, he helped PEPFAR set and meet targets, work that went hand in hand with work by Blandford and his colleague, Centers for Disease Control and Prevention (CDC) health economist Nalinee Sangrujee, focused on nailing down what things cost. As OMB started firing questions at them, the trio realized their work wasn't just useful for guiding strategy; it was likely essential for the program's survival. Knowing what things cost was interesting when money was no object; getting a handle on costs and places to cut them was essential if the funding slowed down or ceased to keep pace with the need. "My job at that point became to show how little we could spend on treatment and still expand," Blandford recalled.

With Birx's blessing, the trio launched a study of PEPFAR's costs—a level of self-examination and evidence gathering in the service of improving the use of resources that, once again, set PEPFAR apart from almost any other American aid. With some deft management of interagency dynamics—and the extra step of getting official government clearance for the survey after some PEPFAR grantees balked and claimed it violated the Paperwork Reduction Act—the CDC-based team launched a comprehensive, country-based accounting of what PEPFAR actually paid for.

While the team worked to clarify PEPFAR's costs, GHI remained murky. The White House had released a fact sheet and a PowerPoint deck after the initial announcement, but it hadn't put anyone in charge, released a strategy, or explained precisely how it would pursue its goals.

No one knew what GHI was, but it was clear that PEPFAR needed to rein in its growth. In June 2009, OGAC—still leaderless after Dybul's ouster—issued its annual guidance statement to the field offices planning for the coming year. The pace was probably going to slow down, the memo said. The funding levels were not going to rise above the figures for the past two years. "In FY2010 and beyond, PEPFAR is less likely to continue scale up of treatment programs in Phase 2, particularly through provision of direct support, at the same pace as in Phase 1, in part because of the significant costs of maintaining treatment for those already supported. Country teams could not plan on additional resources to expand the program, the guidance cautioned, explaining, "In FY 2010, planned country level resources will be essentially the same as in FYs 2008 and 2009."[13]

Beltway insiders had a simpler phrase for "the costs of maintaining treatment for those already supported"; they called it "the treatment mortgage." Such concerns had circulated in the Bush administration. The Office of the Inspector General, in a 2007 review of PEPFAR, fretted that "the US government has in some respects adopted a large population of non-US citizens for whose lives and livelihoods it has varying degrees of responsibility."[14] With Obama in the White House and the subprime-mortgage-associated global economic meltdown underway, inhibitions about referring to humans as burdensome investments disappeared altogether. "Treatment mortgage" emerged from within the Obama administration; several people working at the time remembered hearing that phrase frequently from OMB head Jack Lew. Mead Over, the health economist who'd once called sex workers "epidemiological pumps," dubbed the US commitment to treating people with AIDS in Africa "a ballooning entitlement."[15]

There was no mistaking the racist overtones in this language that made Black Africans with AIDS adoptees and their medication an "entitlement." A mortgage was, of course, a means of acquiring ownership. There was a fear now that in addition to helping these Africans,

America might own them. It was ugly language, difficult to square with the principles and promises of the first Black American president. But in the midst of the economic meltdown, it was precisely the kind of attention-grabbing sound bite that could be used, especially with white intellectuals, to support a new approach. And Obama was surrounded by many such people, who thought that much of the aid system was broken and needed fixing, just as his predecessor had eight years prior.

As Bush had done, Obama revamped the White House organizational chart, dispensing with Gary Edson's position—which sought to link economics and security and included a development portfolio—and bringing on Gayle Smith, a onetime journalist who'd done deep reporting on conflict in the Horn of Africa, as a special assistant to the president and senior director of development and democracy. Prior to joining the White House, Smith cofounded the Modernizing Foreign Assistance Network, a DC-based group that advocated for a new American approach to aid and against the "dual-hatted" role that Randall Tobias had briefly filled, leading USAID and serving as a director of foreign assistance at the State Department. USAID's allies had seen this as destabilizing for the agency and wanted it to have an elevated, independent role separate from the State Department. The call for rehabilitating USAID's leadership was often, though not exclusively, made by groups with ties to the agency's funding. Other more ambitious proposals called for the United States to finally create a cabinet-level Department of Development.

While opinions varied on the solution, there was unanimity about the problem. In 2007, a US-government-convened body known as the Helping to Enhance the Livelihood of People Around the Globe (HELP) Commission released *Beyond Assistance*, a comprehensive review of US foreign aid that opened with a scathing assessment. "Our foreign assistance system is broken. We ignore this reality at our peril."[16] Smith had been one of the HELP report's commissioners. Once ensconced in the White House, President Obama tasked her with conducting a review of development aid and issuing a presidential policy directive, the first such high-level document on the topic.

At the State Department in Foggy Bottom, Secretary of State Hillary Clinton was equally intent on innovations. She had, as First Lady, seen USAID at work in the field and spoken forthrightly about vast gaps in women's health and rights. She launched the Quadrennial Diplomacy and Development Review as a complement to the analogous, defense-focused document produced by the Pentagon, established the first-ever US ambassador for global women's issues, and championed USAID as the world's "premier development institution."

For the second time in less than a decade, American government officials tried to reform development, aid, and health. Development insiders tracked the details, including rumored turf battles between Clinton and Smith over whether development would sit at State or the National Security Council. But in the midst of an economic recession and as the H1N1 outbreak faded away without great calamity, GHI failed to gather momentum. Emanuel told me that activist pushback helped derail it, as did fluctuations in "the consistency of support internal in the administration—with . . . , people being shuffled along, and the White House taking its eye off the ball a little bit."

The initiative didn't have an empowered leader, as PEPFAR did. It was, instead, supposed to be run by committee, much to the chagrin of Dr. Eric Goosby, who, in late 2009, became the next head of PEPFAR. Goosby was an experienced HIV doctor from the Bay Area who'd helped establish AIDS treatment programs in Rwanda and been one of the squad who'd persuaded OMB to fund PEPFAR in the first place. He became, on arrival, both the chief messenger that PEPFAR had to slow down and the program's representative on the GHI "operations committee," which included Rajiv Shah, the recently appointed head of USAID, and Dr. Tom Frieden, the head of CDC.

The committee convened with the frequency of a group that can't get anything done. "We met, honestly, every week on this for months," Goosby recalled. "Every time it got down to what we needed to change, people fell back into their respective allegiances with their programs, their programs retaining all the control and decision making that it had at the moment."[17] The discussions went around and around, while countries—which understood that they were supposed to be developing coordinated plans across agencies and diseases and pooling resources where possible—took the work forward with varying levels of ambition and intention.

"It wasn't that [GHI] was a bad idea," Goosby told me. "It was a good idea that hadn't been socialized. If it had been handled differently, it would have had the impact that the President wanted. He really wanted this because he thought it made sense."[18] Within the AIDS activist community, any energy that might have been devoted to ensuring that an expanded public health effort lived up to its potential was instead diverted to fighting to preserve the American investment in PEPFAR—and to pushing back against similarly scaled-back donor ambitions at the Global Fund.

At the November 2008 Global Fund board meeting, the secretariat's Technical Review Panel—a body charged with evaluating the merit of proposals—recommended funding just over $3 million in new grants. Tripling the funding approved for any prior round, the Fund seemed poised to finally take on the ambitious, large-scale endeavors activists had been clamoring for. A month later, though, the Fund's executive director, Dr. Michel Kazatchkine, clarified that the first phase of grants approved in the new round need to be reduced by 10 percent, with a possible 25 percent cut in the second round, because there wasn't enough funding to cover the full amount committed.[19]

The funding cut came at a time of dynamism at the Fund. Kazatchkine, a committed treatment activist and advocate for harm reduction services and human rights for people who use drugs, would oversee a Global Fund "information note" on the importance of comprehensive harm reduction, and creation of a special fund for proposals centered on gay men, transgender individuals, people who use drugs, and other key populations—areas that received less specific attention from PEPFAR.

The global funding pool was an appealing option for a US administration that wanted to move away from primary responsibility for treatment. In March 2009, the United States announced its largest ever pledge of $900 million for 2009.[20] Even so, later that month Kazatchkine announced a $4 billion shortfall. The Fund's communications team took pains to stress that the gap was not caused by the global economic crisis but rather reflected the growth of the program and the expanding demand. Whatever the cause, the effect was the same. The Fund lacked resources, and other government donors like France, Germany, Japan, and Italy didn't ante up.[21]

At the June 2009 Group of Eight summit in Heiligendamm, Germany, Obama joined the leaders of the free world in a tap dance around the "10 million by 2010" AIDS treatment target that had been written into the communiqué from the previous year's summit in Gleneagles, Scotland. The group said that it would spend $60 billion over an unspecified period, cautioning that even this figure was subject to downward revision depending on the economic crisis of the time. "I understand if they think rock stars can't add or subtract, or spell, or read. But some people around here can," Bono told the *New York Times*.

At the International Conference on AIDS and Sexually Transmitted Infections in Africa held that year in Côte d'Ivoire, activists and scientists alike proclaimed, "AIDS is not in recession," and warned that disaster was not just imminent but already underway. AIDS and human rights activist Paula Akugizibwe excoriated African leaders for failing to control corruption and handed out fake bills with African leaders' faces on one side and "Show Us the Money for Health!" on the other. MSF's Dr. Eric Goemaere detailed ways that countries were already scaling back, as ministries and parliaments staffed by technocrats who'd weathered prior shifts in donor priorities began to reduce their overall budgets, buy fewer AIDS drugs, and open fewer slots in nationally run clinics.[22] The South African newspapers carried stories about people anxiously watching their CD4 cell counts, or those of their children, afraid that when the measure of immune health dropped to the level where drugs were recommended, they would once again not be able to get the drugs they needed.[23]

——— ———

"Mzungu," Peace shouted at my back in July 2009. I'd stopped and turned around on the tree-lined walkway just past Mulago Hospital's main gate. The word gets shouted all the time at white people walking around Uganda, but I'd known it was directed at me.

She had a baby in her arms, a diaper bag on her shoulder. She and I were overjoyed to see each other. "Where are you going?" I asked. When she told me that she was going to the same place that I was—down to the new building that housed the pediatric HIV clinic where Cissy worked—I felt a cold, sick sweat on my skin, despite the sun. This baby she held was a client there. *No,* I thought. No. This was not the baby she had been pregnant with when I last saw her.

We walked down to the clinic, and Peace and I sat beside each other. The new building had a central courtyard, a green lawn, a tap, and a square utility sink. Two staff members washed there and played with the spray, making it arc and create rainbows in the sun. Peace buried her lips in her daughter's soft, curly hair, lifting her chin to explain what had happened in her hoarse, low voice.

The pediatric clinic that treated Apollo had come to their small brick house and tested everybody there. They had told Peace that she had HIV. They had tested her infant daughter. At first, they'd said she did not have it; then they'd said that she did. Adam, the first-born son, named after his father, did not have the virus. She handed me her record book. "NB," someone had written, "client denies the results." When she'd learned that she and her daughter were the second and third generations in that brick house to have HIV—both infected after PEPFAR had begun—it had been more than she could believe.

I was seven months pregnant with my first son that day, and I rested my hands on my belly as we spoke, then reached for the baby girl. She was solid, docile, strong. We looked straight ahead while we spoke, through or around the man sitting opposite us who regarded us with undisguised curiosity. A young girl on my right side, whom I did not know, walked her fingers up and down my forearm, pausing on the single thin hairs that grew out of my moles.

Peace no longer lived in the little brick house. She had gone back to the village where her boyfriend Adam lived. She wanted to be close to him, but he had another woman too. She'd stayed with family while she was pregnant, delivering at their compound when it was her time. I asked her whether she'd preferred the home birth or the hospital delivery she'd had with her first child, also named Adam. I was so bound up in the luxuries of my options for delivering my own child in New York City that I actually asked that question. "The hospital," she said flatly. If she'd given birth in the hospital, then the baby might have gotten the drugs that would have prevented her from getting HIV. She was happy, though, that the baby girl was in a research study. She took out a bottle of medication from her bag. She wouldn't open it for me because the top detected each opening. But she said her daughter was doing very well. She herself had not yet started medication. "What about Adam?" I asked. Had the father been tested? Did he know that Peace had HIV? "He didn't know," she said. She'd only asked him how he might feel about testing someday.

The diagnosis was a blow, but it had not defined Peace, who wore red rubber shoes and a red oversized polo shirt with a short skirt on the day we ran into each other. As she navigated this world of clinics and child care, pickup housekeeping jobs, and a boyfriend with a woman on the side, she'd become more independent and self-assured. When I led us on what I thought was a shortcut from the clinic to the road, she followed, then laughed at me when it ended up at a dead end; she'd known all along. She stayed at the little house in the slum when she came to Kampala. When we rode a minibus taxi from the hospital to the stop closest to her home and to my next appointment, she leaned past me and paid both of our fares. She smiled broadly when she said how much her half brother Apollo loved his niece and nephew, coming home from school each day to find out where they were.

— —

"WHEN I STARTED DOING this work, there were activists and doctors, now there are so many accountants," Dr. Alex Coutinho said when I went to see him early one morning, days after I'd run into Peace. He'd moved down Mulago Hill from The AIDS Support Organisation (TASO) to the executive director's office of the Infectious Disease Institute (IDI), a major treatment clinic, laboratory, and health-worker training project. He'd brought the photos of Emma Thompson and UNAIDS staffer Ruben del Prado with him, though both had faded in the past five years; a photo cube held pictures of his children.

The clinic had 10,000 individuals on antiretrovirals, Coutinho said, and not one more. There wasn't enough money to pay for the drugs and the labs, especially the CD4 cell counts, which were used to establish how sick someone was and the extent of a patient's immune recovery. The IDI had funding from PEPFAR and the Global Fund; he was forever fielding questions about why he'd spent money without obtaining approval. That made sense for trainings, he said, but not for lifesaving medications. You couldn't always wait for someone to allow you to order your antiretrovirals. In the midst of donor efforts to manage the "treatment mortgage," many were doubling down on efforts designed to protect existing investments, including stringent controls and audits to try to prevent misuse of resources. This scrutiny turned up problems that needed fixing and that donors could invoke if they wanted to flatline or reduce funding. To Coutinho and other funds recipients, the controls also made it harder to get the work done. "If I come to your house and you offer me a cup of coffee but then every time I am leaving you check my bag to see if I have taken the coffee with me I am going to stop wanting to have coffee with you," he said.

On that trip I asked him, as I asked everyone, what he thought about reports that Uganda's incidence—its rate of new infections—was starting to rise. The country was an outlier among PEPFAR fund recipients in the region, recording more new infections each year rather than less. I had my own theories about this. In my work for AVAC—the AIDS Vaccine Advocacy Coalition had replaced its full name with the acronym as the organization's mandate grew—I collaborated with advocates and policymakers to hold conversations about how the country could incorporate new prevention tools, including voluntary medical male circumcision, which reduced men's risk of acquiring HIV via vaginal sex by upward of 65 percent. One of the studies had been done in Uganda, by the Rakai Health Sciences Program.[24] The single surgery offered lifelong partial protection, akin to a partially effective vaccine. The procedure was never going to be an easy sell due to cultural and gender norms, patriarchy, and adult men's aversion to health settings. But the Ugandan government and policymakers had seemed to stymie efforts to explore the new strategy altogether—accusing the research team of failing to fully inform them about the study. For his part, President Museveni questioned whether the finding was real at all. Conversations about pre-exposure prophylaxis (PrEP), an experimental approach that offered a daily dose of antiretrovirals to HIV-negative people to reduce their risk, hit a similar wall. PrEP would, if effective, be a tool women could use without asking permission or requiring their husband to accept a latex barrier. Even though the results had not arrived, some policymakers opined that such an intervention would increase promiscuity.

Coutinho said he thought the reports of new infections were overstated and that Uganda would go from being "a wayward child" to a "poster child" again. But he was in despair over the state of the crumbling health infrastructure, describing a government facility in Butiaba, in Hoima District, with no running water or electricity, just a pit latrine. A neighborhood pharmacy in New York City had more supplies than that hospital, he said.

Five years prior, our conversations had often centered on the enormous task of creating AIDS treatment services where none had existed. Now he wanted to keep on expanding that work while also seeing broader improvements in the health system. To do that, though, he needed more money for HIV-specific programs and better Ugandan government leadership. The Ministry of Health's National AIDS Control Program was, he said, "moribund and demoralized." He pulled a piece of paper toward him and sketched a power map of the Ugandan health system, including the Uganda AIDS Commission, PEPFAR, the Global Fund, CDC, USAID, various parliamentary committees, and the Ministry of Finance. He put the Ministry of Health and its AIDS control program in a circle in the center and began to lance the sphere with arrows of influence and manipulation. "She needs to be left alone for a year and allowed to really get things done," he said of Dr. Zainab Akol, the head of the AIDS Control Program. "It's very unlikely that that will happen."

Akol was a long-term presence at the Ministry of Health. I'd met her when she was overseeing a cumbersome drug-donation program for Pfizer's antifungal fluconazole while also running all of maternal-child health. At one dialogue on PrEP, she'd held her head in her hands as though she had a migraine and said, before a crowded room, "Our health system is in shambles." Activists reported that she routinely blocked their efforts to prod her program into action. Coutinho rattled off a series of questions to me about who was responsible for this policy or that program. I pointed to different bodies in the diagram. He nodded. No single agency had control. I'd heard the same thing from Mike Strong, the PEPFAR coordinator at the US Embassy, earlier that week. Strong had listed the Ministry of Health, the US government, and a roster of committees. While neither of them said, explicitly, that President Yoweri Kaguta Museveni's increasingly autocratic regime was behind the apparent inertia, I thought the impact was implied.

Things were going differently in Kenya, Uganda's neighbor to the east. On a trip to Nairobi, I took a taxi on a winding ride through the city's comparatively well-paved streets, through stands of dense, urban forest, to Dr. Jono Mermin and Becky Bunnell's home—they'd left Uganda in 2006 and now headed the CDC and PEPFAR programs, respectively. They'd left when they'd reached the seven-year limit placed on postings in a given country. In Uganda, their Makindye home had been filled with cats, children, and friends, their spare bedrooms occupied by sons of a Ugandan friend of Becky's who'd died many years earlier of HIV. Their Nairobi house had vaulted ceilings and seemed echoingly empty by comparison. When I asked if they were bereft over leaving Uganda and all they'd built there, they said they were, both personally and professionally. They also told me that the health system worked better in Kenya.

In Uganda, the country's decrepit national infrastructure meant that most innovative ideas had to be implemented by a "multitude" of nongovernmental partners working with officials. Ideas grew from pilots to full-scale programs slowly. In Kenya, the government hospital and clinic systems were more mature. Coordinating agencies like the Ministry of Health, the National AIDS and STI Control Program, and the National AIDS Control Council were not without their politics and struggles but generally worked in coordination instead of at cross purposes. In Uganda, Mermin and Bunnell and Ministry of Health collaborators had scaled up delivery of the basic care package over the course of years; in Kenya, they'd teamed up with the Ministry of Health and private-sector partners to deliver it quickly. One program alone delivered testing and the package to nearly 50,000 people in one week.[25]

PEPFAR's efficacy was directly related to national governance, whether the money flowed to the public health sector or not. But behind the stacked-brick walls of the US Embassy on Kampala's Ggaba Road, Ambassador Jerry Lanier and his team felt they had little leverage to get the government to improve. In 2009, the country had failed the Millennium Challenge Corporation's "control of corruption" index for the first time in five years—a fact Ambassador Lanier noted in a diplomatic cable titled "Uganda's All-You-Can-Eat Corruption Buffet."[26] Throughout the year, Lanier and staff members Aaron Sampson and John Hoover dispatched dire, often colorfully titled cables back to the US Department of State. One warned of the "ticking time bomb" of Uganda's unchecked birth rate; another tracked Museveni's "toxic brew of ethnicity and oil" as, in the view of embassy staff and other international stakeholders, he allegedly manipulated the assignment of contracts for drilling rights for the newfound black gold.[27]

Matters were no better in health. "We do not feel the Government of Uganda is showing meaningful commitment to health," another cable said. The embassy did not want PEPFAR money for the "partnership framework" that was supposed to transition the country to "sustainability." "Putting more money on the table now, before we work out the conditionalities of framework money, would send entirely the wrong signal to the Government at this time."[28] In August, a whistle-blower complaint prompted a review of the Uganda AIDS Commission for fraudulent practices.[29] The ambassador and chargé d'affaires had, twice that year, told the government that the United States would not continue to bail it out when it faced the drug stockouts that were a routine occurrence, problems that stemmed from mismanagement of the purchase, importation, and release of medications and commodities paid for by the Global Fund grant that was administered by the Ministry of Health.[30]

"The President's autocratic tendencies, as well as Uganda's pervasive corruption, sharpening ethnic tensions, and explosive population growth have eroded Uganda's status as an African success story," the embassy wrote in a "scene-setter" cable for Deputy Secretary of State Johnnie Carson in October 2009 that detailed harassment and intimidation. Up to a dozen journalists and media outlets had been shut down or charged with sedition in the past year; the head of an anticorruption group funded by the Millennium Challenge Corporation "threshold grant" to help Uganda curb its corruption had himself been threatened to the point that he had fled to an undisclosed location.[31]

For the embassy staff, the directive to halt or slow down AIDS treatment in the name of sustainability and local ownership was a welcome opportunity to show the government that its negligence had consequences. In June, around the time that he'd lamented the lack of coordination, Mike Strong publicly stated that PEPFAR would be capping treatment rolls and that the government needed to find its resources to fill the gap.[32] In October 2009, the CDC dispatched a letter to its partners telling them that they could not start new clients on antiretrovirals unless current clients dropped out of care or died.[33]

Countries had ample leeway in interpreting the PEPFAR directive. An ambassador could have held a meeting with those counterparts and worked out a plan to continue to expand treatment that leveraged other resources or simply chosen not to make the move to cap enrollment a public talking point. But in Uganda, the public health program was also a tool for political negotiation. To a US government team utterly fed up with the Ugandan president and his loyalists, the directive to slow down treatment offered the chance to demonstrate that the United States wouldn't keep cutting checks—at least not for AIDS.

The Ugandan military, known as the Uganda People's Defence Force (UPDF), made up more than half of the African Union

Mission in Somalia troops. The UPDF deployed in 2007, putting itself on the front lines of the country's ongoing civil war, whose violence and turbulence threatened the region.[34] The helicopter crash and subsequent loss of American lives chronicled in *Black Hawk Down* had made direct American involvement in the war a political nonstarter. Uganda's troops were an important proxy—and the embassy knew it. The stream of diplomatic cables critiquing the government also noted the "professionalism of the UPDF [that had] made Uganda one of our primary partners in the fight against terrorism." This partnership couldn't be jeopardized. But if the American government's own AIDS program said to reduce treatment rolls, that was an order the embassy could work with.

During a two-and-a-half-hour meeting with Carson, President Museveni was as charming and freewheeling as ever. He averred that the opposition enjoyed ample political space and freedom to organize but were just like "terrorists in Somalia" insofar as they had no political support. Carson then raised the issue of proposed legislation that would make homosexuality a capital offense. This "Kill the Gays" bill was the brainchild of Ugandan political and faith leaders and an evangelical leader named Scott Lively, who described homosexuality as worse than genocide and "the outer edge of sin against God" and who'd first traveled to Uganda in 2002. The proposed bill had alarmed human rights activists in Uganda and around the world. In the meeting with Carson, the president, who'd spent the past several years consolidating his control over the ostensibly independent parliament, claimed he knew nothing about it.

If Carson showed any signs of incredulity, the meeting notes failed to capture it. Instead, he urged openness and transparency in the elections. The Electoral Commission was packed full of cronies from the National Resistance Movement that anchored what Museveni dubbed Uganda's "one-party democracy." Museveni assured Carson that the commission was free, fair, and neutral. At the end of the meeting, Museveni presided over the signing of an agreement for $245 million in non-AIDS-related assistance from USAID.[35]

As much as the White House and the State Department embraced foreign aid and assistance for health as a tool for diplomacy, the Office of the Global AIDS Coordinator hadn't intended for the embassies to use the new flat funding as a diplomatic cudgel. Capping treatment rolls was a way to contain costs, not corral governments. With encouragement from Goosby at OGAC and Birx at CDC, Holmes, Blandford, and Sangrujee were leading work to figure out how programs could treat more people with the same amount of money. The leadership team recruited Tyler Smith, a twenty-something economist to help implement the analysis. He'd spent much of the next two years on the road, living out of a carry-on bag and developing a thick skin as he cajoled country agencies into sharing their cost data. From a thicket of Excel spreadsheets, the CDC-based team extracted an expenditure analysis that showed what different program partners had spent on the same service—testing, treatment, and so on. Figuring out what things had cost in the past could help do more with limited, if not less, money in the future.

Blandford and Holmes put Uganda on the short list of countries where they'd pilot their expenditure-analysis project, then flew out about a week in advance of a planned visit by PEPFAR head Eric Goosby. The team arrived armed with arguments about why PEP-FAR could keep expanding with flat funding and why this made sound sense if you wanted to control the epidemic. Putting people on treatment saved costs for hospitals and stabilized families and communities. More than half of the people in the nation still didn't have access to AIDS medications. They found the reception from the embassy staff lukewarm at best. Charles Holmes remembered showing Lanier's colleagues slides in the embassy's inner, windowless rooms. One day, as he clicked through a presentation, an embassy staffer cut in. "You can show me anything you want," Holmes recalled him saying. "You're just pissing in the wind."[36] As long as PEP-FAR put money into parallel systems, the government had no incentive to fix the system that it still controlled. It was, yet again, a choice between fighting the virus or rooting out the causes of the epidemic. It was, yet again, nearly impossible to do both things at the same time.

— —

IN AUGUST 2009, WHEN I returned to Uganda for the second time in eight weeks—I was intent on spending as much time there as possible before giving birth—I found more signs of strain in the PEP-FAR program. Rubbing my round belly, I slid into a prime seat behind the bus driver for a trip to the Joint Clinical Research Center (JCRC) clinic, where Sister Natalya worked and Simon was a client. I watched for the black-and-white streaks of colobus monkeys in the forests—thinner than they had been even four years prior. I felt the air thin and sweeten when the bus burst out past the trees and into the thick, low, mistletoe-green fields of the tea plantations; then I grinned as it braked in the dust beside the market.

I arrived, as it happened, the day before the meeting of the Adherence Club, a group that hadn't existed when the program began. I was excited to see what this group would talk about, whether they knew of and were worried about the slowdown in treatment initiations, the caps on enrollments, the global donor retreat. Such stories made it onto the radio in local vernaculars. Taata had heard them in the past. Surely they also knew.

The clinic had a new building now—with a large outdoor seating area edged by half-height walls topped with bars painted the bright *kisanja* yellow that was the color of Museveni's campaign to amend the constitution and remain in office for a third term. Hajjarah, the woman running the meeting, had come to the clinic in 2007 to begin an "outreach" program that brought services into the community, helped reduce the time that people had to travel to get their medications, and traced people who had been lost to follow-up.

Hajjarah was a friendly and tenderly vulnerable woman whom I'd met on a previous trip. One day when the staff bathroom was clogged, the ART team used the bathroom in the private ward. To get there they had to pass a patient who had hepatitis B, a disease that can only be transmitted via bodily fluids. Hajjarah was upset all day. She thought everyone should receive the hepatitis B immunization, that the hospital needed to do a better job of infection control.

The meeting participants seemed attuned to her vulnerability. The audience—nearly one hundred people—called out questions. Was she Acholi? A man asked. They'd guessed by looking that she wasn't a local. She was, she said, and offered a smile. The group was preoccupied with its own identity too. Somehow, its constitution had gone missing. Without it, the members said that they could not be sure they were functioning as planned. Each member had contributed a small amount to join—little more than a dollar—but no one could decide what to spend the money on. Everyone agreed that the members of the group needed income and thought that their membership fees should be pooled to help them launch a project that could bolster their house-hold finances, but they could not figure out what to invest in. Perhaps, someone ventured, it should pay for the writing of a new constitution. Before the meeting closed, without any resolution, Hajjarah took a prevention poster off the wall and read its public service message aloud. Below a picture of a fat, smiling woman, the caption read, "Use con-doms every time." "Is she Acholi?" a voice shouted from the crowd.

Ugandan AIDS activism wasn't dead. It was, in fact, thriving. Lillian Mworeko helmed the International Community of Women Living with HIV/AIDS, and at many of the meetings I convened, she rose with her majestic impatience to ask her government health officials why they weren't preparing to deliver PrEP, the strategy that could prevent HIV, as soon as it was available. Her colleague Margaret Happy had a honeyed voice and, often, a head of thin, swinging girlish braids; she was unafraid of anything, delivering blistering assessments of the gov-ernment's Joint Annual AIDS Review, even when her peers—especially those well favored by the government—urged a more measured tone.

But in Fort Portal, it had been Hajjarah, not the people with HIV themselves, who'd created the Adherence Club, defined its purpose, and launched it with a constitution, the search for which seemed to be a way for the people in the group to explore why they'd convened in the first place.

There was more than enough responsibility to go around. Hajjarah was doing what the JCRC had asked her to do. JCRC was, in turn, navigating the demands of American funders and USAID technical advisors, who had taken over from Amy Cunningham and her commitment to "clearing the way" for Mugyenyi's vision. Cunningham had approached the role with humility, never forgetting, as she said, that she "wasn't a doctor."[37] Mugyenyi wasn't so sure his new USAID handlers—none of whom were physicians either—had the same outlook. "You have officers who were never health providers in control of the most complicated worldwide program... having the same monitoring regulations as if you were looking after a bridge," he told me about that time.[38]

The new USAID team had looked at JCRC's organizational and financial structures and decided that Mugyenyi's treatment empire needed technical assistance. A US-based group called Chemonics received a multi-million-dollar contract to evaluate and provide capacity building to a range of "indigenous" partners including JCRC, TASO, and the Inter-religious Council of Uganda. The project was dubbed AIDS Capacity Enhancement (ACE), and it set itself several tasks, including strengthening JCRC's financial management systems. In a 2009 report, ACE said that it had indeed built JCRC's systems—even as it noted ongoing challenges with filling staff vacancies and convening board meetings.[39]

Before ACE was complete, though, USAID decided that it was time to open its ART contract up for competitive bidding. Cunningham and Rob Cunnane had jumped through a number of bureaucratic hoops to make the initial single-source grant to JCRC in 2003; in 2008, though, USAID decided to revert to its usual practices and then swiftly moved to select a new partner to take over from JCRC. It did so before the ACE evaluation published its findings, before a subsequent review of the ACE project found it had been exceptionally ill conceived. "It appears from the beginning that there was an unclear characterization of what the client and the contractor meant by capacity building," the review's authors reported, noting that the project's aims had devolved to "a computer system development enterprise." They'd sought to buy software instead of sitting with the staff, an approach that "prevented ACE staff from thinking about people as the center of capacity building."[40]

By July 2009, when I'd visited the Adherence Club, the new partner had been selected. JCRC, which had had the largest antiretroviral treatment program in Uganda and was led by a physician with immense political capital within and outside the country, would no longer be USAID's partner in providing AIDS drugs. It would continue to do research, but all of the former JCRC clients would now be seen by a new project called SUSTAIN run by University Research Co., LLC, which described itself as "a global company dedicated to improving the quality of health care."[41]

I was not entirely surprised. In 2005, the first year that I visited the clinic, Sister Natalya occasionally handed me reports from the Ministry of Health, which was technically responsible for the hospital and all of its operations, including the JCRC clinic. One report described the dangerous and inadequate conditions of the laboratory—how there was not a separate room or adequate space for blood draws; another on pediatric treatment declared, "With the current ineffectiveness of [the prevention of mother-to-child transmission] program in Uganda, paediatric AIDS will be with us for some time." She received the judgments but little help in addressing the problems. She said the delegation on the pediatric services had spent most of their time up in the administrator's office, as did the Ministry of Health teams sent for "support supervision"—the government term for mentorship and skill building.

Once, my visit coincided with that of a Kampala-based Ugandan AIDS expert, dispatched to help the clinic do a radio spot on its ART offerings. Sister Natalya had said that she'd visited other clinics and had some ideas about what could be done differently. But the clinics she named—while also funded by PEPFAR—were not funded by USAID. "You have to be real," the visitor had chided Sister Natalya, who lifted her handbag into her lap and clutched it against her. "Leave alone Nsambya [Hospital] and anything funded by IDI [the

Infectious Disease Institute]. Those are not the same as here. Here we have to make do with what we have."

Later, I'd find an evaluation by a pair of Ugandan candidates for master's in public health degrees that confirmed what I'd suspected: the entire adherence program was failing, with the "outreaches" gathering just 2 percent of the necessary information on clients' health and progress and moving forward without any strategic plan at all.[42] I'd find another study that set the program's loss-to-follow-up rate at close to 30 percent—three times what was then an acceptable rate of attrition.[43]

As the head of JCRC and an impassioned advocate, Peter Mugyenyi was deeply invested in the success of the program he oversaw. Neither he nor USAID wanted programs that started people on antiretrovirals and then lost track of a third of them. He'd describe the early years of PEPFAR scale-up as "complete anarchy"—with every program that could put people on treatment scrambling to do so. But at the precise moment when the chaos of an emergency response was supposed to transform into country-owned, "sustainable" programs, USAID made the decision that it was easier to find a new partner than to solve the issues with an existing one, even after it had invested more than $1 million in a capacity-building effort to do just that. In 2008, JCRC clients numbered 40,000 adults and 7,600 children—the largest antiretroviral program in the country.[44] Calculating the cost per person of AIDS drugs was challenging; it was harder still to measure the impact of abandoning a Ugandan partner that had immense standing and social capital within the country. There is no sign that anyone even tried.

This was not the only way the world I'd known five years prior had changed. In March 2009, at around the same time that JCRC lost its funding, the Home-Based AIDS Care (HBAC) program, with its bikes and kits, received a letter from the CDC headquarters' Office of Research ordering it to cease all activities immediately. The letter was the end of a months-long series of document reviews and requests for information from the Atlanta-based Institutional Review

Board (IRB), which had taken a keen interest in whether it had reviewed and approved final versions of the study's social and behavioral data collection tools as they evolved.[45]

Mermin and Bunnell had by then left the country, but when I asked people who'd remained in Uganda, some wondered if the investigation wasn't payback for their boundless energy and ambition. None of the Ugandan team, including James Mugeni, could tell me what precisely the accusations or findings had been. (Mermin and Bunnell told me that a subsequent high-level CDC review of the HBAC investigation determined that there had been no ethical violations at all and no justification for closing the study.)[46] Jim Campbell, who'd delivered the news to the HBAC field officers and research counselors, hadn't said any of this, of course. But James Mugeni would always remember what he'd said. "If a child stole a cookie from a jar, you didn't kill them for the crime."[47] He couldn't explain the severity of the injunction.

I knew that if I wanted to, with enough reporting and, for CDC, FOIA-ing of documents, I could eventually understand and explain JCRC's loss of funding and HBAC's precipitous closure. But the specifics seemed less important than the pattern. In both cases, programs designed and implemented by Ugandans and Americans and implemented with American funding were dismantled with little apparent regard for what would be lost as a result. More than a decade after HBAC's closure, the Ugandan CDC staff still winced at what had happened to their program. Peter Mugyenyi retreated to a large hospital he'd built on a hill in Lubowa, his large executive office hung with photographs of himself and President Bush. PEPFAR was uniquely suited to pay for programs that sought to "build the future" but had few safeguards against internal processes that broke trust or dismantled innovation.

When I moved to Uganda in 2004, I intended to write a book about the beginning of PEPFAR—and I'd met people who had a similar sense of wanting to see a historic turning point. "I didn't get to see the Berlin Wall come down, so I came here," a professor on sabbatical from a prestigious US university said to me. But I had missed the chance to write a story focused solely on the beginning, the end of the mass death, the first flush of joy of a return to life. At first my question had been whether this unprecedented public health response would succeed; now I wondered if it would survive as funders' attention wandered, agency personnel turned over and favored efficiency over history, and interest in innovation seemed to give way to an acceptance of mediocrity. I also had to accept that even if I answered all of these questions, I still would never be able to understand precisely why Maama Apollo and Taata had lost their baby or why, in May 2009, Taata himself had died.

Cissy texted me the news when I was in America, close to the end of my first trimester. By the time I ran into Peace and learned about her daughter's HIV, her father had passed away. She hadn't been able to explain why, casting her eyes down and moving on when I asked for details. When I went down to the home with my translator, Maama Apollo hadn't been there to explain either. Instead I heard the story from her elder daughter, who'd recently arrived from the village in which Maama Apollo had left her some years prior. The house had been emptied out, as is traditional when a Ugandan family is in mourning. We pulled a bench across the courtyard and sat by the latrine with its dented metal roof; a hand-painted advertisement for an evangelical church leaned against it. The daughter pulled a loose thread from her dress and tried to work it into a cat's cradle while she spoke.

He had not been feeling well, she said, and all his children had tried to help him. When they'd asked what he wanted, he'd asked, over and over, for beef. He'd once told me that he didn't miss any foods—he'd had whatever he wanted for all those years as a chef. "We can't bring beef today," his children had explained. "Maybe the next day." But the next day he didn't respond at all to his oldest son; he just lay there with his face to the wall. "Did he want chicken?" He'd nodded yes, then rolled over again. Now he's just resting, they'd thought; now he's just asleep. But Stella, the bright-eyed girl who loved to play clapping hand games with me, had gone to rouse him, and he had not woken up at all, not even when Apollo cried, for he was sure that his father was just sleeping.

Now, Apollo followed his mother everywhere. When he asked for chapati money—one hundred shillings—and did not get it, he'd argue back that his father used to give it to him, then ask for Taata to be returned. A line of ducks walked through the oppressive heat; a cloud of flies buzzed around my ankles. Stella wandered into the courtyard. When she used to misbehave, he was the one who always forgave her. "Who will do that now?" she wanted to know.

Taata had been buried in the same home village to which he'd brought his newborn daughter three years prior. A mighty storm swept through on the day of his burial—a great, violent wind that had brought a huge tree down amid the mourners. I imagined it as a vestige of the whirlwind that had once swept mercy into their country, their home, Taata taking leave with an elemental power, or a manifestation of the community's collective grief. It was none of those things, though. The tree had nearly killed Maama Apollo when it fell. It was the weather of a random and capricious world in which some people died and others survived for no apparent reason.

——— ———

PEPFAR in Uganda was a solution to the problem of keeping people with HIV alive when their own government did not care to try. In America, it was a workaround for the enduring ambivalence about foreign aid that made efforts by turns competitive, ineffective, and fragmented. Gary Edson, Jay Lefkowitz, and Senators John Kerry and Bill Frist had all determined that the program needed to live in the State Department to give it stature and ensure impact that they were not convinced USAID could deliver. But even after the program's performance proved the wisdom of this idea, USAID had not abandoned the notion that this effort belonged wholly under its control. A USAID-run PEPFAR would help reinscribe the agency's status and solve the problem of fragmentation posed by the fact that America's most successful aid program sat in the Department of State.

These arguments returned to the fore in November 2009 when USAID finally acquired a leader. Dr. Rajiv Shah was a dynamic young physician and health economist who'd erected ambitious African agriculture and vaccine financing initiatives while at the Bill & Melinda Gates Foundation. Appointed USAID administrator on

November 9, 2009, just days before the earthquake in Haiti, Shah was plunged into the chaos of massive humanitarian relief within his first week. When he looked at the broader US development effort, he saw a system that urgently needed reorganization. "Having seen the way our programs worked on the ground and in country, they just looked incredibly scattered and unorganized to me. And so I believed they should be restructured," he told me. With the full support of the "smart power" administration, he pulled a range of agriculture projects housed in five or six different agencies into a program called "Feed the Future" that had a unified strategic vision, targets, and goals and so managed to bring in more funding than any single project could on its own. Shah credited Feed the Future with catalyzing funding from other countries that saw what the United States had achieved and bought in.[48]

It was a familiar sequence for a country that was incapable of overhauling its aid architecture: aggregate agencies, coordinate actions, repackage a newly ambitious program as an inspiration to other governments. By embracing strategic realignment as a substitute for structural change, the United States dealt with its own dysfunction in much the same way that PEPFAR dealt with a country like Uganda.

Feed the Future was a model for getting "better organized and more result-oriented and more efficient in our operations," Shah said. "I thought we could bring that to our health work and to probably half a dozen other portfolios." He'd come to this conclusion based on the disorganized lay of the land, not because of the agency's grievance over not having been chosen as the home for PEPFAR. "Frankly, I hadn't lived the histories of people and different communities that fought over certain bureaucratic things," he said. "I didn't have a wound."

This put Shah in the distinct minority within his agency. Lois Quam, who arrived in 2012 to head the Global Health Initiative, encountered deep-seated PEPFAR-related angst at the agency. "It was hard for them to move on and have a discussion about [the question] 'Where do we want to go?'" she said. "The discussion would float back to decisions that had been made."[49] Shah wanted to move forward because he'd come in with fresh eyes, but USAID career staff who worked on PEPFAR wanted the program to move under its roof because of the past. These mixed intentions, along with the HIV/AIDS funding reduction and the talking points that suggested AIDS investments were excessive, siloed, and unsustainable, meant that efforts by Shah and USAID-influenced legislators to consolidate global health within USAID looked very much like a threat to the program.

The fact that these efforts had been underway before Shah arrived with his fresh eyes didn't help at all. In August 2009, the House Foreign Affairs Committee released, for comment, a concept paper on completely overhauling foreign aid, starting with the repeal of the 1961 law that created USAID and rebuilding from the ground up. The committee envisioned an aid approach scrubbed clean of earmarks and directives, focused on outcomes and impact, and centered on reducing poverty. It also proposed that USAID play a central role in this brave new world by assuming a "supervisory role" over PEPFAR, chairing the Millennium Challenge Corporation, and taking a seat on the National Security Council. The proposal married heavy lifts like legislative change with revisions of organograms; it came, too, at a moment when USAID had been without a leader for nearly a year, with reported candidate Paul Farmer dropping out after months of negotiation, around the time that the paper was released.[50]

With Gayle Smith at the White House and Hillary Clinton at the State Department, the Obama administration did not lack for savvy, committed development experts. But the fact that each undertook major overhauls while the key posts remained vacant heightened a sense that political goals were also in play. Even after Shah was appointed, Clinton's and Smith's parallel strategic-planning exercises in the development realm raised eyebrows. "State is adamant about retaining oversight of development policy and that the Secretary of State may become personally involved in advocating for that position—motivated in part by a desire to amass as many budget resources under Foggy Bottom's umbrella as possible," one story reported.[51]

Concerned about the true motivation for development overhauls and strategic reorganizations like GHI, AIDS activists argued that PEPFAR—a singular success—ought to be left alone. "Make global health a priority in any revamp of foreign aid. Protect the power and independence of the Office of the US Global AIDS Coordinator. And don't mess with Lantos-Hyde, better known as PEPFAR II," ran a letter signed by the Global Center for Health Policy, Treatment Action Group, RESULTS, and others in late 2009.[52]

Fighting for an independent PEPFAR was part of a broader fight for continued, and expanded, HIV-specific funding. In New York, Sharonann Lynch gathered stories about how AIDS investments were improving other health services and outcomes and packaged them into "Punishing Success?," which had all the hallmarks of MSF's masterly communications shop, starting with the cover image of a woman in one of the Treatment Action Campaign's signature "HIV Positive" T-shirts burying her face in her hands. The subtitle, "Early Signs of a Retreat from HIV/AIDS Care and Treatment," told a reader everything she needed to know.[53] Peter Mugyenyi did a whirlwind lobbying trip in Washington, DC, meeting with Gayle Smith, Physicians for Human Rights, and anyone else who would listen to explain that slowing down treatment would imperil his patients and the program. The ACE report on capacity assistance to JCRC had noted the executive director's frequent travel. In this case—and perhaps others—the US government's own threat to PEPFAR had compelled him to hit the road.

Felix Mwanza, the Zambian AIDS activist who'd gotten the Treatment Advocacy and Literacy Campaign back on its feet, joined a Nairobi meeting convened by Paul Zeitz's Global AIDS Alliance. At the group's request, he dispatched a letter to President Barack Obama explaining the deleterious effects of the funding cuts. And at the International AIDS Conference in Vienna in 2010, activists hounded Emanuel and other US representatives wherever they went, denouncing the US retreat on AIDS.

The work paid off. The *Boston Globe* and the *New York Times* both took the bait and ran prominent stories on the consequences of the scaled-back financing.[54] Within days of the *Times* article, PEPFAR issued a new communiqué to the country teams telling them to continue expansion of ART.

In addition, groups sought to reframe the conversation about sustainability. MSF's Dr. Gorik Ooms teamed up with Paul Zeitz and Brook Baker to popularize a concept of "diagonal" development, a direct rejoinder to the accusation that HIV programs were "vertical," focusing on a single disease. A focus on doing one thing, like treating HIV, could have benefits across the health system. Pharmacists trained to track antiretroviral stocks accurately would apply the same expertise to other medications; centralized laboratories that ran CD4 cell counts and viral loads could provide other services. Prevention of vertical transmission programs, which ran in antenatal clinics, brought infusions of resources and staff to programs with a broader mandate and mission. Tuberculosis was a major cause of mortality across HIV-endemic countries, with stand-alone TB programs often in woeful disrepair. Linking HIV and TB services and improving the quality of both was yet another way to have a knock-on benefit.[55]

Using various figures from international estimates of the per capita funding needed for governments to take over and own health services, including ART, for their citizens, MSF's Ooms demonstrated that no government could do so without additional, reliable infusions of aid. Sustainability wasn't possible without sustained aid. "The conclusion is always the same," he wrote. "More national and international financial commitments to health care are needed, and sustainability—if narrowly defined as independent from international aid—is an illusion."[56]

To maximize diagonal impacts, disease-specific programs needed to be connected to other health services, particularly in the public health sector. The dismal hospital that Coutinho had described in Butiaba wouldn't ever improve its services if AIDS treatment facilities remained in shiny clinics across the road. But the public health sector also had to be invested in the process. In South Africa, Dr. Francois Venter had watched as the PEPFAR-supported treatment program put "more people than [he] thought was humanly possible" on antiretrovirals in the first five years. In 2008, when the directive came to begin transferring patients into public-sector facilities, with a commensurate shift from direct services to technical assistance for government facilities, the effort "ran straight into a wall," Venter said. "We underestimated the institutional lethargy" in the public health system. That lethargy kept government officials taking tea with the hospital administrator instead of working with Sister Natalya to re-design clinic patient-flow and triage systems; it kept Sister Natalya from trying her own innovations or arguing back when yet another expert told her to "be real." On the PEPFAR side, partners that had been paid handsomely to provide ART in parallel clinics sometimes didn't work particularly hard to hand off their patients, since doing so meant a loss of income.[57]

As an effective, disease-specific program that filled in the gaps in weakened health systems, PEPFAR was still relevant in its original form. But that didn't stop USAID from trying to bring about whole-sale change. From 2009 to 2012, the agency kept up a sustained effort to consolidate global health, including PEPFAR, bypassing propo-nents of other approaches and seeking out allies on Capitol Hill, some of whose home states housed major USAID contractors.

Both Quam and Goosby raised flags to allies within the State Department. "We have indications that our colleagues in USAID are shifting the venue for our global health discussions from the inter-agency GHI process led by State to the Congress," Lois Quam wrote in an email to "S" (Secretary of State Clinton) in late 2012, citing a new legislative requirement that the State Department work with USAID to evaluate whether PEPFAR should move into USAID. "It is commonly believed, by key stakeholders, that these reports came at the request of USAID despite USAID's protestations to the contrary."[58]

The following week, Shepherd Smith and fellow Evangelical Kay Warren used their meeting with Clinton to obtain assurances that the program would stay where it was and that the congressional reports requested wouldn't be used to justify a future move. It was an instance of the "strange bedfellows" solidarity around PEPFAR that united queers, anarchists, and conservatives. Clinton loved contraception, women's health, and bodily autonomy. She was not from Smith's party, but she had the power to help protect the program that he believed in.

Shah's bone-deep conviction that things worked better when they were coordinated also didn't wane. In November 2012, he advanced another proposal for consolidation, prompting more concerns at the State Department that the White House might take up his proposition.[59]

Years later, Goosby was still exasperated by the "circuitous, behind-the-scenes" maneuverings. "They tried to do it three separate times," he said of USAID's attempted takeover.[60] While USAID's attempts to move PEPFAR failed, they also drained energy and momentum. Instead of focusing on innovation or expansion, the most organized constituency for global health in the United States poured energy into keeping PEPFAR where it was and explaining why AIDS-specific funding was still needed. "That's what precludes PEPFAR from being the transitional, catalytic program for expansion in all countries that it should be," Goosby said of political jockeying about its agency home.

When I asked Shah about the November 2012 memo to consolidate global health, he didn't recall it specifically, but he did remember what he'd been thinking. "Look, if we can come together, we all care about the same things, and America can elevate its leadership. If we stay fragmented and subdivided, we're both basically allocating limited resources to different subpriorities within health, and we're totally under-optimizing what America's role in the world could be as pandemic threats and infectious diseases become more of a reality in a connected world."[61]

In the coming years, the costs of America's fragmented and politicized inaction in the global health sphere would become excruciatingly obvious, with much attention paid to how the Donald Trump administration failed to fund and therefore weakened Obama's Global Health Security Agenda (GHSA). Launched by a coalition including the World Health Organization and the US government in response to the West African Ebola outbreak in 2014, this "multilateral, multisectoral" initiative sought to unite more than forty countries in work to build efforts to prevent, detect, and respond to infectious disease threats. The United States itself committed to invest more than $1 billion per year over five years to help countries meet GHSA targets.[62]

The GHSA did not seek to build primary health systems or do the kind of foundational health work that the Global Health Initiative had proposed and that PEPFAR and Global Fund investments provided with disease-specific programs. These investments were not explicitly designed to address biodefense, but they inarguably did, by strengthening laboratory infrastructure, putting supplies on the shelves, and training staff in clinics. These simple steps built public trust in the medical system, so that people were more likely to seek services when ill. This improved the chance of diagnosing and treating both familiar ailments and entrenched pandemics, as well as emergent outbreaks.

With its community-led and community-embedded response, the HIV field also had valuable lessons in how to address the stigma, discrimination, rumor, and mistrust that swirled around, and often hampered the response to, new diseases. During the 2014 Ebola outbreak in West Africa, CDC-funded and Bill & Melinda Gates Foundation–funded projects helped contain a Nigerian Ebola outbreak after a Liberian American lawyer named Patrick Oliver Sawyer flew from Liberia and disembarked in Lagos, Nigeria, while gravely ill with the hemorrhagic fever.[63] PEPFAR-funded laboratory and testing resources also helped contain Ebola outbreaks in Uganda in 2007 and 2012.[64] Yet the gulf between AIDS and Ebola was such that infectious disease experts watching Ebola unfold were moved to point out the undervalued lessons the former offered the latter. "Oscar Wilde said that to lose one parent may be regarded as a misfortune, to lose both looks like carelessness. Ignoring insights from HIV/AIDS relevant to other epidemic responses would be more than careless," wrote Dr. Kevin De Cock and Dr. Wafaa El-Sadr.[65] Their warning would go largely unheeded.

By the time the GHSA was launched, the Global Health Initiative had quietly expired via a 2012 blog post on its website, replaced by a new State Department Office of Global Health Diplomacy (OGHD), with PEPFAR head Eric Goosby installed at the helm.[66] Almost immediately, the OGHD encountered the competition for primacy of leadership that had helped derail the initiative it sought to salvage. The Department of Health and Human Services (HHS) had long had an Office of Global Health Affairs; on the day that OGHD was created, Obama's HHS head, Kathleen Sebelius, created a new post, "assistant secretary for global affairs," and appointed veteran health expert Nils Daulaire.[67] A high-level panel at the National Academies of Sciences, Engineering, and Medicine later concluded that the fuzzy mandate and lack of health-specific training for foreign service professionals all meant that "the OGHD has not been as targeted and effective with its efforts as many had hoped."[68]

Overall global health diplomacy work under Obama did, however, notch some successes. Ambassador Jimmy Kolker, who'd helped launch Uganda's PEPFAR program, succeeded Daulaire in the HHS role, where he sought to ensure that rigorously researched, evidence-based American positions featured in diplomatic discussions at the World Health Assembly. "Our ability to be the best informed and most influential delegation has disappeared," Kolker told me in late 2017, less than a year into the Trump administration.[69] "But during the Obama administration, we made a point to be that."

The Trump administration undeniably wreaked lethal havoc. But it also had not inherited a cohesive system. An honest reckoning had to attend both to what had been there to destroy and what had not been created. Neither GHI nor the OGHD were, in and of themselves, a tragic missed opportunity. But there was something tragic in how difficult it was for an administration intent on following the science and investing in global health to unify and expand investments in ongoing and new pandemics, basic public health abroad, and security at home. In failing to figure out how to help others, the country had also lost a chance to help itself.

When I asked Gayle Smith about GHI, she said, "I think it was an attempt to do some things, and I'm glad we attempted it. Bits of it worked, bits didn't, but it was not the driver of policy or the budget." Yet Secretary of State Hillary Clinton had repeatedly called GHI "the next chapter in America's work in health worldwide."[70] The fact that, as Smith rightly stated, it had not driven policy or budget decisions was why that chapter remained unwritten.

Smith also pushed back on the idea that the Obama administration had flat-funded PEPFAR. "I would look at the budget over all of the fiscal years and where we ended up on treatment, and the difference between when we came in and when we left," she told me. "It was a dramatic increase in treatment, and a dramatic increase in funding," she said.[71] PEPFAR funding had hit an all-time high in FY2010 and an all-time low in FY2013. While funding levels climbed back up in subsequent years, US funding for PEPFAR in FY2016 was lower than it had been in FY2009.[72] But Smith was right about the dramatic increase in treatment. It had been the activists who made it happen.

CHAPTER 11

THE END OF AIDS

E MILY, DO YOU SEE who it is?" Sister Natalya asked me when I'd walked down the hall of the otherwise empty Joint Clinical Research Center (JCRC) clinic on February 2, 2011. She stood above a thin, seated young man in a windbreaker whom I didn't recognize. "It's Simon," she declared. "Don't you see?" It was a phrase she used often, a rhetorical question that marked when the world had, in some way, for better or worse, met her expectations. I'd delivered my first son in December 2009 and hadn't been back to the clinic since that August trip when I'd visited the Adherence Club. I hadn't tried to find Simon on that quick trip, but if I had, I would have failed. He had, at some point in 2009, dropped out of care. He had just returned to the clinic that afternoon, Sister Natalya said. It had been two whole years.

I nodded and tried to make the young man sitting on the bench turn into Simon. In the past two years, I'd nearly been undone by sleep deprivation and struggled to find a balance between writing, being a mother, and doing my job. I'd been determined to return to Uganda, though, traveling with our son for the first time when he was ten months old. If I could make the daylong airplane voyage, I'd reach compounds with nannies who fussed over our boy and tied him to their back, guest bedrooms, and meals I didn't have to cook.

On those trips I returned to a place that felt like a second home and to a version of myself I struggled to locate in New York. But the trips were few and far between, and in the intervals, events unspooled in ways I struggled to make sense of. Now I stared hard at this young man.

"Don't you see," she said again and smiled.

"Simon, it's so good to see you," I said. I embraced him, and he felt like bones. He did not look at me; his eyes did not light up, and his slightly scheming grin did not crack his face. He had a small furze of hair on his lip, a denim jacket hanging off his frame, his pants falling down from his waist. He'd come with a groundskeeper from the church where his friend the reverend worked. The clinic was closed, but it was clear he needed care. He had a dry cough and an air of exhaustion. Getting to the clinic was still a struggle for him and so we agreed I would pick him up from the reverend's the next morning.

The next day when we arrived at the office where Hajjarah, the clinic's outreach coordinator, worked, he paused, waiting for me to follow him in. We had scarcely taken our seats before she started lecturing him. "You have dependency syndrome," she'd said. She used the local language, but this she said in English. She held a thin metal spine from a hanging folder in her hand with a scarf wrapped around her fist so that it looked something like a fencer's épée. She sliced the air as she spoke.

"Kids can get a dependency syndrome and not be able to help themselves," she said to me. At the Adherence Club, she'd said that people who weren't taking their drugs should not be members anyway. She had seemed overwhelmed that day. Perhaps that was why she now seemed so very angry. She wanted Simon to know he could not count on me—I'd never provided him with any material support, I protested—or on his friend the reverend, she went on.

"He may get other orphans," she said to Simon. "His money may run out, or he may go away."

"This kid is terrified of people leaving him. No one is giving up on him," I said, and hoped he understood me. "Can we figure out what he wants to do?"

Hajjarah posed the question, and Simon began to talk, a volley of rapid, husky vernacular that sounded at once exasperated and defeated. When he stopped, Hajjarah replied in English. Earlier, he had told her he was eighteen, but now he said he wanted to go back to school—where he hadn't advanced past the equivalent of sixth grade. "Do you want to be like those old people who'd gone back to school when Museveni had finally launched UPE [universal primary education]?" she asked him, then pulled a blue ledger labeled "Nonadherent Clients" over to her. She declared that Simon would sign a contract with her stating that they both agreed he would take his medications.

Simon's next appointment was with the doctor, who spoke with him for some time. He reiterated what Hajjarah had told him, though in kinder tones. You could not always count on people, he said. Benefactors didn't stick around. He said he knew so many people who needed help, who wanted to stay on their medications, unlike Simon. The doctor's face twisted, and his long, slender torso grew stiff as he spoke. It pained him that Simon had squandered so much assistance. He asked him about his favorite football team and where he went to church. Simon spoke in a low rumble of words that I did not understand. The doctor nodded. Then he looked directly at me and said, "There seems to be some mental retardation here."

"How can you tell?" I felt something uncoiling inside of me, a knot of resistance toward something I'd deduced but had not wanted to know and a strange, sad relief at an explanation for why Simon no longer smiled or had canny ideas and hardly spoke at all. In children, HIV races to the brain, causing a range of detectable changes even in kids who take antiretroviral therapy right away. Learning delays, emotional issues, depression, anxiety, fatigue, attention problems—children with HIV in Africa had all manner of challenges compared to their HIV-negative peers, but it was hard to tease out the contributions of the virus versus the conditions they'd grown up in: witnessing the loss of one or both parents, dropping in and out of school, suffering chronic pain.

I could see the face of the boy I'd met six years earlier in this young man, but his personality was utterly changed. I sat there hating how Hajjarah had spoken to him and hating, too, what the doctor had to say, and then hating myself as well, for my sorrow was not only for Simon but for myself. Before I could stop it, a piteous thought crossed my mind. As my trips had grown shorter, I'd become conscious of where I spent each minute and with whom. Now, for an instant, I wondered to myself if I'd made the wrong decision when I decided that Simon would be one of the people I'd follow for the duration of my time writing about AIDS in Uganda.

I banished the thought so quickly I could perhaps omit it in the re-telling of that day and say instead that once the doctor offered his opin-ion, many things made sense: how days and sometimes hours after seeing me, Simon called to find out when I was coming back, how he did not seem to remember our conversations, how he had always moved and spoken with a logic that was unlike any I had ever seen.

But Sister Natalya had asked me to see what was in front of me, and so I did not banish my flash of disappointment. I'd watched American AIDS experts lose patience with this country that had once been the model for responding to the epidemic. I had listened to my fellow citizens declare that treating AIDS in Africa was creating a le-gion of dependents. Politics and economics drove such declarations, but so, perhaps, did some aspect of national character. My self-pitying pique was part of a national reflex.

In the clinic that day, I wondered if Simon could have been hurt by all of the help he had received, as Hajjarah implied. I considered whether the surfeit of fortune that left him with a local Ugandan benefactor and an attentive *mzungu* friend was the reason why he refused to learn a job or endure the barbs of children in order to stay in school. The argument against foreign aid was that it precluded local solutions. If Simon had been like so many other children with HIV who had no one to step in and pay school fees or even simply pay attention to them over a plate of pork, would he have acted differently? It seemed unlikely. The virus had biological, psychological, and social effects—he was living with all of them. The idea that this life would be easier if he had received less atten-tion hardly made sense. But the support also hadn't been sufficient.

What could have been done? What else could *I* have done? I'd begun grappling with those questions in earnest after Peace delivered her baby with HIV and Taata died. When I went to visit Peace and Maama Apollo on trips back with my son, I found the two women at odds. Peace was not Maama Apollo's biological daughter. Each was vexed by the other— her presence in or absence from the house, her contributions to or generosity with the household income. They did not have enough, and living with HIV was not enough to bond them. Peace drifted away, spending more time in the village close to Adam. There, the answer to my question was relatively simple. I looked at Olivia, Maama Apollo's daughter from her first partner, now growing into a young woman. I would pay for her school fees, I announced. I had failed Peace, I thought. I would try again, just like my country—an altruist with the luxury of making mistakes, trying again, losing interest, rebidding the contract, or deciding that a different child needed school fees or help.

But Simon did not need material help. The reverend was a kind, constant, and generous man. He clothed and fed Simon, paid for school fees and supplies. He was patient with Simon's fits of anger. The reverend was the one who explained to me that Simon had once tried to knock down the home of the two cousins who I'd seen taunt him one day on the verandah, that he sometimes even chased this man of the cloth with a knife. Still, the reverend offered him a gardening job, a place to live. There was nothing that Simon needed that I could buy.

"The drugs are confusing my head," he said to me a few days after the visit with Hajjarah. We sat together on the grounds of the church, green hills billowing around us.

"When you are awake or asleep?" I asked. He looked confused.

"Thoughts or dreams?" I tried again.

"Dreams," he said.

"What are the dreams?"

"I don't know."

I left promising him to remain in touch, urging him to take the reverend's help of a simple job. That night he called me and asked when I was coming back, and I explained that it would not be for some time. He called and asked the same thing the next day.

Sister Natalya herself was busy handing over clients to SUSTAIN, the new ART initiative that was setting up its clinic up the hill. "SUSTAIN says it has come to strengthen us, but in fact they have come to weaken us," she and her colleagues quipped, chafing at the extra paperwork.

Country ownership was an antidote to dependency syndrome but only when it suited funder needs. Simon, the nurses, and the countries they came from had not been asked whether they agreed with the diagnosis or the cure.

In early 2011, it seemed quite possible that the years of ambition in fighting AIDS in Africa were over. The pills that had once seemed so miraculous had proved their worth, and their limitations. But there is a peculiar potency in medications, which shift meanings even as their active ingredients remain the same.

Sister Natalya sometimes handed me "Daktarin," the grooved plastic sheet with the chute on one side, and asked me to fill little plastic bags with the chalky white antibiotic Septrin that each client was supposed to take. I was always happy to, though the pills I thought most beautiful—and which were too precious for me to touch—were the antiretrovirals, brightly colored capsules with a glycerin shine. The clinic's generic antiretroviral Efavirenz was pumpkin colored, with a gleam that made me think of magic fables and nursery rhymes. The pills were Jack's magic bean, the riches of the king in his counting house. The box said the hue was Lake Quinoline Yellow, and on long afternoons while Sister Natalya pushed pill packets through the window and shook bottles to see how many pills were inside, my mind wandered, and I made the lake a place in a magic world where the pills did everything one could dream of.[1]

ARVs alone could not help Simon. But a few months after we spoke of his dreams, a game-changing research result showed that the pills had heretofore unknown powers that could help revitalize the dream of defeating AIDS.

— —

IN 2005, A US-FUNDED trial run by the National Institutes of Health HIV Prevention Trials Network (HPTN) called HPTN 052 had begun working in nine countries, ultimately enrolling 1,763 "serodiscordant" couples in which one member of the pair was

HIV-positive and the other HIV-negative. For the purposes of the trial, a couple was a pair who had been having sex at least three times a month for the past three months, with plans to keep having sex and no intention of moving away.[2] Half of the people with HIV would start antiretroviral treatment when their CD4 cells were between 350 and 500; the other half would start when national guidelines indicated: at 250 when the trial began.

As with all prevention trials, both participants were counseled, on every visit, about how to avoid HIV transmission, given condoms, treated for sexually transmitted infections. The investigators knew that some people would still get HIV from their partners, and they wanted to find out if people who were on antiretroviral therapy were less likely to pass on the virus, a phenomenon known as "treatment as prevention."

At each meeting, the data review board looked at rates of HIV infections in both trial arms. After the April 2011 meeting, they'd called the lead investigator, Dr. Mike Cohen, and his team. The rate of transmission between couples where the person with HIV started treatment right away were so much lower than the rate of transmission in couples where the person with HIV was waiting for treatment that it was unethical to continue the study as planned. Everyone in the trial who had HIV needed to be offered antiretrovirals right away—and the world, or at least the people in the world interested in fighting HIV, needed to decide what to do with the incontrovertible proof that antiretroviral treatment was prevention.

It was new evidence for a field suffering from "AIDS malaise." The Barack Obama administration had flat-funded PEPFAR for three consecutive years. In November 2010, the Global Fund's third replenishment round ended with $11.6 billion in pledges and projections—a 20 percent increase over the 2007 round but more than $1 billion short of the most modest need estimate from the "Resource Scenarios 2011–2013" report presented at the preparatory meeting.[3]

PEPFAR had maintained or expanded its treatment rolls, but the program didn't have an overarching target, as it had when George W. Bush launched it in 2003, and some programs, like Uganda's, were still decidedly unambitious about increasing the rate at which people newly diagnosed with HIV started treatment. Ambition and efficiency went hand in hand. As US Global AIDS Ambassador, Dr. Eric Goosby had overseen the switch from air- to sea-based delivery systems and intensified use and purchase of generic medications. Clinics allowed clients to be seen by nurses instead of doctors, and the expenditure-analysis work had helped countries identify ways to save costs based on local approaches. All of this made it possible to do more as funding stayed the same.

But the specter of the treatment mortgage had not dissipated, and the annual toll of new infections remained unchanged between 2009 and 2011. The HPTN 052 data were precisely what was needed to reignite ambition.

Almost immediately, leaders within PEPFAR and in the activist world began looking for ways to use the data to their advantage. Dr. Deborah Birx shot off an email to John Blandford asking him to calculate the number of lives saved and infections averted if the effect seen in the HPTN trial—a 96 percent reduction in the risk of transmission—was applied across PEPFAR programs. Blandford pulled an all-nighter in a Kenya hotel room and came up with a set of figures that he'd use over and over in the coming months.[4]

At the Office of the US Global AIDS Coordinator (OGAC), Ambassador Goosby and Dr. Charles Holmes decided that they wanted to bring the question of how to implement "treatment as prevention" to the PEPFAR Scientific Advisory Board (SAB), an independent group Goosby had established in order to seek and obtain guidance and mandates on precisely these types of issues. The World Health Organization (WHO) would also review the data and update its antiretroviral treatment guidelines accordingly. The most recent version recommended initiating people at a CD4 cell count of 350 or below. The trial suggested that starting people earlier would reduce new cases; the people who started right away also had less tuberculosis and better overall health outcomes, and so it was likely that the WHO would adjust its guidelines. But the WHO could be slow to act; Holmes and Goosby wanted the SAB to weigh in so that PEPFAR could act fast.[5]

The activists, too, saw an opportunity. Ever since Obama's intention vis-à-vis the Global Health Initiative and PEPFAR had become clear, the Northeast Corridor crew of activists had been working on ways to fight back, including amfAR's Chris Collins, Matthew Kavanagh, Paul Zeitz, Sharonann Lynch, and Jennifer Flynn, now the managing director of Health GAP. They were joined, too, by Regan Hofmann, a director at the UNAIDS advocacy office in Washington, DC, and a woman living with HIV; Christine Lubinski, a savvy communications pro working for the Infectious Diseases Society of America; and Leigh Blake, a platinum-haired Brit with working-class roots who'd raised the first real money for the Gay Men's Health Crisis with the star-studded "Red Hot" albums back in the 1980s.

AVAC, the organization I worked for, was also invited. AVAC worked on the full range of so-called primary prevention strategies that reduced risk in HIV-negative people. Voluntary medical male circumcision was one such tool; so were pre-exposure prophylaxis and male and female condoms. The HPTN 052 result offered another prevention tool—people with HIV could prevent the risk of onward transmission if they had access to and were able to take antiretrovirals that reduced their viral load below the limits of detection.

I'd joined AVAC in 2005, on my return from Uganda, at the invitation of its executive director, Mitchell Warren, who'd helped promote the female condom in South Africa and had an infectious enthusiasm about prevention, a topic that had interested me since my days at IAVI. At first, there'd been a clear distinction between my research-focused day job and the writing on AIDS treatment scale-up that I fit in during early mornings and weekends. But as new strategies leaped from trials to public health programs, I'd returned to the activist world that had become, for me, more a social scene than a professional setting. The fight to maintain global coffers like PEPFAR and the Global Fund was now a fight to secure funding for primary prevention along with antiretroviral treatment. HPTN 052 said that treatment was prevention—and so the distance between my advocacy work and reporting life grew even shorter.

Returning to the activist meetings, I found many things unchanged. I recognized the aural mash-up of a high-stakes poker game and a surgical operating theater—the conversation on conference calls still fast-paced, epigrammatic, highly technical, and bound by conventions: everyone said his or her name before speaking, even though most people on the call had known one another for years. "This is Matt, Paul, Sharonann." Conversation went on over a cacophony of clacking keyboards, a volley of suggestions, rejections, restatements, refinements.

On the calls, I marveled once again at the discipline and breadth of expertise of my friends and colleagues. They were tightly focused on figuring out how to parlay the new science into demands that would compel the Obama administration and European governments to reverse the funding retreat and take decisive action. As I had years prior, I felt ill equipped to contribute. I did not know political insiders who could carry messages into the White House—"What about Valerie Jarrett?" someone would say. "Who knows her?"

I also felt ill at ease with the emphasis on treatment, even though I understood the strategy and science behind arguing that the HPTN 052 data represented the chance to reinvigorate the AIDS response. Antiretrovirals were now "treatment as prevention," a remedy with two benefits for the price of one. But the emphasis still seemed to come at the expense of primary prevention for HIV-negative people. Rates of new HIV diagnoses in adolescent girls and young women, people who used drugs, gay men and other men who have sex with men, and transgender women were all persistently high. Worldwide, AIDS programs were better at treating people than preventing new HIV diagnoses.

While I wondered about the trade-offs of arguing, yet again, that AIDS treatment would change the world, some longtime AIDS activists voiced worries that the new finding would be used to valorize long-term heterosexual partnerships like those of the couples who'd been in the study. On the Health GAP listserv, Sean Strub, longtime AIDS activist and founder of *Poz* magazine, wrote back with a lengthy, footnoted analysis of why switching from treatment for people living with HIV for the sake of their health to treatment for the sake of prevention potentially violated that individual's rights to choose when to start treatment. "It astonishes me that so many advocates who have worked so hard to protect the rights of people with HIV, specifically, and to advance a self-empowerment movement more generally, are blind to the very slippery slope represented by this degradation of respect for the rights of individuals and patient autonomy."[6]

The movement had fought for a world where people could have safe, pleasurable sex with partners of their choosing, with minimal risk that they would get HIV, and for assurance that if they did, they would be treated with antiretrovirals and dignity, not stigma and blame. Now donor-imposed scarcity had forced an activist strategy focused primarily on the drugs alone.

It was a painful choice—all of the activists involved knew that pills were not a complete solution for a plague driven by hate that had many ways to kill. In January 2011, on the same trip when I had seen Simon for the first time in two years, Milly Katana and I had driven out of Kampala in her tidy blue Corsa, passing a giant Chinese factory with red and gold lions at its gate and taking a side road that wended through gently rolling green hills. In recent years, Katana had earned a master's in public health and pivoted from being a professional "person living with HIV" to being a public health professional. She didn't see the categories as mutually exclusive, but it was important to her to have the academic credentials increasingly required by the funders paying for the AIDS response.

"We are looking for the person who has died," she'd say, each time she asked for directions, without specifying a name. We were looking for the funeral of David Kato, a leading Ugandan gay rights activist who had recently been murdered. The police claimed that a member of his household staff had bludgeoned the slender man to death— that it was a domestic dispute, a robbery gone wrong.[7] But in the context of the country's homophobia, this strained belief. It was pervasive, frightening. Katana wanted to find the funeral without overtly revealing her destination.

We'd stood that day beside a grave in a crowd thick with white-skinned European and American donors and allies, faces flushed and jaws clenched, some holding giant flower arrangements over their heads for a modicum of shade. By the time we arrived, the condolence message from President Obama had already been read, the mourners had already tackled a clergy member who'd begun to urge homosexuals to repent, and the villagers had refused to bury the activist's body, leaving his comrades to lower the small form, wrapped in a green sheet, into the ground.

Less than a month prior, a visibly nervous Kato had shared the dais with two of Uganda's most ardent homophobes, Ugandan pastor Martin Ssempa and David Bahati, a member of parliament, at a debate over the legislation proposed by the pastor and the parliamentarian. The "Kill the Gays" bill—about which Museveni had averred ignorance in his 2009 meeting with American diplomat Johnnie Carson—called for capital punishment for homosexuals and proposed jailing people who knew gay, lesbian, or transgender people and did not turn them in. While Kato had rebutted their remarks, Bahati had reacted with broad, attention-grabbing expressions; the activist's voice had been nearly inaudible to the assembled crowd.[8]

The climate for LGBT individuals in Uganda had been getting steadily worse since 2002, when a virulently homophobic Evangelical named Scott Lively arrived in the country looking for partners in antigay persecution. As the Ugandan LGBT rights group, Sexual Minorities Uganda (SMUG), laid out in a lawsuit against Lively accusing him of crimes against humanity, the pastor had urged Ugandan faith and political leaders "to arms to fight against an 'evil' and 'genocidal,' 'pedophilic' 'gay movement,' which he likened to the Nazis and Rwandan murderers, ignit[ing] a cultural panic and atmosphere of terror that radically intensified the climate of hatred." Life had been difficult for LGBT Ugandans before Lively arrived, but most had not felt a sense of mortal peril.[9] "For us as a community, we really saw what it means to have imperialism in the present day whereby we [LGBT individuals] are called a foreign import, yet they are using foreign language and culture to discriminate against us," said Richard Lusimbo, a Ugandan gay rights activist and SMUG staff member at the time the lawsuit was filed.[10]

PEPFAR's relationship to LGBT Africans was complex and, to many, deeply unsatisfying. The program did not directly tackle the colonial-era statutes that criminalized sodomy and/or homosexual identity. These laws kept many same-sex-loving people in the countries where PEPFAR operated far from health services and wary about revealing their identities. Nor did the program, with its biomedical bent, have a clear and consistent approach to offering so-called key populations prevention services that were culturally specific and locally endorsed and that addressed multiple needs and priorities, including housing, income, freedom from state-sanctioned violence, and more.[11]

PEPFAR did support prevention and treatment programs for lesbian, gay, and transgender people and other marginalized groups. Ambassador Goosby had, early in his tenure, affirmed the program's commitment to working with and for these groups and had also begun to speak affirmatively of harm reduction to prevent HIV in people who used drugs. In practice, PEPFAR's prevention work with people who used drugs remained unambitious and relatively minimal. With LGBT individuals, there was more tangible work.[12] It also paid for studies that helped quantify the epidemic in gay men and other men who have sex with men (MSM), as public health experts liked to say. One such study in Uganda found a 12 percent HIV prevalence rate among Ugandan MSM—-roughly double that for the general population.[13] Estimating rates of HIV in MSM and other stigmatized or criminalized groups was and remains difficult: people do not disclose identities or behaviors that could get them arrested or abused in a health setting. But the data that did exist all pointed to the same disproportionate rate of infection, driven by many factors, including human rights violations, lack of ready access to condoms and lubricants, and a dearth of HIV prevention and treatment programs tailored for LGBT Africans.[14] People weren't likely to go to clinics if their identities, or the behaviors that put them at risk for HIV, were criminalized.

When it came to the proposed antigay legislation, the United States worked behind the scenes to intervene. The American Embassy staff met with Bahati and his allies prior to the debate to carry the message that notable Evangelical Rick Warren was, like the American government, deeply opposed to the bill.[15] The ambassador sought and obtained assurances from President Yoweri Museveni that he wouldn't sign such a bill into law, and when the legislation kept moving through Parliament, he went back and asked again.

But PEPFAR itself didn't always exercise the kind of proscription it sought from the Ugandan president. It had, for years, given millions of dollars to the Inter-religious Council of Uganda, a group that provided antiretrovirals to thousands of Ugandans while its leaders spoke openly in favor of the homophobic legislation.[16] For Lusimbo, the shift in funding was as much about who lost as who won. "The Bush administration [took] away the resources from people who can do something to impact the community or society and gave [them] to the big groups—the Evangelicals and faith-based organizations who totally changed the conversation."[17]

The US-based activists working to figure out what to do about HPTN 052 knew to their core that homophobia and human rights violations were nearly insurmountable barriers to providing universal treatment access; they knew, too, that every person's experience with antiretroviral medications was unique. They were not, and never had been, naive. They also knew that HIV treatment alone was insufficient to bringing about an "end to AIDS"—a notion that Dr. Anthony Fauci proposed in an influential 2011 editorial in *Science* magazine. "The fact that treatment of HIV-infected adults is also prevention gives us the wherewithal, even in the absence of an effective vaccine, to begin to control and ultimately end the AIDS pandemic."[18]

But "wins" depended on clear asks, targets, and disciplined messaging. Up against the ropes for the past several years, they saw the "treatment as prevention" finding as too much of an opportunity to bypass in the name of nuance. I knew they were right, but I soon dropped off the calls anyway. By the time I left, Sharonann Lynch had dubbed work on increasing non-US contributions to the Global Fund the "Step Up" campaign. The American effort was dubbed "Getting to O."

— —

THE NEXT TIME I encountered Lynch was in July 2011 in Rome at the International AIDS Society's pathogenesis meeting. I arrived with Liam, our son, and our nanny and installed all of us in a yellow-walled apartment off the Piazza del Popolo. I was, as usual, exhausted. But I was also elated. Days before arrival, a trial called Partners PrEP had found that a daily antiretroviral dose reduced HIV risk in both women and men in heterosexual serodiscordant couples.[19] I'd been working in HIV prevention for six years, working for and with women living with and at risk of HIV for that entire time. This was the first evidence of a strategy they could use on their own. If a woman chose to conceal her pills, she would not even need her partner's permission to protect herself from HIV.

I had been dimly aware that the WHO was planning to introduce guidance on serodiscordant couples at the conference and had had a passing thought about how useful it would be if that document also recommended pre-exposure prophylaxis (PrEP). When I encountered Lynch in a plush hotel common area, where every glass-topped table seemed designed to gouge my toddler's head, she told me that the guidance wasn't going to be released after all. I'd exclaimed, "Oh, that's great," or something to that effect. I'd genuinely meant it. Guidelines took time to develop and even more time to implement at the country level. I thought that if PrEP could be added to the serodiscordant couples guideline, a delay of a few months was worth it. Before I'd finished my sentence, Lynch's eyes had narrowed to slits, and I knew that it was not, in fact, great at all.

The serodiscordant couples guideline had, like all other WHO documents, been developed via a formal, independent external review. When the news broke from HPTN 052, the WHO had updated the guidance to include a recommendation that the HIV-positive partner in a couple receive antiretrovirals immediately. It was a huge shift—one that opened doors for immediate policy changes while longer deliberations about what to do with 052 got underway. The emerald-green document had been printed; a Rome event for its release was in the official conference book. But then, at the last moment, the release had been cancelled. The guidance would not be issued. Dr. Gottfried Hirnschall, a beleaguered WHO staffer, explained that the sentence on treating serodiscordant couples had been entered in haste and not subjected to formal review. He told *Science* magazine's Jon Cohen that "key partners" had raised concerns about the process.[20]

At the meeting, rumors swirled that one partner in particular had thrown its weight around. It seemed the Bill & Melinda Gates Foundation (BMGF), a major funder of the World Health Organization, had intervened, calling WHO and urging that the guideline release be delayed. To anyone following the BMGF's public pronouncements and investments over the years, the rumor had the ring of truth. Both Bill and Melinda and the scientists who worked for them had been saying for years that "it was not possible to treat our way out of the epidemic." They usually followed up this statement with an assertion about the importance of primary prevention—that could be used by HIV-negative individuals, particularly women and adolescents, to reduce their risk of acquiring HIV. "I remember discussions between us [BMGF] and WHO about those guidelines," Geoff Garnett, a BMGF deputy director for global health said, arguing that BMGF didn't have "authority" to get the guidelines scrapped. The generous funder had voiced concerns, though. "We probably did say, 'What are you doing producing guidelines based on evidence that hasn't gone through [review] process?'"[21]

AVAC received significant funding from the Bill & Melinda Gates Foundation, as Lynch knew. When I said that it seemed important to consider how PrEP could fit in, given the massive rates of new infection in women, she'd replied that PrEP could hardly be adopted as a panacea or even a large-scale program, given how many people with HIV still needed antiretrovirals. The strategy wasn't intended for universal coverage, I argued back. The frustration I'd felt on the activist calls over the near-exclusive emphasis on treatment began to well up. I had grown accustomed to the ways that primary prevention for people who did not have HIV was relegated to a subheading or a bulleted demand far down on activist agendas. It wasn't that people didn't care, just that the resources were scarce and the politics treacherous.

It was, in a way, ludicrous to demand a biomedical solution like PrEP for a gay man like David Kato, who was both at risk of HIV and unable to survive within the confines of his home. Syringe-exchange and harm-reduction programs hadn't ever been taken to scale in Eastern Europe and Central Asia, where the epidemic was raging. The little blue pill that was a single dose of oral PrEP would never be a panacea for the gaping holes in funding and rights for the community-led solutions people wanted and needed. It was, however, useful for some people. A crucial first step was figuring out who needed PrEP because of their HIV risk—and ensuring that they were able to learn about and perhaps choose to use this strategy. This focus on the small segments of the population who'd take an antiretroviral to avoid getting HIV was wholly different from the principle of universal access that dictated everyone with HIV should be able to take antiretrovirals for treatment. PrEP wouldn't be for all HIV-negative people—but people who were skeptical about its utility sometimes made it seem like its proponents wanted the blue pills proffered to every HIV-negative person on the planet and then used this ludicrous proposition to argue against the strategy. "I wish you'd stop saying that everyone in the world needs PrEP," I said to Lynch. I was standing now, holding a glass of wine that I was about to drain. Liam watched me warily, holding our son on a sofa with a swooping back. "I bet you do," she'd replied. We wouldn't speak to each other again for over a year.

—— ——

TO LIVE WITH A virus or to work within an epidemic is to tack back and forth between the personal and the political. A person gets HIV from an act of proximity, if not intimacy. These individual acts become an epidemic due to forces far beyond individual control. Lynch and I fought then, as we would in the future, because each of us was, in her own way, deeply frightened for reasons that lay beyond us. At that particular moment, she had seen that if the activist movement's slogans did not take hold and their campaigns did not yield wins, then the other side's insidious new logic for supporting global AIDS surely would.

In June 2011, a month before Lynch and I squared off in Rome, the AIDS world's power brokers, including UNAIDS, the World Health Organization, and a predominantly white, male array of public health experts, had rebranded the AIDS response. After two years of talk of treatment mortgages and entitlements, the most visible leaders of the global response offered a rejoinder. The document, "Towards an Improved Investment Approach for an Effective Response to HIV," proposed an approach it dubbed "the investment framework."[22] The document looked supremely scientific. Just as Dr. Anthony Fauci and Dr. Mark Dybul had done nine years prior when they developed the plan for PEPFAR, the Investment Framework Working Group had surveyed the available data on and costs for a whole range of HIV strategies. The group looked at biomedical tools and at the structural interventions that, contrary to Republican fears, build literacy and financial independence, not onanism. It organized all of these tools into a set of core services and "critical enablers" and found a way to put all of these elements into a single graphic that, with its giant oval wrapped around small eggs alongside a rounded square, had the packed density of a text-filled bento box. Its specificity about where and how to spend resources was a tonic after years of rhetoric about and funding for abstinence-until-marriage programs. Antiretroviral treatment was important, as was male circumcision. So, too, were human rights—the need to include, listen to, and improve the health of people who use drugs, men who have sex with men, and transgender people.

The investment framework was well researched, evidence based, and, at the same time, thick with ideology. Like the activists' tight focus on treatment as prevention, the new framing reflected the prevailing conditions of skepticism and scarcity. The AIDS response was no longer a matter of moral duty, global solidarity, or a contribution to national and regional health security. Now, in a shift from "emergency to sustainability," it was an investment, and the funders were savvy businesspeople. HPTN 052 was the hot technological breakthrough. It was time to be a smart investor. If you spent more now in the ways that the authors suggested, you would, over the long term, save money. It was a smart retort to the treatment mortgage, which had already turned donors into investors.

When Lynch and I faced off in Rome, we both knew that the revolution that the anticorporate AIDS-drug-access movement had sought to catalyze would be a long time coming. We'd been left in a world where the individuals and groups paying for the response had license to use language and advance the expectations of capitalist sharks. This included weighing the cost-effectiveness of antiretrovirals for treatment in HIV-positive people against antiretrovirals for prevention as PrEP.

The Bill & Melinda Gates Foundation had paid for the Partners PrEP trial, which had found that a daily AIDS pill reduced the risk of sexual transmission and was scheduled to present its findings for the first time. It had paid, too, for modeling that sought to inform decisions about how PrEP should be used. The foundation's vast resources notwithstanding, it liked to think of itself as paying for innovation, not taking things to scale. This modeling had looked at serodiscordant couples, the same group that had been enrolled in HPTN 052. It asked whether it was more cost-effective to put the HIV-negative partner on PrEP or to put the HIV-positive partner on treatment, whether or not he or she was medically eligible.[23] From an investors' perspective, such a question was perfectly reasonable. But the Rome AIDS conference wasn't a shareholders meeting, and many participants were appalled. "Economics has long been described as the dismal science, but it is hard to think of a more dismal proposition than to delay giving ART to people already infected with the pathogenic HIV virus in order to give the drugs to HIV-negative individuals instead," wrote Dr. Nathan Ford, Lynch's colleague at the Médecins Sans Frontières (MSF) Access to Medicines Campaign.[24]

Yet the dismal science was now the organizing framework for thinking about AIDS. "Every dollar spent is an investment, not an expenditure," a UNAIDS "toolkit" on the investment framework explained to funders. "Investment delivers returns. Returns multiply over time." The framework had helpful questions like "Are you happy with your return on investment to date?" It had warnings too: "If you don't invest fully, you will have to pay more later and keep on paying forever," read one bullet point. Another stated, "Emotional investments do not pay off, nor do investments that are spread too thinly."[25]

When the *Lancet* quoted an unnamed UN official as saying, "AIDS is not an exceptional disease—it is an exceptional opportunity," the metaphor might have seemed to have passed its breaking point. "Integration" with other health services meant you got more bang for your buck.

The *Lancet* article decreed that "the politically astute and charismatic Michel Sidibé," the head of UNAIDS, was in a prime position to guide the AIDS response toward integration, to help investors see the "opportunity."[26] Sidibé did not disappoint. He would, in his speeches, lift up critical issues of human rights for LGBT individuals, harm reduction for people who use drugs, and the crisis of violence against women. "Funding sustainable health care is a moral obligation, a right not a luxury," he'd tell participants at a Vatican conference on AIDS.[27] But five months later, his agency's issue brief carried, in its opening pages, a "return on investment" table that presented infections and deaths as the returns, alongside the cost associated: "12,200,000 infections (US$ 2450 each)." Funding was a moral obligation; investors had a right to see their projected returns.[28]

These investor-oriented documents were notably vague on what the world's major funding source for fighting AIDS should do. The United States was, in 2011, the single largest contributor to the Global Fund and the single largest funder of HIV programs in the world, paying for an estimated two-thirds of the global response. Yet no one had assigned the American people a dollar figure or a treatment target that would place it in the investment vanguard.

Getting the American government to ante up more funds seemed unlikely. But with HPTN 052, getting the government to agree to try to put more people on treatment seemed feasible. "Let's just ask for what we want," DC-based activist Matthew Kavanagh thought. Throughout August 2011, he, Lynch, Paul Zeitz, Leigh Blake, and others worked to figure out a concrete demand. Kavanagh, who had gotten to know John Blandford and Deborah Birx in the context of his

DC work, would from time to time call Blandford and ask for help figuring out just how much treatment PEPFAR's fixed pot of money could buy. Blandford, who couldn't divulge government data, would tell him, "Well, Matt, you know there's a lot of public information. If I were in your position, I'd probably look at this report. You know you probably could back calculate from that."[29] Kavanagh, a whiz with spreadsheets and evidence-based arguments and a tendency to add the interrogative "right?" at the end of his fact-packed sentences, looked at Blandford's sources and worked out a plausible ask. The program could, with no new money, aim to put six million people on antiretrovirals by 2013. Right? This was, as it turned out, almost exactly what the PEPFAR team had concluded. Right.

To meet this goal, PEPFAR would have to double the pace at which it started people on antiretrovirals. But if treatment was also prevention, then some of the prevention dollars that had been locked up in abstinence-only programs could be moved over to this new, evidence-based approach. The Republicans had always loved antiretrovirals; Katy Talento had presciently argued that treatment had preventive benefits way back in 2008.

In late 2011, the Scientific Advisory Board gave its approval for PEPFAR to "embrace" the 052 findings and offer treatment to all individuals with HIV, regardless of CD4 cell count.[30] But even with SAB approval of "treatment as prevention" as a PEPFAR strategy, the program still needed political support. No scientific funding or advisory board could compel the US president to support the new target, and without his endorsement, the critics of the approach, including USAID and a reportedly unchastened Bill & Melinda Gates Foundation, would continue to claim that expanding treatment rolls was a bad, exorbitant idea.[31]

In late August, Leigh Blake delivered the goods. For the past several years, she'd been working with Alicia Keys and the NGO they'd co-founded, Keep a Child Alive. She'd decided that it was time to move on to a new endeavor, though, and had brought Paul Zeitz on to take over her role. Then 052 had happened, and she'd decided that getting this campaign across the finish line would be her last hurrah. She'd written a letter on the issue and gotten it signed by people whom candidate Obama wanted to write him checks for reelection: Morgan Freeman, Queen Latifah, Bono, Keys, and others. When Keys got an invitation to perform at an Obama fund-raising event at the Gotham Club—tickets topped out at $38,500 a head—she and Blake asked for a meeting with the president in the Green Room before Keys went on stage.

Blake had rehearsed the script with Keys and knew what she had to say, but on September 20, she'd been so dazzled by Barack and Michelle Obama that she'd bungled her lines. "You've really fucked up my retirement, Mr. President," she blurted out. "I was supposed to be padding around on terra cotta tiles in my retirement home in Spain," she told him. "Instead I became an American citizen, just so I could vote for you." Obama laughed, said it had been a wise decision, and leaned in for a fist bump.

Blake watched as Alicia Keys—due to perform downstairs in moments—tried to cut through the giggles and get back to point. Her lines were the most important. Would the president scale up treatment, would he support a goal of PEPFAR funding for six million people on antiretrovirals by 2013, would he look at the letter she'd brought, the celebrities. She couldn't let Leigh Blake's giggles overtake the meeting. Finally, Keys handed the president the letter. He looked at it for a few beats. "This looks interesting," he said, as Blake recalls. He told Gayle Smith, the journalist turned development expert working on the National Security Council, to follow it up.

"*Asante sana,*" Blake said to the president at the door. It was "thank you" in Swahili. "*Karibu,*" he replied. Then Keys went downstairs and brought down the house. On stage, the First Lady mused, flirtatiously, that it had been like a date night, and "Who knew what could happen?"[32] Obama bounded up with a twinkle in his eye. Who knew indeed? The activists had gotten to O.[33]

—— ——

WHEN THE PEPFAR HEADQUARTERS shared the proposal that the US government set a new goal of treating six million people with HIV beyond its borders by 2013, Hillary Clinton and her people were interested in what they saw. The year 2011 marked thirty years since the beginning of the American AIDS epidemic—she'd make a speech around World AIDS Day. She asked for OGAC to help provide the text. As they knocked around conceptual framings and ambitious goals, a concept clicked into place. You could take all of the recent scientific findings, put them into practice, and aim for "an AIDS-free generation."

The carefully phrased concept held up to scrutiny: AIDS is the syndrome of medical conditions caused by untreated HIV; it is not the virus itself. A generation is a stratum in the layered structure of society; every generation also comes with a time stamp, including future ones. You could leapfrog over Taata, Peace, and even Apollo and aim for the generation that included Apollo's children to be free of AIDS.

The concept met the criteria of two key groups: OGAC didn't want to say anything it couldn't back up with numbers, and the secretary of state didn't want to give a speech for the sake of talking. Goosby team member Laurie McHugh worked on a draft of the speech, then sent it over to Clinton's speech writing team; they bounced it back and forth, taking care to ensure that the claims held up. Meanwhile John Blandford and Charles Holmes found themselves defending the proposal to USAID staffers who seemed to Blandford to be intent on opposing the expansion, regardless of the data. But the data held up—and swayed the secretary of state. "It was the bottom line that made it real," McHugh recalled.[34]

While Clinton's and Goosby's teams were hammering out the AIDS-free-generation speech, the White House was also getting ready to go public with the provisional commitment that Keys and Blake had secured at the Gotham Club. At a follow-up meeting with Gayle Smith, Paul Zeitz walked through the details, emphasizing that because treatment worked as prevention, PEPFAR could, in theory, move prevention funds into the treatment category without technically depleting the budget. Both conversations incorporated primary prevention, as well, especially voluntary medical male circumcision, as the WHO hadn't yet recommended PrEP.

On November 8, 2011, with her long hair loose, Hillary Clinton took the podium at the National Institutes of Health to commemorate three decades of its work fighting AIDS. America and the world had, she said,

> a historic opportunity . . . to change the course of this pandemic and usher in an AIDS-free generation. Now, by an AIDS-free generation, I mean one where, first, virtually no children are born with the virus; second, as these children become teenagers and adults, they are at far lower risk of becoming infected than they would be today thanks to a wide range of prevention tools; and third, if they do acquire HIV, they have access to treatment that helps prevent them from developing AIDS and passing the virus on to others.[35]

It was technically true, theoretically feasible, and the first time that the United States had laid out a milestone beyond simply showing mercy in its fight against HIV. The AIDS world thrummed with renewed ambition and with the clear emphasis on evidence-based prevention. It was a vision that had been missing for some time.

Activist celebration was heartfelt—Lynch called it the best speech she'd heard on AIDS—and short-lived. The new US proposal lacked a time frame and a budget. Then, not two weeks later, the Geneva-based secretariat of the Global Fund announced that it was cancelling the upcoming "funding round"—the period in which it reviewed and made new grants to countries. The round had opened in August, but country contributions hadn't come in as expected. "We cannot at the moment encourage in good faith an expansion of these programs," Christoph Benn, the Fund's director of external relations, told the media.[36] Dr. Tido von Schoen-Angerer, the MSF executive director who'd been asked by Ezekiel Emanuel to choose between treating diarrhea and treating AIDS, said, "There's a shocking incongruence between both the new HIV science and political promises on one hand, and the funding reality that is now hitting the ground on the other."[37]

There had been warning signs all through September. Michel Sidibé, the head of UNAIDS, had steadfastly demurred when activists asked him to take a prominent role in demanding new, ambitious targets and funding commitments. "It would be wonderful if you and your team are able to identify other countries that might be ready to voice their support for this effort, and then communicate that to the White House," amfAR's Chris Collins wrote to Sidibé on September 23. Health GAP staffer Asia Russell had also reached out, just prior to a trip to Africa. "Would it make sense to raise this with leaders in South Africa while you are there this week? It might be a very useful opportunity."[38]

None of this triggered action. The investment framework quantified the surge in resources required for low and lower middle-income countries—a jump from roughly $16 billion per year in 2011 to at least $22 billion by 2015. But every activist knew an ask without a target wasn't a real ask. They wanted Sidibé to be clear and specific—to use his stature to urge countries to ante up. But he did not. Instead, the Global Fund adopted a new, more regulated approach to grant making, unveiled in a report titled "Turning the Page from Emergency to Sustainability," reflecting the findings of a high-level committee convened to address concerns about financial management and fiduciary responsibility.[39] The committee had, however, expanded the mandate of its review from management to underlying mission, as Asia Russell, who'd mastered the intricacies of the Fund, noted with alarm, writing that it "should have looked at a narrow set of governance and audit questions, but its members leveraged the environment of crisis . . . [to promote] the idea that the three diseases were no longer 'emergencies', and that it was time to abandon core tenets of the Global Fund's approach, such as allowing countries themselves to request funding based on what they actually needed rather than on what donors agreed to provide."[40]

Indeed, the report stated that the Fund had, in its early years, a culture of "treatment at any cost." The notion of "country ownership" had covered for all manner of ineffective activities. Now the costs had to be brought under control and country ownership linked to accountability. To this end, the report proposed—and the Fund adopted—a "New Funding Model" in which countries were told that their funding "envelope" required them to explicitly state how the grants would be spent and which strategies and programs would be prioritized. The past years of "blue sky" proposals, which could be fully funded or rejected, hadn't provided enough stability; country ownership hadn't always led to strategic, grassroots-endorsed action. Countries had hired consultants to write the proposals; governments had come to see the shining star of "the new multilaterals" as donors like any others.

Like the investment framework, the New Funding Model had elements of strength. It called for greater strategy and specificity, an emphasis on human rights, transparency, and greater inclusion of the people most affected by HIV. These shifts reflected lessons learned; they had the potential to make a difference, but their rationale—improving efficiency, moving to sustainability, shifting to a world where, rates of infection and AIDS deaths notwithstanding, HIV was not an emergency—undercut the principles.

"UNAIDS is bullshit useless. That is my assessment," Lynch wrote one day in the midst of the "running file" where she tracked every meeting, email, and personal communication on her campaigns. An activist had reported back on a UNAIDS meeting. "I said over and over and over that they need to be MAKING MOMENTUM HAPPEN not waiting for it to happen, but it seems not to have taken root."[41] Without UNAIDS pushing countries to step up, many demurred. When activists queried UK development officials, they heard that the country would consider a big commitment but wanted to hear what the United States had to say first.

But when the United States did speak, there was no new money involved. On December 1, 2011, President Barack Obama stood on a George Washington University stage and announced that PEPFAR would put six million people on antiretrovirals by 2013. This was a doubling of the rate of treatment initiation—and an ambitious target that came with no new money. It was the beginning of PEPFAR's new reality, one governed by and responsive to the tools of twenty-first-century corporate management—data, spreadsheets, performance trackers, impact evaluations. From 2010 on—as flat funding became the norm—it became the program that boasted, year after year, about how it did more with the same amount of resources by finding efficiencies, a factory for saving human lives that upgraded every year. After a 2013 peak in spending, global investments would level out—never reaching the $22 billion milestone set for 2015. Presented with abundant scientific evidence and a clear timeframe for action, governments and other funders chose not to pursue epidemic control. The people who bore the brunt of this failure of imagination were individuals like Simon, who struggled to make sense of the world, or comrades of David Kato, who risked death by naming their identities. An HIV response focused on efficiency could not be relied on to pay for approaches that encompassed both medication and stigma, mental health and social conditions, even though Simon, David, and many others needed such offerings to thrive.

President Obama stood with Bono and Alicia Keys on stage. Paul Zeitz, Matt Kavanagh, Sharonann Lynch, and Leigh Blake were spectators. Kavanagh made a point of choosing a chair close to Eric Goosby, figuring correctly that the president would stop to greet him. "Mr. President," he said, "Thank you so much. A year ago, we were protesting you, now we're here celebrating you. We really thank you for your leadership."

As Kavanagh recalled, Barack Obama pulled his hand away from Kavanagh's grasp, stepped away, then rocked back on his heel and pointed a finger. "You shouldn't have been protesting."

"Mr. President—" Kavanagh was delighted that the protests had registered with the president. If Obama had professed not to know about them, then Kavanagh wouldn't have been succeeding at his job. "We appreciate what you're doing now, but at the time..."

The president cut him off. "You shouldn't have been protesting. That's not why I did this." Then he walked away.[42]

When it came to the domestic AIDS epidemic, President Barack Obama would prove far more of an active champion, with the Affordable Care Act providing pathways for Americans with HIV to obtain coverage where they had previously struggled, since insurers classified the virus, along with cancer, asthma, and other health issues, as a preexisting condition. Prior to the ACA, these conditions impacted eligibility for and the cost of coverage. The Obama administration also cleared the waiting lists for the AIDS Drug Assistance Program that subsidized payment for antiretrovirals for people living with HIV and launched the first-ever National HIV/AIDS Strategy, which provided a long-overdue national approach to the entrenched epidemic.[43]

Yet Leigh Blake had reason to weep, as she did, on the train home from the 2011 World AIDS Day event. She was heartbroken about the absence of the activists on the stage. She and her fellow travelers had worked hard to secure the new commitment and deserved a spotlight on their work. The arms-length distance continued after that night—with the president taking positive steps, keeping the program alive, but doing little else to bring the plague war and the potent activist movement that was ready to fight for so many of his principles closer to the fold.

In 2012, when the International AIDS Conference came to Washington, DC, for the first time in decades, the president declined to attend, even though he himself had made it possible by lifting long-standing restrictions on entry into the United States by people living with HIV with non-US passports. The following year, in December 2013, he'd sign the PEPFAR Stewardship and Oversight Act of 2013, which reauthorized the program for another five years. Unlike the 2008 reauthorization, which brought significant changes to the prior law, the 2013 version was largely a "cut-and-paste" continuation of the past bill. Lawmakers on Capitol Hill once again hailed the program's remarkable progress; Obama signed it into law in his office with little fanfare. Going into the 2013 fiscal year, he requested $4.5 billion for the program—an 11 percent decrease from FY2012.[44]

At the end of that same year, PEPFAR reported that it had, in spite of flat funding, exceeded the 6 million treatment target, reaching a cumulative total of 6.7 million people on antiretrovirals as a result of PEPFAR support. This was a fourfold increase from the figure at the start of the Obama administration. PEPFAR also reported that it had come close to reaching the cumulative target of 4.7 million voluntary medical male circumcisions. Launched at the same time as the 6 by '13 goal, the target of 4.7 million voluntary medical male circumcisions didn't make it into Obama's speech, a sign perhaps of a perennial aversion to a public emphasis on this sensitive but highly effective preventive procedure, for which PEPFAR was the primary source of funding.[45]

By the end of 2013, the program had proved that it could survive and perform in the absence of a hands-on advocate in the Oval Office. But both PEPFAR and the broader AIDS response, including the Global Fund and UNAIDS, had taken a risk. Successfully rebranded, the global AIDS pandemic response had survived in no small part because it had promised it would bring the need for such large investments to an end. As promising as "treatment as prevention" was, and as persuasive as the models were, this outcome wasn't guaranteed. Still, investors had been told what they wanted to hear. Now it was up to the architects of the response to deliver.

CHAPTER 12

MADAM AMBASSADOR

N o one knows that story," Dr. Deborah Birx, retired colonel in the US Army and head of the Global AIDS Program of the Centers for Disease Control and Prevention (CDC), said to Secretary of State John Kerry moments before he swore her in as the next head of PEPFAR. As the crowd laughed, he swiveled toward her and raised his palm, then dropped it into hers in an awkward high five. "I've got news for you," he said, turning back to the crowd and wagging a finger. "They're about to."

Around me, the people packed into the Benjamin Franklin Room at the State Department laughed again. I watched her hold her hands loose and dutiful, like the churchgoer she was and always had been, as he explained how she had lost a lot of blood during the birth of her first daughter and her obstetrician had ordered a transfusion. Birx had read a report on a new blood-borne virus, though, and so, Kerry explained, "literally, just before she passed out from pain, Debbi screamed: 'Do not let them give me blood.'" Around me, the crowd chuckled once more. It turned out she could have received HIV-contaminated blood that day, Kerry said. That was why she had such a personal connection to AIDS.[1]

I had not yet begun to interview people about Birx, having conversations in which assessments of her acumen often veered into stories about the emotions she evoked or displayed—making this person cry, giving that person nightmares, offering public dressing-downs. It would be three years before I'd be glutted with such tales, offered freely and confidentially in the interstices of interviews. Even so, that day I thought that some of the laughter at the screaming scientist—from people who had, moments before, been taking selfies with their cameras aimed toward the stage—was knowing. As Kerry offered this story about her personal connection to AIDS, the most relevant link wasn't the transfusion but her gender. He laid her laboring body on a gurney for all of us to see. Even with her medical degree and her list of credentials, she lived in a world that would never let her forget the body she was born in.

—— ——

At first, Birx hadn't wanted to lead PEPFAR at all. Sandy Thurman, Bill Clinton's AIDS czar, had talked her into it. They'd met years prior when Birx, then in the military, was invited to Thurman's office to talk about Clinton's LIFE initiative. Thurman ran late. Alone in her well-appointed office, Birx, looking at the refined furniture, decided not to take a seat. She ended up waiting for an hour. "I just stood there in my uniform, not sitting down. Because I was like, 'That's an antique, I can't sit there and wait for this person.'"[2] When Thurman finally arrived and Birx did sit down, the two found they had more in common than an appreciation for fine, old furniture. In their markedly different ways—"I'm more Southern," Thurman would say—they both had little patience for complacency in the face of AIDS. After their initial meeting, they became fast friends and frequent collaborators. In 2013, Thurman was back in Atlanta, when she told Birx it was time for her to throw her hat into the ring for US global AIDS coordinator. Birx responded that Thurman herself was the one for the job. She had a velvet glove for every occasion. But Thurman's sense of strategy was greater than her ego. She had a solid enough sense of her own value that she played the role that was needed, not the one with the greatest visibility. She did the flowers for weddings and made sure that, when needed, official functions had enough "lubrication" to make the event congenial—and therefore conducive to building relationships—even if it meant paying for it herself. She kept her eye on the prize and, when called for, shone behind the scenes.[3]

Thurman wanted Birx to become the next head of PEPFAR because of how she worked: hard, humbly, through the weekend and overnight. If Birx asked for an analysis, and a team said they couldn't do it, Birx did it herself, often with her assistant, Angeli Achrekar. Birx had found Achrekar like Thurman had found Birx, by homing in on the quality of her work on a CDC PEPFAR country team that had, after Achrekar's arrival, started to submit reports that were strong and clean. Birx had plucked Achrekar up and brought her to work by her side. "I always look for amazing women who don't know how amazing they actually are," she told me.[4]

Thurman was paying more attention to the program's bottom line than the boosterism about ending AIDS. When Eric Goosby left the position in late 2013, he'd staved off multiple USAID takeover attempts and led the team that helped craft and launch the AIDS-free-generation strategy. Under his leadership, a flat-funded program found cost savings and efficiencies that allowed it to not only meet but exceed the "6 by '13" target. He and his team also established the Scientific Advisory Board and ushered in an era of inclusive language on women's sexual and reproductive health and rights, harm reduction, and prevention for so-called key populations, including gay men, transgender men and women, and sex workers. He'd also run an office that many staff members recalled as exceptionally warm and friendly—right down to the red Muppet named "Nomo" awarded weekly to someone who deserved recognition.[5]

But for all these successes, Goosby and his team had not been able to address enduring challenges with tracking PEPFAR agency spending at the level of the partners who provided services on the ground. At least part of the problem sat with the way that USAID awarded and tracked money within global health, beyond PEPFAR funds, Goosby's deputy director Julia Martin explained to me. (These funds included money from the President's Malaria Initiative, a Bush-era,

USAID-run effort that also notched considerable success.) The agency created centralized "mechanisms" at the headquarters level that a USAID country program could "buy into"—essentially using some of its country-level funds to pay for the services from partners who'd gotten the centralized funds. Not only did this keep USAID funds in the coffers of the predominantly US-based groups that ran centralized projects, but it also meant that these mechanisms sometimes pooled PEPFAR and non-PEPFAR money. That, and the fact that delays in spending funds could sometimes cross fiscal years, made it hard for the PEPFAR headquarters staff to get a clear picture of centralized PEPFAR funds that were unspent or that had been committed or obligated for specific country activities but not expended.

Tracking how much PEPFAR money was left in a given mechanism was challenging, to say the least. The CDC did not have an equivalent for "obligating" funds; it also had far less experience and grant-making infrastructure than USAID, and so experienced its own challenges. By the time Goosby stepped down in late 2013, the problems with this system had come home to roost.

The problem became public on April 12, 2012, when crack science reporter John Donnelly broke the news that the program had $1.5 billion in unspent "pipeline" funds.[6] All government programs carried some money in reserve as a buffer against the vicissitudes of appropriations, economic fluctuation, and contracting delays. But this pipeline was twice as big as what would be expected for a program like PEPFAR. When the story broke, activists who'd argued that flat funding hurt the AIDS response lost a talking point overnight—why expand the global envelope when there was so much money sitting in reserve? Goosby was honest about how hard it was for the program to track funding. "To be frank, all of that raised the question of how much money is in each country, and where's the money? Our ability to understand that is quite complicated," he told Donnelly, explaining that the Office of the US Global AIDS Coordinator (OGAC) had to "force" agencies like the CDC and USAID to explain "what they are doing as the money moved down to programs."[7] PEPFAR had defined itself by its ability to manage aid better than any American effort in history. Now it looked an awful lot like its fumbling, inefficient predecessors.

From the outside looking in, the program had a clear mission and the proven ability to meet ambitious targets with limited funding. But at least some of that ambition had been realized by the intentional use of agency pipeline funds that had accumulated over multiple years, well above the threshold of what groups needed as a buffer for unanticipated events. Those excess pipeline funds helped bump up yearly budgets that would drop back down when the pipeline ran out. To continue expanding the treatment rolls, the next head of PEPFAR needed to solve the problem of figuring out what was being spent where, by whom, and for what with even more specificity than the program had sought in the past.

Birx loved data—she always had. It helped her get control of a situation or a problem and control the way people saw her. She'd brought hundreds of slides to the Bush-era AIDS czar Dr. Joe O'Neill to explain why the Department of Defense had to get in on PEPFAR's ground floor, because she brought hundreds of slides to everything.[8] She'd had to work twice as hard for as long as she could remember. "I came out of the hard sciences and there were just no women. It was a horrible place," she told me one day. "I was downgraded for a better performance all the time. If there was an honors project, I got the B-plus, the guy got the A."[9]

Data helped to show the world as it was, not as people wanted it to be. In the years that Birx ran the CDC's Global AIDS Program, she'd seconded John Blandford and Nalinee Sangrujee to PEPFAR's DC headquarters to do the cost-effectiveness study and expenditure-analysis work that started to shed light on where the waste was in the system and how the program could do more with the same amount of funds.

Leading PEPFAR would give Birx exponentially more control over how data were gathered and used to make decisions. She acceded to Thurman's suggestion that she throw her hat into the ring and then followed Thurman's lead as she; Cornelius Baker, a Black, gay, HIV-positive AIDS advocate and health expert; and a core group of DC activists launched a campaign to secure the position. Thurman made the people she believed in family. Growing up, her mother had cajoled her and corrected her and loved her into ladyhood with the nickname "Missy." Thurman had other nicknames for Birx, including "Birxy" and "Madam," but Missy was the one she used most of the time.[10]

The first problem Thurman and Baker tackled was that it didn't seem like Birx was the White House pick. There wasn't a formal process for selecting the next PEPFAR head; the position remained a presidential appointment, subject to congressional approval, as it had been the day that George W. Bush put Randall Tobias beside him in the Oval Office. But the short list was an open secret. Dr. Nils Daulaire, head of the Global Health Council and a close friend of fellow Vermonter Senator Patrick Leahy, was by many accounts the White House favorite. Dr. Chip Lyons, head of the Elizabeth Glaser Pediatric AIDS Foundation, was also on the list, as was Jen Kates, an incisive leader at the Kaiser Family Foundation. Kates, in particular, was a savvy, deservedly admired activist ally. Daulaire, on the other hand, had steadfastly taken a conservative stance on drug company profits and patent law. He simply couldn't be put in charge. As one activist would tell me later, as much as anything, the consensus was that "it couldn't be Nils."

Everyone loved Kates, but she wasn't a physician or a researcher. The last battle for AIDS funding and targets had been won by scientific argument; the activists needed another medical professional in the game. They also appreciated Birx's ability and willingness to play the inside-outside game, sharing information. As an activist accustomed to being shown the door at critical moments, Paul Zeitz had been impressed by her willingness to work with him and his allies. He'd met her at a key meeting related to HPTN 052 guidelines. While she was in the room, she kept the activists outside apprised of what was going on. "She was texting us, 'This one is not with us.' . . . Someone who knows how to do that is brilliant. We knew as a movement we would have access to her, she was sophisticated—she knew that's what you're supposed to do in a powerful government position," he said.[11]

Thurman and Baker organized a listening tour for Birx, holding dinner parties, making phone calls, letting folks know it was okay to support her, that it wasn't betraying Kates to back Birx. Birx's boyfriend, Paige Reffe, helped too. A former Clinton advance man, Reffe would sit at the long table when the activists and the campaign team came to their home in DC's quiet, leafy Cleveland Park neighborhood to weigh in on strategy. He figured she needed to pull out all the stops.

When Reffe realized Birx would be on a plane to brief President Bush on the CDC's work on his postpresidency "Pink Ribbon Red Ribbon" initiative, focused on cervical cancer and HIV, he told her she had to ask him to put in a good word for her at a wreath-laying in Tanzania where he'd overlap with President Barack Obama for a day. She balked—then followed through. She'd waited until the end of her briefing, then set down her papers and made her ask—a bold, personal move that left the room in shocked silence. The former president grinned. "Let me get this straight, Debbi, you want me to bend down with the wreath and whisper, 'Pick Deb?'" She did, and he agreed, Birx reported to Reffe. "Let me get this straight," Reffe countered. "He called you Deb?" He was amazed, though not surprised, at the degree of affection his partner elicited from some of the world's most powerful men.[12]

The former president did weigh in in her favor, as did President Jimmy Carter and a range of other high-powered activists who succeeded in their goal of making Birx seem not "impossible" but "inevitable." After her nomination was announced in March 2014, the White House personnel office staff told Paul Zeitz they'd never seen that kind of mobilization for a candidate for a comparable position.[13]

It was a level of effort that matched, and underscored, the power of the person at PEPFAR's helm. Every USAID administrator put his or her stamp on the agency with a catchy phrase for its direction, one or more signature initiatives. But it was hidebound, earmarked, and stuck on a mid-level rung of the political decision-making hierarchy. No slogan or innovation lab could ever change that. By contrast, PEPFAR had been designed to protect its leader's autonomy—the direct line to the White House, the anomalous placement in the State Department, and the ambassador-level position all enshrined in the authorizing law.

Birx might have demurred at Thurman's initial overture, but by the time she secured the nomination, she and Achrekar had a master plan that they planned to roll out over the first twelve to eighteen months on the job. The pair told me that all changed in early 2014, when they flew to Washington, DC, for a briefing on the program's finances before Birx's confirmation and realized that they'd need to accelerate—or abandon ship.

—— ——

"MOTHERFUCK IT," BIRX SAID to Achrekar in a State Department bathroom in March 2014.

"You don't have to do this," Achrekar replied.

Moments earlier, they'd both excused themselves from a detailed budget briefing Birx had requested from the current PEPFAR team. They'd had one budget update, but it hadn't been sufficiently detailed, so they'd flown up with the dark chocolate they brought to sweeten the moods in their marathon meetings and sat down for another briefing. When they'd seen the details, they'd walked out of the room.

Birx and Achrekar said that the reports they saw showed that the program's current rate of expenditure was going to send it over a fiscal cliff. PEPFAR was about halfway through its financial year, with $3.9 billion left to spend. But the burn rate for the first two quarters put the program on track to spend $4.3 billion by the end of the year— and the difference was money the program didn't have. They recalled that Julia Martin had been part of the meeting. When I asked her about it, she said she didn't recall the specific event but agreed that some of the pipeline funds had been put into recurrent costs, particularly for treatment scale-up. "In 2014, the concern was, when that pipeline has been used...how do we continue with the program at this heightened level of expenditure?" she told me. "That was a completely reasonable question and something to plan against."[14] (Goosby, who'd left OGAC by that point, said he'd had no way of getting a clear picture of that time. "The culture wasn't one where I'd get a phone call saying, 'Hey, let me run this by you.'")[15]

Birx, Achrekar, and Thurman all said that it was clear the program wasn't only going to overspend in FY2014; it was also on track to be overbudget in FY2015, based on the country plans that had already been approved.

"Debbi, look, you're not confirmed yet, we can walk," Achrekar said in the State Department bathroom. They both knew that they'd do no such thing. To turn the program around, they'd need to introduce, in a matter of months, a series of changes that would have been unpopular if they'd been phased in over a matter of years; they'd have to take on the implementing partners and USAID. No amount of chocolate would sweeten the conditions they'd impose. They would also need to be sure that Secretary of State John Kerry and his deputy, Heather Higginbottom, knew the changes that were coming. They knew that even though they functioned as a unit—they liked to say they shared a brain—the world didn't see them this way. "We knew," Birx said later, "that they would accuse me of everything."[16]

Birx, Achrekar, and Thurman arrived at the PEPFAR offices in Washington, DC, on roughly the same day in the spring of 2014. As Thurman had once recruited Birx, Birx now returned the favor, asking Thurman to join her team as the chief strategy officer. Right away, they began implementing their plan. All of the country teams had already had their country operational plans (COPs) approved by the acting PEPFAR coordinator who'd stepped in after Goosby's departure. The country ambassadors had signed off and communicated the commitments to their government counterparts.

Birx told me that she warned Secretary of State Kerry that she was going to make a lot of people unhappy—and then she did, cabling each country to tell them that their plans were not approved and that they'd have to come to Washington, DC, for a planning meeting at the Madison Hotel. When they arrived in May 2014, each country team was assigned to a room, with a member of the headquarters staff designated as the chair. Over the course of nearly a week, the chair walked the teams through a detailed survey of what PEPFAR was paying for and how this related to the country's epidemic. At that meeting, the country teams learned that every plan now needed to be based on data from sites and the subnational units (SNUs) that made up every country—states in the United States, districts in Uganda, provinces in South Africa. Per Birx's instructions, the country teams had to explain how many people were testing positive at every site, how many people were receiving antiretroviral treatment at each site, and how much HIV there was in any given SNU. The money would follow the epidemic, not prior patterns. If PEPFAR was paying for a program in a place where there had been one or two HIV-positive diagnoses in the previous year, it had to stop. USAID and CDC, which had never before been required to share programmatic data with each other, now had to account for their numbers.

As the chair of the Kenya review, Thurman realized that hundreds of PEPFAR-funded sites were not seeing any people with HIV at all. Julia Martin guided the Zambia team through the Birx-mandated process. She helped staff comb emails and contact colleagues back in country to find proxies for the data they lacked, swapping in HIV among pregnant women for overall prevalence, for example. She helped them figure out which sites and subnational units needed more resources and where thresholds of incidence or prevalence indicated that PEPFAR should withdraw its funding. This process was called "geographic prioritization."

In the Zambia room, when the exercise was over, the CDC director rose to address Martin and the assembled room. He said that people would die as a result of the decisions the team had been forced to make. This was not what the country wanted, he warned. Women would not get services in the rural vertical transmission programs PEPFAR planned to leave. They would pass HIV to their babies, who would also die.

Martin worked to remain composed. "I got emotional. It was excruciating, and I felt responsible," she told me. "Not for people dying," she explained, but the feeling of responsibility that you get when you've lived and worked in a place. I'd met her in 2004 when she was one of the original staff members at the Infectious Disease Institute in Kampala. "I worked in Uganda for nearly five years, unpacking boxes, putting together formularies, giving out drugs, going to funerals." Martin knew what it meant to be loyal to an institution and embedded in a country. She also completely supported the work of getting country teams to prioritize specific geographies—a strategic shift known within PEPFAR as "the pivot." "I felt that what we had been asked to lead was right. I still do to this day," she said.

As Thurman watched the process unfold, she knew that her decision to back Birx had been the right one. "No one would have had either the intellect or the intestinal fortitude to move as fast as she did," she said. She'd watched Birx make decisions that angered not only the agencies and the country staff but ambassadors and country government officials, many of whom had urged PEPFAR to invest in geographies with low HIV as a way to deal with other health issues facing their constituencies. "Very few people who have come into public service—very few folks I have ever known in government— would be willing to do what she did. Maybe General Patton or somebody like that. But outside the military I don't think I know anyone else who would have been willing to make those decisions."[17]

Birx's next steps inspired equally strong emotions. She swept into OGAC with a demand that headquarters be able to see what was happening down to the clinic level. Goosby had said how hard it was to track spending; she said that had to be fixed. When Mike Gehron, a computer systems expert who'd helped build and evolve PEPFAR's data collection and sharing systems heard her demands, he "felt the hand of God." He didn't mean this flippantly. A man of deep faith, he told me that he had been urging the program for years to find a way to allow the information collected at the site level to flow seamlessly from the sites to the implementing partners and thence to the agencies, the US embassies, and finally the Office of the US Global AIDS Coordinator. He'd built a version of this system in Tanzania, after listening to agencies and partners explain how hard it was to take data from multiple sites, each with its own reporting system, and pull that together into aggregate reports. He'd suggested that PEPFAR use a version of his Tanzania platform, known as PROMIS, across all its countries and that it start looking at site-level data regularly throughout the year.[18]

His suggestions hadn't been taken up during the Goosby era, perhaps because regular, headquarters-level oversight of site-level data ran counter to the notion of country ownership.

Irum Zaidi, a CDC epidemiologist, had provided data-analysis support for PEPFAR teams as a "strategic information officer" from the program's inception. Like Gehron, she too had noted missed opportunities in gathering and using information from PEPFAR-supported sites. "There wasn't a full understanding of how the data could be utilized," she said of the early years. "There was not…a full understanding of [whether] it is our responsibility to use the data or if that's just the host country government['s responsibility] and they need to respond."[19]

The move to gather and use information at headquarters was a marked shift for the program. Since its inception, PEPFAR had compiled its annual reports to Congress through a painstaking process by which individual subgrantees, or "implementing partners," pulled the information from the clinics and programs they funded and submitted those reports to the agencies that funded them, which in turn aggregated those numbers and reported them to the embassy, which rolled those numbers into a single country-level report submitted to Congress.

This wasn't a seamless process, as Gehron had seen when he'd worked in Tanzania. Sites keyed in data from paper records, sharing them in formats set by their implementing partners. The partners then entered that data into the PEPFAR software system. It was choppy and inefficient, and it meant that someone sitting in Washington, DC, could not possibly know what was happening in a given PEPFAR-funded clinic. For a program that prioritized country-owned systems, this didn't matter.

Americans poring over data from health clinics in sovereign countries thousands of miles away ran counter to the principles of sustainable development. But, as the preceding decade of expanding treatment rolls and mounting HIV infections showed, the pandemic wasn't a development issue; it was still a health emergency. Doing development work and ending plagues required different strategies. And the AIDS world had promised "investors" would tackle the latter.

It was a perfect moment for Birx, who prized the "visibility" that data afforded into program performance, to take PEPFAR's helm. Even a few years prior, her desire to track the program's funds in exhaustive detail would likely have triggered resistance. The more information you asked for, the more you asserted ownership of the program. Now, though, she moved forward with a PEPFAR-specific modification of a hugely popular open-source health information software platform called District Health Information System (DHIS), which many countries where PEPFAR already operated used to gather health information. The PEPFAR version, called DATIM, wasn't owned by national governments like DHIS. For PEPFAR, it would mean that piecemeal data analysis, like the work Julia Martin oversaw in 2014, would be a thing of the past. Eventually, country teams and headquarters staff would be able to see how the remotest clinic was functioning.

As a complement to building DATIM, Birx and Zaidi, whom Birx hired as chief epidemiologist, undertook to reform the annual planning process. "I don't want a book," Birx had said at one meeting—meaning the lengthy, narrative-based descriptions of annual plans. Tyler Smith, the health economist who'd worked as a deputy for John Blandford and the expenditure analysis team, thought he knew what she meant.

Starting in mid-2014, Smith—now promoted to a "special advisor" position—undertook a grueling, breakneck revamp of the entire annual planning process. No more process and priority conversations captured in lengthy, narrative documents but a set of complex calculations executed by planning "modules" that Smith and his colleagues built. The modules guided teams in which data to collect, then guided them through the process of "cleaning" the data so that it could be used for the complex calculations that would help guide program direction. As Smith worked on the new tools, he frequently found himself in the office of his colleague Tracy Carson, an OGAC staffer who'd help Smith "think through all the angles" on a particular problem.

Along with Carson and Zaidi, Birx's principal deputy Mark Brown—who'd been Ambassador Goosby's director of management and budget—undertook the delicate, diplomatic work of selling the new process to the agencies. To do so, they had to reassure, even as they asserted control. CDC, USAID, and other agencies had previously been solely responsible for managing the performance of their subgrantees, or "implementing partners," and had had considerable leeway in setting annual targets and selecting locations for the program to work. In the new approach, far more people would be able to see how different groups and, by extension, different agencies were performing; decisions once made at the country level would be guided by the new planning tools.

To change the course of AIDS, the new system needed new targets. Granular data and standardized decision-making tools do not, in and of themselves, change the course of a pandemic. Counting how many doses of a vaccine are distributed in a given geography does not show whether people in that place are protected, unless there is a target set for the percentage of the population that's been immunized. When treating AIDS was about preventing death, the treatment targets showed the magnitude of the mercy. If the goal was an AIDS-free generation or a better return on investment, different milestones mattered. In late 2014, UNAIDS obliged, with a set of targets that it proclaimed would not just lead to an AIDS-free generation but would, in fact, lead to the end of the AIDS epidemic.

"Ending the AIDS epidemic—four words that hold so much hope and promise," the agency announced in a document laying out its "Fast-Track Strategy" in 2014. "We can say these words with confidence—we will end the AIDS epidemic by 2030." When the reader flipped past the clock-strewn cover—no time to lose!—she learned that "fast-track" meant spending money on a core set of targets in a "fragile five-year window." It was the investment framework in an investor's prospectus format—glossy, visual, distilled to three core goals: identify 90 percent of people living with HIV, ensure that 90 percent of those identified were on treatment, and ensure that 90 percent of those were virologically suppressed, or "90-90-90." The other "targets" were a cap of 500,000 new infections among adults and zero discrimination.[20]

A few months later, a follow-up document displayed return on investment in dramatic, Seurat-esque graphs: a swelling curve of red dots showed the numbers of AIDS deaths and infections if the world took no action; a diving line of blue dots showed satisfying downward trends if "Fast-Track" was implemented. The purple overlap indicated the five-year window, from 2014 to 2020, in which an infusion of resources and ambition would determine whether the curve went up or down.[21]

The Fast-Track Strategy tied targets to impact—the end of the AIDS epidemic—for the first time in the pandemic's history. But there was science, as well as politics, at play in how the plan was introduced. The trio of core goals—"90-90-90," "500,000," "zero"— sat together at the bottom of the second page as though a matching set. One needed to know nothing at all about AIDS to understand that they were not the same at all. "90-90-90" was measurable, catchy, compelling; it was a set of actions. On the other hand, "500,000" and "zero" were goals. The text offered a list of prevention strategies, including male and female condoms, male circumcision, harm reduction, sexual and reproductive health information, and family planning, that also needed attention, but it did not specify targets, costs, or distribution. Doing something unspecified with these strategies and meeting "90-90-90" could reduce new infections from 2.1 million to 500,000 per year.

UNAIDS wanted funders to pay for the blue wave and suggested that this would happen if they bought and paid for "90-90-90," even though the agency knew—and had the numbers for—the other targets that had to be met to make that line slope down. It was an open secret, especially within the HIV-prevention-focused world that I worked in, that spreadsheets at the UNAIDS building on Avenue Appia in Geneva held the figures for every single parameter, projections for how many circumcisions, pre-exposure prophylaxis (PrEP) users, condoms, and changes in levels of discrimination would be needed to achieve epidemic control. UNAIDS just hadn't put any of them into the public document.

The omission led to elision. Within a matter of weeks, "90-90-90" was synonymous with ending AIDS. UNAIDS accelerated the conflation. On December 1, UNAIDS published a document titled

Ending the AIDS Epidemic: Achieving the 90-90-90 Goals; on December 10, its press release bore the title "BRICS Health Ministers Adopt the UNAIDS Fast-Track Strategy to End the AIDS Epidemic," when in fact the health ministers from Brazil, Russia, India, China, and South Africa had "agreed to endeavor to achieve the 90-90-90 HIV treatment target by 2020."[22] Every document was scrupulous in noting, somewhere in the fine print, that other things had to happen too—and equally consistent in leaving that which was vague and therefore unactionable. UNAIDS waited nearly a full year before releasing targets for primary prevention, stigma reduction, and discrimination that were core elements of its modeling.

For Birx, whose team had reportedly helped steer the Fast-Track Strategy, the "90-90-90" targets—issued by an independent agency—were just the sort of marching orders she'd come to appreciate after years in the military. In late December 2014, the Office of the Global AIDS Coordinator launched "PEPFAR 3.0," which was, in many ways, the American interpretation of the Fast-Track Strategy. The document taxonomized the program's previous decade. There had been the emergency phase and the sustainability phase. The next five years would bring the "most challenging, but exciting, phase yet... Sustainable Control of the Epidemic." The text was breathlessly ambitious and marked by the idiosyncratic capitalization that was also a feature of Birx's voluminous slide decks. "We have to shift the way we do business. We can best control the epidemic by pivoting to a data-driven approach that strategically targets areas and populations where we can achieve the most impact for our investments."[23]

With its emphasis on impact, data, and efficiency, the new PEPFAR strategy spoke investor-ese perfectly. It was, in that sense, an extension of the rhetoric that had refashioned AIDS as a subject for a business case. It was different, though, in that this strategy was tied to money and a new emphasis on data and "visibility" that could be used to tie funding to performance against targets. PEPFAR *was* the investor; the clinics and partners were subsidiaries. And Birx, at the helm, was the CEO.

The staff at the OGAC office reacted to the flurry of changes in different ways. More than one staffer who'd worked for Ambassador Goosby marked a change in the office atmosphere. Nomo the Muppet disappeared. Thurman and Baker kept candy on their desks and joked that they offered "pastoral care" in their offices for people who'd been stung by Birx's impatience or demands. It felt, to one staffer, like Birx was firing off ideas faster than the team could implement them, "like throwing spaghetti at the wall."

The AIDS activist Paul Zeitz had attended Birx's private swearing in at Ted Kennedy's office—and joined Birx and her family for dinner at Delmonico's steak house afterward. Then he'd taken a position on her staff, where he found the early freewheeling atmosphere exhilarating. "I had her wind at my back," he'd recall. Working with deputy Jenny Ottenhoff, Zeitz launched a major PEPFAR initiative on children's treatment and repurposed a tranche of PEPFAR funding as seed funding for a data-use initiative to support the new UN "Sustainable Development Goals," targets that replaced the Millennium Development Goals in 2015.[24]

Women's health advocates also appreciated the new energy. Birx and Achrekar had started thinking about what to do for adolescent girls and young women even before Birx had gotten the job. Achrekar had started her public health career working on adolescent health; she'd earned her PhD looking at the implementation of "Saving Mothers, Giving Life," a maternal-health initiative that emerged from the confusion of the Global Health Initiative and went on to achieve many of its goals. They scoured the literature looking for evidence about what actually reduced risk. When Birx encountered the Population Council's Judith Bruce, a social scientist who'd spent years analyzing the factors that put young girls at risk and the things that could help them, she'd marched up to her and said, "I have a lot to learn." She was particularly interested in the Population Council's "Girl Roster," a tablet-based app that could be used in a given geographic area for door-to-door surveys that asked if a girl lived in the home, how old she was, if she was in school, living with her parents, in a sexual relationship—Bruce seethed at the use of the word "marriage" for girls below the age of majority. The app told you who was where, what a girl's risk was, what she needed. It was exactly the kind of granular data that gave Birx confidence.[25]

Birx wanted to know about the Girl Roster because she wanted to do something big, at PEPFAR, for women and girls. Nina Hasen, a petite, no-nonsense behavioral neuroscientist was, by the time Birx arrived, the technical advisor for prevention. She'd been hired with no HIV background because, her supervisor later told her, HIV was easy to learn, and she needed someone like Hasen, who could manage difficult humans. Hasen loved the Goosby years—they were the most satisfying of her career. She'd felt his strong support for human rights and been thrilled when he'd given $6 million to the gender technical working group. She had worked with other members of that group, including PEPFAR staffers Daniela Ligiero and Nomi Fuchs-Montgomery, to thaw the chilling effect of Bush-era PEPFAR. Yes, they kept telling programs, you can use PEPFAR money to train staff in providing contraception—then you just need to find another funding source for the relatively cheap supplies.[26] Hasen, Ligiero, Fuchs-Montgomery, and others did what Birx and Achrekar had done: they scoured the literature for evidence of what worked. But, Hasen said, it wasn't until Birx arrived that the picture of PEPFAR's "big" push on adolescent girls and young women crystallized into a new, multimillion-dollar initiative.

Birx, Achrekar, and the OGAC team dubbed it "Determined, Resilient, Empowered, Mentored, and Safe" (DREAMS). Birx sold DREAMS to the Office of Management and Budget (OMB) the way she'd once sold vaccine strategies that she wanted to put into clinical trials. You needed a little of this immune response, a little of that one—she could do that with a pair of shots. She took what she'd learned, with a Girl Roster–type approach in a central role, and sought $300 million for a new initiative that would reduce new HIV infections in adolescent girls and young women by 25 percent in two years and 40 percent in four. She picked the targets because of the magnitude of the problem, not because she knew it could be done.

"We couldn't do weeny," she said to me. "We thought it was more important to really put out there what was really needed as a goal rather than what was achievable."[27]

OMB balked—not at the package of services, which included community-change curricula, gender-based violence prevention, youth-friendly spaces, school fees, and microfinance, as well as bio-medical services like testing, condoms, and PrEP, but at the price and unweeny targets. When Birx and Achrekar heard no, they just asked for another meeting.

"You just kept going back?" I asked them one afternoon. Yes, they said. That was what they'd done.

"We're unrelenting. We're unrelenting," Birx replied.

"No is never an option," Achrekar said.

"No just means that we go back and do the same thing all over again," Birx went on.

"Different data, more data," Achrekar agreed.

Eventually, OMB had agreed to their proposal, and so on World AIDS Day 2014, when Birx might have heralded the program's new data-focused planning or its revamped strategic planning process, she focused instead on a multi-million-dollar program that was the first significant, evidence-driven effort to reduce HIV in adolescent girls and young women. For the previous decade of PEPFAR's existence, feminist implementers had worked to make the program do as much as it could without drawing excessive attention to an issue that many believed was Kryptonite to Republican support. Birx and Achrekar hadn't done it alone or invented it overnight, but this massive investment also had their will and determination in its DNA. That day when they'd described their work, they spoke in overlapping sentences, smiling wide and somewhat private grins. When they said "unrelenting," they savored it. They weren't sorry at all.

———   ———

IN 2013, YVETTE RAPHAEL had been suffocating. Her job kept her tied to a desk, doing the necessary but dry work of monitoring and evaluation. The same damn hard worker who she'd always been, she

got it done, but she chafed. Raphael, who got her nickname Sjambok, or "The Whip," because of her "zero filter for bullshit," didn't
ever try to conceal her dissatisfaction. At work she'd tuck her chin,
narrow her eyes, purse her lips, and get the job done. She had good
managers, though. They saw that she wanted to do more and arranged for her to give a talk to the organization's board of directors.
She spoke not about her day job but about the issues facing women
and girls—the work she was most passionate about. Raphael didn't
hold back. "I gave a real-life feel. I talked about the underworld of
the HIV field, what theory could not describe."

In the underworld, rape and sexual violence were an all-day,
every-day problem, as was a patriarchal system more invested in protecting the perpetrators than securing justice for women. At about
the time that Raphael lectured the directors, her comrade Prudence
Mabele launched a guerilla art campaign. She'd applied red paint to
women's undergarments, using everything from toddler nappies to
granny panties. It looked like blood; on closer inspection, the red
stain was writing that said, "Stop Rape." On Valentine's Day 2013,
she walked through the former women's prison on Constitution Hill
and hung one hundred pairs.[28]

"How about you become the link to the South African AIDS
sector?" Raphael's managers proposed. The sectoral system afforded a
single forum for all governmental and nongovernmental actors.
Sjambok had a platform. "Bam!" she said. "A department of health
person would call me instead of some of the management." As she
became "larger than life," she knew what it must look like to the
outside. The management—including a new Black female director
who became a mentor to Raphael—never tried to rein her in. But she
imagined what people were thinking. "We have created a monster."

Raphael used the word "monster" over and over when she described her ascent from mid-level manager to high-profile activist.
With each advancement, "I was a new monster," she said. At one
point, she said, "I even became a villain." The word gave her control
over the worst stereotypes the world has for strong Black women.

"When I say 'monster,' it's to make me feel better for feeling badass," she said. "It's like Serena Williams on the court. How the fuck do you expect her to serve?"

"Yvette, put this on," Prudence Mabele said to Raphael in June 2014. She was about to join a panel of the PEPFAR implementers meeting in Durban, South Africa. Mabele had swooped up to where Raphael was standing alongside Cornelius Baker, whom Sandy Thurman had corralled into joining PEPFAR to build better linkages with "community"—the catchall term for activists, advocates, people living with HIV, feminists, and human rights defenders who had defined the AIDS agenda from the beginning of the epidemic to the present day. "It was a bright yellow T-shirt." Raphael was nervous, scared of "this Deborah Birx." "She shoved this into my hands. 'You wear it now.'" Raphael pulled it on. When she took her seat on the panel, she saw the same yellow shirts on activists scattered throughout the audience. "Fund Civil Society Now," the shirts read. As Baker and many others had noted, a decade after its launch, precious little of PEPFAR's money went directly to local groups. When she collected herself, Raphael wasn't all that surprised. "Pru would always pull the weirdest stuff out of her head."

For his part, Baker was taking note of who was and wasn't in the room. It wasn't the most well-attended session at the meeting, but he could tell from the questions and comments who understood the importance of working with activists and who was going to be an obstacle.

Not everything had gone precisely as he planned, though—it never did with Birx. Baker and Thurman had flown to Johannesburg for a meeting on the day she'd addressed the entire program. It was the first time the hundreds of staffers had assembled since many of them had undergone the stringent COP revision at the Madison Hotel. Birx immediately warned the room that the pace wasn't going to let up. She said that while she'd been at the CDC, staff scores on work-life balance satisfaction surveys had gone down. She expected the same to happen now. If you worked for her PEPFAR, you needed to work harder than you'd ever worked before. To some veterans, this felt like an attack. Thurman and Baker returned to find some PEP-FAR staffers in tears. It wasn't the first time that they'd done damage mitigation after something Birx had said; nor would it be the last. That was how Missy was. If you believed, as Baker and Thurman did, that her strategy for controlling the epidemic was sound, then she was worth it. As that strategy rolled out, her allies, enemies, and the wider world, would draw their own conclusions.

CHAPTER 13

OUR WORK IS FAR FROM DONE

S HOW ME HOW YOU do things," Cissy asked the nurse in charge of an adolescent clinic in the West Nile region. It was mid-2014. Her job had changed because the Ugandan PEPFAR program had changed. After years of projects funded by the Centers for Disease Control and Prevention (CDC) and USAID jostling alongside one another in the same districts and sometimes even the same health facilities, the program had undertaken an effort called "rationalization" in which each agency and each partner took over the entirety of specific geographic areas. After rationalization, Cissy's organization had been assigned responsibility for new districts, including West Nile, where it was supposed to support government clinics in providing high-quality services.

That day, she watched as the nurse asked the teens, who were all living with HIV, to open their patient record books, the little side-stapled examination notebooks with rough-pulped covers that clients carried with them. They were flimsy, and their covers grew suede-napped with wear, so that some people made newspaper covers for reinforcement, as I'd once made paper covers for school textbooks years and years before.

Within a clinic, the little book carried messages from the counselor to the nurse to the pharmacist or lab tech. A prescription in the pages told the pharmacist what to dispense. Only health professionals were supposed to write in these books, but as Cissy watched, the nurse in charge of the teens told them to check their pages and see when they'd last had a CD4 cell count. Those who needed a new measure of immune strength had to then write down, in their books, that the test needed to be done. Many of the teens had been in and out of school their whole lives. They'd had sick days and whole terms or years when their families had paid fees for other children thought more likely to survive. Now, the teens labored with their writing, bending over the papers, holding their faces close to their pens. Finally, the lab technician came out of his office to see if he had any work at all to do that day.

On the same trip, Cissy encountered a mother and her daughter, who had a huge goiter growing from her neck. For years, the mother had brought her daughter's clinic record book but not the child herself, saying each time that the girl was unwell or that it cost too much to transport the two of them. She'd begged for refills and received them, duly noted in the pages each time. But the clinician hadn't seen the girl, hadn't weighed her or adjusted the pediatric dosage to account for her growing body. She'd been underdosed, the virus stronger than the drugs. The goiter showed the damage that had been done.

Cissy's new role was coach, cheerleader, and counselor to her underpaid government counterparts. She had to make them want to run programs with the love and rigor that she'd brought to her own work. If she didn't, some of those adolescents might not get the care they needed; the girl with the goiter might not recover. But she herself was also at risk. In the new "visibility"-oriented PEPFAR, with data flowing from clinics to implementing partners to agencies to the Office of the US Global AIDS Coordinator (OGAC), failures registered at the highest level. If the adolescents mis-entered their lab test requirements, the source data were corrupted. The notations from those small books that were copied into ledgers, then entered into computers, then fed into DATIM would be wrong.

Cissy told me these stories one afternoon in 2014 while I sat with my feet curled under me on the taut belly of her beige sofa. The Virgin Mary was still on the wall, but there were far fewer shadows than when I'd visited for the first time, fourteen years prior. Her children were grown, each filled with presence and beautiful personality. She had grandchildren, too, and it was for their sakes that she'd stopped talking about living with HIV anymore. Stigma was rampant. She didn't want them to be teased. She was worried, too, about what would happen to her family if she was too public about living with HIV—and she was right to be.

In February 2014, just a few months before Birx took over PEP-FAR, a Ugandan nurse living with HIV named Rosemary Namubiru inadvertently stuck herself with a cannula while trying to place an IV line into the arm of a squirming child. She'd later say that she bandaged herself, then picked up a new cannula and kept on trying. After she and a colleague eventually succeeded in placing the IV line, the child's mother—who'd say that Namubiru used the same cannula—demanded to know Namubiru's HIV status. Namubiru, who'd worked in Kenya for twenty-nine years, had recently learned that she had HIV—she thought she'd acquired it from a patient. But when she revealed her status, she was arrested, while television cameras rolled, and charged under a section of the Ugandan penal code that criminalized "doing a negligent act likely to spread infection of disease." Namubiru, who was held for several days before a judge saw her, was tried and convicted—even though the child had not acquired HIV. When I went to visit Cissy, Namubiru—who had so much in common with my gentle, large-eyed friend—was still in jail.

A day prior, I'd worn a *gomesi*, the Buganda traditional dress, for the first time. I'd made the flying four-day trip for a friend's wedding, keeping it absurdly short so that I could return to my unweaned second son. He was born in 2013 when his brother was just over three years old. During my maternity leave, I had, for a time, ceased to try to work and write and parent at the same time. I'd luxuriated in walks with my older child, carrying my newborn strapped to my chest, close to my heart. We asked each other questions and stood for as long as it took to satisfy our curiosity: What made the dump truck spin or the bee walking through the grass choose to fly? For the first time since I'd become a mother, I felt I was giving it my full attention—which is to say, I felt I was doing it right.

The feeling vanished the moment my older son started school and I went back to work. The boys felt far away from me, and I felt empty, enraged, unable to let go of them or of my own ambition. Sometimes, at work and at home, I roared. It should not be so hard. Liam told me that he and I were doing this together, that we both were doing a good and loving job of raising our sons. I listened and let his words sink in like a balm. But on whirlwind work trips, I studied Yvette Raphael and Deborah Birx, both women with children, careers, and assertive personalities. I wondered if women who got called monsters by the world or by their innermost critics did better by embracing the appellation or ignoring it. I wondered, too, if any of us really had a choice.

When it came to dressing for the wedding itself, I found myself ill prepared. Milly Katana, who'd long told me my wardrobe was immature, found a tailor who could make traditional garb that fit on the basis of a cell phone selfie. She met me at the church and pushed me into a storeroom where she wrapped me in what seemed like endless layers of cloth—the *kikooyi* that went beneath the flowing dress. The garment I'd thought would be light felt heavy, constricting. I could take it off whenever I wanted to, but Museveni's government was also taking steps to police women's attire too. Just weeks before Namubiru's arrest, the 2014 Anti-Pornography Act, informally known as the "mini-skirt law," imposed new standards of decency in women's dress. Mobs grabbed women deemed to be violating these standards and humiliated them in the street.[1]

Women going to work and people living with HIV lived in fear of capricious persecution. So did Uganda's vibrant community of lesbians, gays, and transgender men and women. In February 2014, President Yoweri Museveni had signed the Uganda Anti-Homosexuality Bill into law, after repeatedly assuring the American ambassador and other diplomats that he wouldn't. At the signing ceremony, Museveni waggled his cigar-sized pen at the audience and said that he wasn't afraid of losing funding. NGOs were "running up and down" doing things he didn't really understand. Uganda didn't need foreign aid anyway.[2]

Four days after the signing, activist and staffer at SMUG Richard Lusimbo woke up to find that a tabloid, the *Red Pepper*, had outed him and five other Ugandan gay activists, using pictures and selectively edited text from a photo essay that a gay American named David Robinson had, with their permission, printed in the *Advocate*.[3] Lusimbo wasn't publicly out when he did the interview. "I was really naive, and the truth is, I think that was one of the reasons I did it because I'd never given an interview to a media house or anything," he told me. There was another reason too. "It felt good," he said.[4]

I wasn't surprised that Lusimbo had done the interview. I knew of the in-between life of gays and lesbians in my own family, my own personal life—and in the lives of many of my friends in Uganda. I knew plenty of white American gay men who had steady Ugandan boyfriends who stayed at their houses on the weekends, sleeping in the same room, waking shirtless to make coffee in the morning, passing their clothes on to the Ugandan house staff to clean. There were house parties and known bars and clubs for both gays and lesbians. Although not flaunted, the life was still there to find. You had to want to try.

After Lusimbo was outed, the "hatred messages" started pouring in. He turned off his phone and shut down his computer, relieved beyond words that he was flying out of the country to a human rights conference in San Francisco the next day. Other LGBT Ugandans who didn't have a ticket out found themselves in mortal fear and peril. Many fled toward the Kenyan border in hopes of escaping violence from strangers and their families.

Sara Allinder, the PEPFAR coordinator at the time, found out that Museveni had signed the law when she got a call saying, "Come to the front office." She'd walked into the ambassador's suite and watched with senior American embassy staffers. The reaction was blunt. "What the fuck?" In the months that followed, Allinder and her team scrutinized PEPFAR's programs to see if any of them would put Ugandan LGBT individuals and staff working at PEPFAR-funded clinics at risk if they continued operating, and they began to look at actions that could convey the full force of American disapproval.[5]

The United States came up with a set of small but potent punitive actions, including putting a set of Ugandan officials on a "no visa" list and removing funding from the Inter-religious Council of Uganda (IRCU), the religious grantee that had held a "Thanksgiving" rally in December 2013 when the law had first been signed.[6] To the many LGBT rights activists who'd been raising concerns about the group for years, the decision was grievously overdue. They'd been complaining loud and long enough that the US Office of the Inspector General (OIG) had, in 2013, conducted an audit of the group.[7] It had turned up only one potentially problematic document, though, and USAID/Uganda had respectfully suggested that even that was not, in fact, a problem.[8] The IRCU's Thanksgiving Day parade, held two months prior to the law signing, also hadn't been cause for severing ties, since the event hadn't been paid for with PEPFAR funds.

Whether or not IRCU paid for the *kisanja*-yellow placards denouncing sodomy with American money hardly seemed to matter. Under the Mexico City Policy (MCP), no group receiving American money could talk about or advocate for abortion, even if it did not use American funds to do so. Yet one could promulgate hate speech and cash American checks, provided you kept the homophobia in a separate budget line.

American activists wanted the IRCU defunded, and they wanted homophobic leaders held to account in every nation. In Uganda, the activists wanted the same thing. But they also understood that the bill signing was a manifestation of both homophobia and political strategy. Museveni signed the Anti-Homosexuality Act (AHA) shortly after another story about oil-related corruption had emerged. In the months prior, the country had taken a series of steps that provoked donors and allowed the president to rally the Ugandans most affected by graft and corruption around the need to resist outside meddling in the country's culture and principles.

"Museveni's political longevity, and his increasingly brutal methods of holding on to power, are crucial to understanding the current AIDS response in Uganda.... As most Ugandan human rights activists will tell you, the decision to jeopardise the nation's health has everything to do with power and nothing to do with medical science," warned SMUG executive director Frank Mugisha.[9]

Before returning to Uganda, Lusimbo stopped in Nairobi for a conference on African sexuality and gender identity. He attended an electric reading by Binyavanga Wainaina, a Kenyan literary lion who'd recently come out as gay in an essay in which he grieved about having held the secret back from his mother.[10] At that meeting, Lusimbo gave another interview that, when published, would prompt reconciliation with his family and launch the beginning of a fully-out life.[11] He unblocked his social media and stopped even trying to hide. "The only way to meet these tabloids...to beat them, was to live my truth."

In August, Uganda repealed the law on a technicality.[12] Museveni's point had been made. Lusimbo celebrated with fellow activists in a jubilant rainbow-colored parade in Entebbe.[13] He had his truth and a clearer view of how America operated too. He'd watched the embassy staff walk a delicate line, offering behind-the-scenes support without taking the critical stances of politicians in DC. Compared to President Barack Obama and Secretary of State John Kerry, both of whom had condemned the law, Americans in country "were a bit retreating."

The United States was a complex ally to say the least. With its HIV funding, people like Cissy were tasked with the exceedingly intimate work of making sure that people with HIV learned their status, started treatment, and took it so that their virus became undetectable. The "90-90-90" goals depended on reaching specific coverage levels—a wholly different endeavor from making treatment available so that people who knew their status could take it if and when they wanted to. But as PEPFAR zoomed in to focus on individuals and the precise measure of virus in their blood, the program eschewed a full-throated effort to uproot the stigma, discrimination, and homophobia that had helped put the virus there in the first place. The program was careful about when and how it denounced homophobic legislation.

The program was also careful about how it approached services for people who use drugs, another stigmatized group where criminalizing laws and state repression hampered public health work. "PEPFAR was quite attuned to political dynamics and very careful," said Daniel Wolfe, the director of the International Harm Reduction Development Program at the Open Society Institute. Contaminated injection equipment was not a major source of HIV infection in most of the program's initial fourteen focus countries, but it was in both Vietnam and Ukraine, which created a formal partnership with the US government AIDS program in 2011. Wolfe saw the program's caution pushing the envelope in what it could provide and advocate for as a "missed opportunity," likely reflecting valid concerns that eagle-eyed, anti-harm-reduction members of Congress would raise questions.[14]

Such political balancing acts had personal consequences. Cissy could help the nurse at the adolescent clinic come up with a better system for logging CD4 cell counts; she could counsel the mother about why she had to somehow find the money to bring her daughter in to see a doctor. But she would think long and hard before she shared her own experience of living with HIV with anyone beyond her inner circle of colleagues and friends.

I made my visit to her in May 2014, before the AHA was repealed. While we spoke, Lusimbo and his comrades lived in fear for their lives, and Namubiru sat in jail. PEPFAR, the Global Fund, and UNAIDS had all bought into a treatment-centered plan for controlling AIDS. For all the UNAIDS talk of achieving zero stigma and discrimination, this new campaign would test the degree to which the course of an epidemic could be changed while the world that had created it meted out new forms of discrimination, undertook incremental improvements, or—most often—remained unchanged.

— —

To achieve epidemic control in the countries where PEPFAR worked, Birx and her colleagues at the Office of the Global AIDS Coordinator developed an orientation guide that introduced a fictitious country, "Dataland." At a September 2015 meeting, PEPFAR coordinators received an orientation in the new process. A slide titled "Drill Down Across the Cascade to Monitor Impact" showed a set of looping arrows linking three different dashboards that would, henceforth, be examined quarterly. Dashboards worked like a long tracking shot. The first showed Dataland's country-level progress against targets; the next tracked progress by district or subnational unit. The final one tracked "within district." It didn't show every clinic but a comparable dashboard for Uganda would show West Nile, Cissy's organization, and how well it had performed. The charts all used stoplight color schemes. Groups that were on track—at 50 percent or more halfway through the year—were coded green.[15]

The quarterly reviews were part of an elaborate, data-focused system that also looked at financial expenditures and results from site-monitoring visits—every site was to be visited at least once a year, with follow-up "remediation" visits if issues emerged on a standard scoring sheet. Each piece of information would help "triangulate" to an explanation as to why a target was being missed. Perhaps a site-level visit would find something amiss in record keeping, or a financial review might locate an underspend. Coordinators were to "ensure team comes together for data review, data interrogation and data use."

These verbs embodied Birx's bone-deep faith in information. If you looked at it, asked it questions, and used it, you could not fail. It wasn't just PEPFAR coordinators who were invited to Dataland. In 2015, when Birx and her team decided to launch in-person planning meetings to review data and develop the plans for the next year, activists got invitations too.

On May 14, 2015, I yanked myself out of the quicksand slumber that follows an overnight flight and stumbled through the hallways of a hotel appended to the Frankfurt airport until I found the meeting room, fluorescent lit and crammed with round tables, where the opening session for the 2015 PEPFAR regional planning meeting was already underway. Birx stood at the front of the room; she'd begun speaking by the time I slipped into my seat. I looked up at a slide showing a map in which the continent of Africa had been replaced with a giant, engorged human heart. I adjusted my vision. In the "cartogram," each landmass was shaped according to HIV prevalence in the population: the relatively low-prevalence West African countries collapsed in, with a slight bulge for the Gold Coast; the Horn of Africa was also flat and thin. Southern African, bulging at the bottom, was the mightiest ventricle of them all.

Birx looked around the room and beamed. Addressing the activists, she chirped, "We're so glad you're here." I swiveled my head around to see whom else she was talking to. I spotted Asia Russell and, with his dreads piled high in one of his mushroom-cap Rasta hats, Chamunorwa Mashoko, an erstwhile Zimbabwean fashion designer and DJ turned AIDS activist. As I scanned the room, I didn't see Maureen Milanga, Russell's colleague at Health GAP.

Milanga and Mashoko were core members of the African AIDS activist squad that had pushed PEPFAR to involve civil society and, eventually, invite them to these meetings. They began demanding access well before Birx took the job. Mashoko began writing to his PEPFAR coordinator asking to see and review the country plans in 2009. Felix Mwanza, the gravel-voiced, bomber jacket–wearing Zambian activist did the same. So did Maureen Milanga, a statuesque Kenyan human rights activist who'd joined Health GAP after a stint at the AIDS Legal Network, and Ugandan AIDS activists, including Lillian Mworeko, Margaret Happy, and Ken Mwehonge. These and other African activists worked alongside and in coordination with Asia Russell, who'd relocated to Kampala, and Paul Davis, who had spent a few years in Kenya.

Many had spent years tackling their own government and taking on the Global Fund. Mwehonge had overseen national surveys of drug stockouts; Mwanza had been instrumental in ensuring that the Zambian government listened to people with HIV as it developed its programs.

But taking on America and its funding hadn't been a given. American embassies in African countries are fortresses of rock and cement. In Kampala, cars cannot stop in front of the gates, and visitors surrender almost all of their possessions to security guards before entry, as if entering a prison. (In 2013, I appeared at the US Embassy in Kampala for an activist meeting with my unweaned four-month-old son strapped to my chest in a cloth carrier, and he was almost deemed unallowable, as he hadn't been put on the pre-submitted list of participants. Margaret Happy would have her antiretrovirals taken away at a different meeting.) Trying to gain access to the physical buildings was tiring and humiliating; once attendees were inside, the meetings often felt the same. Mwehonge took over the PEPFAR brief at the Coalition for Health Promotion and Social Development from a colleague who had "felt a fool" at the meetings where incomprehensible data flashed by on slides thick with acronyms the participants could not understand.[16]

Nor had the embassy teams been particularly willing to let activists see their plans—especially ones that were not finalized. But in each country, the activists kept up a steady drumbeat of letters and emails to the local staff and to the headquarters team in Washington, DC. In the final months of his tenure, Ambassador Eric Goosby had dispatched a cable to the field offices instructing them to begin a process of civil society engagement.[17] Goosby's 2013 cable included guiding principles but not a step-by-step procedure for what "engagement"— a tired, nebulous word in the development vocabulary—actually meant. Birx and her team filled in the details, with activists demanding open doors and data-sharing. With Cornelius Baker and Sandy Thurman also urging expanded community engagement and emphasizing the importance of engaging the ambassadors, the in-person meetings became a key venue for both making plans and building personal connections.

For Health GAP's Maureen Milanga, that first meeting in Frankfurt was a matter of establishing her right to be there. The PEPFAR coordinator had been enormously resistant to her participation, making her wait in the parking lot in front of the embassy for a copy of the draft plan, then delaying in writing Milanga's visa letter—which was why she hadn't made it to Frankfurt for the start of the meeting. But Milanga was hard to deter. She had been raised by a single mother, a French teacher, who urged her students to act with independence and flout the formalities of the classroom that persisted as holdovers from the colonial era. An early mentor had given her a book on human rights; the next day, she'd asked Milanga if she'd read it. "Good, now you're going to teach these people," her mentor had replied, then propelled her into a room filled with rural Kenyans displaced by postelection violence. She'd led the training that day and hadn't looked back, going on to work with LGBT Kenyans who were often left out of both the PEPFAR and Global Fund planning processes.[18]

I sat next to Milanga during the deliberations in the room where the Kenya country team and PEPFAR staff gathered to walk through their plans with civil society looking on—and contributing. To Milanga, it was crystal clear why she and the other activists needed to be there. "The country operational plan [COP] meetings were not about just accepting what was being funded by PEPFAR, but were about having a true discussion about what was good for the program and what was good for communities and what was worth investing millions of US taxpayer dollars on."[19]

In the room next door, where the Zimbabwe plans were developed, Chamunorwa Mashoko brought a deep-seated analysis of postcolonial dynamics to the work and thought the United States would do well to consider the impact of history on the present pandemic, including how white Rhodesian colonizers' seizure of land and enforced changes in Black African diets impacted health. While he sensed hesitation among the PEPFAR team, he never doubted his right to be there. "To me it was like a date that went wrong but concluded well," he said. "When you are first engaging with institutions that have not included you in their activities for about twelve or thirteen years…and now you are coming in…those PEPFAR guys were not sure if we understood what we were talking about."[20] Those PEPFAR guys doubted whether Mashoko and other activists had a grasp of the abbreviation-laden lingo of their data sheets and strategic plans. The reason the date concluded well, at least as far as Mashoko was concerned, was because they did.

Even before the activists had secured invitations to the country planning meetings, they'd secured sections of PEPFAR planning documents and started studying up on the budget codes and indicators that populated those tables from Dataland. "It was [like] they were at a dress rehearsal, like we weren't even there," Lusimbo said. He listened to Asia Russell and watched Lillian Mworeko and Kenneth Mwehonge—they'd come to call themselves "the triumvirate"—in action. He started printing out the slides at home, making notes, raising his hand when the lights went up. There were no stupid questions.

Mashoko, who'd lost family members to AIDS, had become an AIDS and sexual health educator for students at the university where he taught. He'd told them things about their bodies other people wouldn't utter. At the end of the 2015 Frankfurt meeting, he gave a speech explaining to PEPFAR staff why civil society would keep demanding to be included. He was gentle but firm and, that day, very proud of what he'd won.

— —

MWEHONGE HAD ALWAYS BEEN a charmer and an organizer. When his mother, seeking to get him out of the house for a while, sent him to get water, he returned much sooner than she'd expected. He'd just asked his friends to help him. In college, though, he'd taken up with a young woman whose late father had been a Tanzanian soldier and politician with deep loyalty to Museveni. Through her, he'd met ministers and visited the State House. He realized that these "big people" were just like everybody else. You could talk to them and make jokes without a problem. Once he'd figured that out, he'd had no problem talking to anyone—which was why, when the Ugandan activist team needed someone to approach Ambassador Birx at the reception during the 2016 planning meeting at the Hyatt Rosebank Hotel in Johannesburg, he'd been the person the triumvirate sent to pose a demand.

Mwehonge had sidled up to Birx at the reception on the open patio, threading between long tables with hot trays of canapés—little cigarillos filled with cheese, miniature pies brimming with ground beef—and cold trays of desserts, bars sliced on the bias, lime and lemon and chocolate trapezoids. There was a problem, he told her, while the servers orbited with trays filled with glasses of wine. Uganda's pre-exposure prophylaxis (PrEP) treatment target was simply too low. "What do you need?" she'd asked. Three thousand new people on PrEP, he'd replied, just as the activist group had agreed. She'd get it done, she said. The next day, it became clear that she had. When Mwehonge approached the door of the Ugandan meeting room, the PEPFAR coordinator and Ugandan health officials were waiting outside. "Ken, what have you done?" they demanded.[21]

What he'd done was precisely what Sandy Thurman and Cornelius Baker had hoped he would—not Mwehonge, in particular, but anyone and everyone going to the receptions they'd had to work so hard to institute as part of Birx's PEPFAR program. Both had sat on city AIDS planning councils in the United States and knew that civil society needed to be a formal part of decision making. They also knew that the best work happened between people who had a sense of connection and that connection didn't arise in conference rooms. It happened over a glass of wine at the end of the day—which was why, for a time, they'd bought the wine with their own money, pushing carts up and down the aisles of Woolworths to buy candles too, because, Baker said, "you need ambiance."[22]

When Felix Mwanza arrived at the 2016 planning meeting, he realized that "PEPFAR at the national level is different from PEPFAR at a global level." In country, he'd found his attempts to engage with the staff blocked or met with hostility and skepticism. In the Rosebank, where a rose-tinted art photograph of a South African township was the only indication of being on the continent, he found allies in the American leaders. That year, he said, "we looked at the data they presented and we looked at the gaps. Most importantly, it was the undermining of treatment targets." Combing through the country's massive Excel data sheet on targets and progress, known as the Data Pack, Matthew Kavanagh had noticed that the program planned to put fewer people on treatment in the next year than it had in the prior reporting period. Mwanza pushed back, finally taking his issues to the top. "I had to walk to Ambassador Birx's office and present issues that [were] in the best interest for people living with HIV. She came and told them if they do not include or revise targets or figures, they should forget signing the COP."[23]

I'd been in the room with Mwanza that day, standing beside him dutifully, when Birx said to us, "Stay here, so people don't see us walk out together." She'd clipped out on her low, sensible heels. We'd looked at each other without speaking. Birx was about to force the Zambian treatment program to add 60,000 treatment slots to its rolls—because we'd asked her to. It was thrilling to wield such power—and one of the ways that the bilateral US program differed from the Global Fund. Here, decisions could be made by a single person; with the Fund and its multistage consultative planning process, it was seldom possible to do such rapid course correction. The funding mechanism that met so many activists' core requirements was, in many ways, less susceptible to activist intervention; the bilateral monolith was permeable to activists who could speak the language of Dataland.

High-stakes pitches to Birx herself were a last resort. Many more changes happened in the planning rooms as the activists lobbied government, PEPFAR, and Global Fund representatives to listen to their concerns and take action accordingly. The fact that it was a PEPFAR-convened meeting didn't stop activists like Maureen Luba, a petite, quietly unstoppable Malawian activist—who'd later become a colleague at AVAC—from urging her fellow citizens in government to adopt a universal-access approach to antiretrovirals or pushing policymakers to commit to adopting PrEP guidelines. In the planning meetings one could—and did—demand what was essential, from whoever could deliver it.

The freewheeling space for activism contrasted with the explicitly pluralistic structures developed by the Global Fund, which mandated that country coordinating mechanisms (CCMs) be established in all countries seeking funds.[24] The CCM had been designed to support country-based participatory planning and priority setting for external aid. By 2014, this once-revolutionary concept had become something of a bureaucratic arena, with elaborate processes for electing civil society representatives that sometimes led to the exclusion of vocal activists and unapologetic champions of LGBT rights.[25]

The Global Fund also didn't collect and share the kind of information that PEPFAR did. The Global Fund secretariat did not seek or publish reports on what specific Global Fund grants or subgrants in country had paid for; nor did it seek to track actual performance against targets. When a grant recipient was slow to disburse funds, that usually triggered an alarm at the national or secretariat level. But moving money fast wasn't a proxy for whether the money had been well spent. It was far harder for activists to discern what specific problems were and even harder to demand and secure immediate solutions.

Under Birx, PEPFAR shared more of its country-level performance data than it ever had. Activists also began to come with their own data, in the form of "People's COPs," which reflected in-depth, on-the-ground assessments by civil society of what was working and what was missing.[26]

But as time went on, the trade-offs also became clear. Activists had enormous influence within the system, but the system was, for the most part, still governed by PEPFAR's priorities—which rested on achieving specific targets that were critical to "epidemic control."

Most country plans centered heavily on progress toward the "90-90-90" goals, which meant that activists focused on these too.

To live in Dataland was to accept an American program that wielded immense influence over policies in sovereign countries. To be eligible for PEPFAR funding, countries needed to adopt "universal treatment" that offered antiretrovirals to people the day they tested positive. Starting in 2017, they were required to support testing protocols that traced the partners and contacts of people testing positive for HIV—an approach known within the PEPFAR landscape as "index testing." The PEPFAR Fiscal Year 2019 Country Operational Plan Guidance stated that countries had to find at least 50 percent of new HIV-positive adults through index testing and testing of individuals with tuberculosis.[27] If you tested everyone, you spent a lot and didn't always find new cases; if you just tested people's contacts, you paid for fewer tests and found more people needed for "the first 90." In the world of optimizing investments, the proportion of people with HIV identified after a testing push was called "yield."

Index testing was high yield; it was also hard, delicate work. You couldn't tell contacts how you'd gotten their name, because the index client might be the sex worker they used, or their wife, or their john. Done without discretion, index testing put the people who'd shared their contacts at risk of violence, stigma, and loss of shelter or financial support. Programs striving to meet their targets ran the risk of cutting corners and putting people with HIV at risk; as the program rolled out, activists compiling reports confirmed their fears. Seventy-five groups would sign an open letter calling for a halt to index testing targets until there were assurances that the programs were safe.[28]

Birx and her team would briefly pause index testing, and modify the approach, but the strategy remained central to the program. "We're never asking with a USG hat on, we're asking from the standpoint of 'here's the data,'" she'd say.[29] The data were also the basis for the "planning letters" she and her team sent to countries each year. Running to twenty pages, they laid out precisely what the programs were supposed to do. Poor-performing countries got dropped back to "maintenance funding" or called to the carpet for failing to use American money well. In 2019, South Africa's letter said, "Despite a significant infusion of resources by the U.S. government especially over the last three years, progress has been grossly sub-optimal and insufficient to reach epidemic control, including the targets of the Surge Plan."[30]

No other global health program used data the way that Birx's PEPFAR did. The President's Malaria Initiative, a USAID-led initiative launched by President George W. Bush and viewed as an overall success, shared intermittent performance reports and posted its grant agreements on its website. Once a country received a Global Fund grant, the only information available to activists seeking to track progress was the amount of funding obligated and disbursed to prime recipients. Data on targets, performance, geographic coverage, and population disaggregates simply wasn't available. "This level of global health data is unprecedented and PEPFAR deserves praise for its transparency," an amfAR report declared.[31]

In the years that PEPFAR pursued, and then intensified, its biomedicalized strategy, incidence went down. The number of people acquiring HIV every year decreased. In South Africa, overall incidence rates dropped by 40 percent between 2012 and 2017.[32] The Rakai Health Sciences Program investigators calculated a 42 percent reduction in incidence between 2006 and 2016.[33] A review of incidence in eSwatini (formerly Swaziland) also found a 43.57 percent reduction.[34] Findings of such consistency across countries with different health systems and economic and urban-rural demographic profiles offer confidence that what's observed is actually happening. In all of these cases, authors attributed declines to the massive expansion of antiretroviral treatment (ART) coverage and voluntary medical male circumcision that occurred in this period.

For antiretroviral therapy and male circumcision to have a population-level effect on incidence—meaning reducing rates in communities, not just risk in individuals—many people need to be reached. In South Africa, Francois Venter found the "90-90-90" slogan immensely useful as a goad and goal for provincial health authorities. Returning to the question of whether the targets had been reached helped him bring focus to conversations about what an adequate effort looked like. When, in 2018, the PEPFAR program in country started missing its treatment targets—a function of many factors, including a deteriorating health system and inadequate investments in human resources and record keeping—Birx and her team threatened to cut funding. A "February Frenzy" ensued that got 100,000 South Africans onto treatment—many of whom had been lost from care.

By the time PEPFAR triggered the "Frenzy," it wasn't America's program. The South African government covered 80 percent of the costs of the largest antiretroviral treatment program in the world. It wasn't America's program, but PEPFAR's relentless focus on hitting targets had a national effect. "While many observers have credited PEPFAR's innovation and accountability for keeping the South African HIV response focused, they lament PEPFAR's relentless push toward numbers and targets in pursuit of epidemic control, which they claim fails to grasp the complexities and nuances of the health system or the broader context of poverty, violence, and migration," one independent report said. "However, many feel any reduction or removal of PEPFAR support would be problematic, potentially creating a vacuum of services, particularly for members of key population groups."[35]

PEPFAR was intense, unyieldingly target driven, and insistent that the data—not any specific individual—dictated decisions. In the regional planning meetings, the level of information was so fine grained that one had the sense of being in the place itself, not an anonymous conference room. I loved those meetings precisely because of that uncanny sense of being very close and at the same time having a bird's-eye view. At the Joint Clinical Research Center (JCRC) clinic or on the back of a motorbike, PEPFAR disappeared, replaced by the agency, the partner, the nurse, the man on the bike. The trick of detailed data is to make it seem like you are seeing everything. On PEPFAR's public dashboards, I could track progress on ART in the district where the JCRC clinic sat. It was almost like I was there. But data do not equate to truth; they are only as good as the source they derive from—the soft-covered record books with entries made by adolescents, the ledgers flopped open in Sister Natalya's lap. I needed to go back to the clinics and see how they looked up close, now that I was able to see them from afar, and in 2018, I did.

—— ——

IN MANY RESPECTS, TORORO was as I'd left it—Tororo Rock was still a flat-topped haunch silhouetted against the sky; on Uhuru Road the top branches of the trees in a colonial-era *grande allée* intermingled in a wall of green. The branch road to Tororo Hospital was still unpaved, the single-story, cement-walled buildings connected by walkways roofed with corrugated metal so that it was possible to move back and forth when it rained. At the Tororo building of The AIDS Support Organisation (TASO), thorny bushes flowered purple and orange at the base of the walls; the open-air waiting area was scented, sweet and thick, with the aroma of human bodies that had slept in close quarters, walked long distances, worn their best clothes.

But the Rock Classic Hotel, where everyone had stayed back in the day, had been overtaken as a headquarters for Chinese engineers, builders, and investors. The white expats now segregated up the hill to Green Meadows, where I'd met, over breakfast, an earnest woman with lank blonde hair who was one of the only American lawyers in the world representing Ugandans who'd gone to the wars in Iraq and Afghanistan, suffered horrific wounds, and received no worker's compensation or assistance from America. She arranged video conferences with judges and took statements from men in shacks who'd lost their sight or their limbs.[36]

Tororo, like the rest of Uganda, had been drawn into global events—wars, competition among globalizing powers. And TASO Tororo was deeply enmeshed in the PEPFAR machine. On that visit, I found the program in the midst of a "surge" led by the medical director, Dr. Rebecca Amongi, a curvy, supremely confident mother of three.[37] When she'd first taken the post, she'd gotten verbal reports from the monitoring and evaluation staffer. She liked numbers on paper that she could look at, but she hadn't made a fuss until the USAID-funded agency managing TASO's Tororo program had complained that her site wasn't performing. Dr. Amongi told me that she'd dispensed with the oral reports and started using the PEPFAR "dashboard," which showed the daily and weekly totals, the PEPFAR targets, the same data that Birx saw in DATIM. Now her team was out in the field all the time, testing people, starting them on treatment, getting the contacts from the "index clients," and following them up. They'd improved so much so fast that they'd come in top-ranked among all the TASO sites. The executive director said he and other leaders from the Kampala headquarters would come and slaughter a goat to eat in celebration of the accomplishment. Her colleagues emailed to find out how she'd done it.

When she invited me over to her house on a Saturday afternoon—juggling her youngest while he nursed and flipping back and forth between phones—I got a glimpse of how she'd turned the program around. She made one phone call after another, tracking down a staffer whom she'd sent into the field because she didn't think the contacts of a person recently diagnosed with HIV had been traced and tested. This was the "index testing" that was core to Birx's plan for epidemic control. Dr. Amongi couldn't let anyone give up, because then her numbers would drop, she'd miss targets, and Tororo wouldn't be on top the next time. She put down the phone and told me that if she wasn't convinced by the field officer's update, she would follow him out to be sure the testing had been done.

In all my years of visiting with people paid to execute PEPFAR's plans, from the global AIDS ambassador to the bike-riding field officers, I had taken for granted that the program's mission and approach shifted depending on whether I was in Uganda or America. The ideology had never been as bad in the field; the sense of urgency had sometimes been greater in DC. I had never before seen a Ugandan health professional doing exactly what I'd heard a PEPFAR head demand.

After visiting Dr. Amongi, I traveled to the town where Simon lived. I'd only been away for five years, but more seemed to have changed. Unlike in Tororo, the town's grand aisle of trees on the boulevard leading to the colonial-era government buildings had not been allowed to stand. The great, shaggy-barked giants had all been cut down. The grassy green bowl of a meadow that I'd used as a shortcut between the main road and the dirt path to the guesthouse was ringed with metal fence, a concrete structure halted, mid-construction, in its center—dingy, gray, and bare. Off the back porch of the little wooden house with the thatched roof that was my favorite room, I saw lights winking in the village along the ridge. It had finally been electrified.

The Joint Clinical Research Center (JCRC) clinic, where Sister Natalya and I embraced, then stood back, clasping each other by the shoulders, then embraced again, was completely empty, as though it were waiting to open or had been shuttered for years. The benches still stood in the open waiting area with the yellow bars; not a single one was occupied. The lab was locked, the equipment inside covered, unused. JCRC was still running research studies; while I was there, she'd see one client, a child with his mother. I wondered if she missed the busy days. She shook her head. "We worked so hard."

I'd left her and walked up the hill, threading past the thick-walled private clinic, and a new multistory main building with electronic doors. I reached the ART clinic, which was now run by a PEPFAR-supported Ugandan group that had replaced the group that had replaced JCRC. I'd let the staff know I was coming and meandered around, meeting people who worked there, until I settled down in a chair opposite a clinic staffer named Lydia, who'd been there since the first days when JCRC handed off its clients and who was in charge of follow-up and outreach—an updated version of Hajjarah's job.

She sat opposite me and reeled off from memory the "cohorts" she was keeping track of—groups of clients who'd been in care for twelve, twenty-four, and thirty-six months. She knew the retention rates for each cohort. She had to report this information into DATIM, where it could be viewed by the PEPFAR team in country and the leaders in DC. She knew when people's twelve-month visits were coming up, and a few days prior, she began to make calls. Please remember to come in, she said. "So that my retention remains high." The prior quarter, one cohort had been at 80 percent; this quarter, she'd gotten it to 97 percent. PEPFAR measured virologic suppression, so she also followed up with people on ART whose viral loads had started to climb. At any given time, she was working on tracking ninety people down, sending PEPFAR-funded staff out into the field, and relying on government-funded, community-based health workers whom PEPFAR had paid her team to train.

After that, I'd gone to sit in a clinic room. I hadn't been in one for several years. On the quick trips I'd made with one or both children traveling along with me, there hadn't been time to pull up a chair and sit until I faded into the background of a doctor's day. Now, my sons were older. I tested their patience and the energy of Liam and our nanny, Ben. But when they swam into view on my cell phone at night, wheeling around in Cadman Plaza, eating popcorn and ice creams, ignoring—as they should—my pleas to talk about the day, I knew that it was all right for me to be away.

The clinic room was big, airy, plain. The doctor had a desk, a wall of shelves beside her; the client's seat was a straight-backed chair. I sat down, and the doctor greeted me, then turned toward a woman wearing a black, gauzy head scarf and matching dress. She was small-boned, petite. The formal intimacy of the doctor-client exchange was still the same. The women exchanged greetings, discussed the client's health, whether she'd had fever, cough, or fatigue.

But then the conversation changed to a script that had been written in America. The doctor wanted, with some urgency, to get the woman's permission to test her husband as well. It just wouldn't work, the slender woman said. It just wasn't possible. The doctor asked if perhaps they could go out to her home on a day when she herself would not be there, maybe a market day. Could they park at the edge of the property and say they were doing a health fair?

"No," she said, stiff and small. I asked the physician why the woman had such concerns. She relayed the question, and the woman's body softened as she began to weep. Her husband beat her. She was not yet twenty. She had not told him she had HIV.

Under PEPFAR's index testing guidelines, every program had to have a referral system for people at risk of domestic violence. Lydia came into the room and stood by the corner of the table. No, she said, the referral system was not yet in place. They did not have a partner in the community. The doctor had spoken for a few more moments with the young woman in her black, gauzy veil. They would not try to test the husband for now. When the woman left, the doctor turned to me and said how interesting the exchange had been. Usually, she did not take the time to ask her patients such personal questions.

"I don't find anything impossible. We eventually get to 'yes,'" I'd heard Birx say in a podcast interview.[38] There was a scientific rationale for every yes she obtained. But the relentlessness was cause for pause. There were no data on how hard a country, clinic, physician, or person living with HIV could be pushed to do something faster or differently.

As I spoke with Lydia, I noticed a distinction between the targets, which seemed to come from the outside, and the data, which they embraced and owned. I found the same thing with Abisagi Nampijja, the HIV and tuberculosis information officer assigned to show me around the Rakai Health Sciences Program (RHSP) when I arrived in Kalisizo.

Like Lydia, Dr. Amongi, and Cissy, Nampijja spent a good portion of her time ensuring that her government counterparts provided quality services to people living with HIV. Clients still came to the Rakai clinic for services. As we talked in her office, I could see women and babies sitting on benches through her open door. But the majority of clients were now seen at government facilities, where she relied on local staff and district health teams (DHTs) to work with her to solve problems. It was hard, she said. The district health officers didn't always provide the funds allocated for the clinics; they didn't always show up for events. But once she got a DHT member on her side, anything was possible. Bringing the data back to the people who served the community got them excited, involved. It was the opposite of what Sister Natalya had experienced years prior—when she'd been told that her clinic was failing, without being given a chance to review the findings or suggest a solution.

"If you're on good terms with the people down [at the community level], then you're good," Nampiija said. She loved to bring data back to the DHTs and ask them what they thought was causing a loss of TB patients or a drop in HIV retention. "If you get people who are really interested in what they do—ahhh," she let out a long, delighted sigh. "It makes everything very exciting. When you get DHT members and district focal persons, with even the little money they get [paid], you see how passionate they are when you tell them about performance."

In Rakai, Tororo, and Fort Portal, the groups providing the technical assistance were all "indigenous," Ugandan-run organizations. In 2018, Birx had announced that 70 percent of all PEPFAR funding had to go to indigenous groups within thirty months.[39] These groups weren't the government, but they also weren't American. They chafed at the targets, but they loved the data and conveyed that enthusiasm to government counterparts who worked in a system that was shockingly unchanged.

In Rakai, I'd prevailed on a head pharmacist to take me out to Kasasa, where I'd been on one of my first trips in 2005. The pharmacist spent her days fixing errors caused by mismanagement at the government-run National Medical Stores (NMS), which had taken over the supply chain a few years prior. PEPFAR Uganda now required all of its partners to get their drugs through NMS; it also paid staff at nongovernmental organizations like the RHSP to troubleshoot the problems with an underfunctioning agency that sent out oversupplies to one place and left stockouts in another.

The pharmacist had her laptop open in the van, working while we drove, and I tried not to interrupt her. She walked me in to meet the local government health worker who ran the antiretroviral clinic. She sat in a barnlike room—a new building had been erected on the property—with a wall of shelves behind her. While the health worker chatted with the pharmacist, I looked at the color-coded folders in their neat stacks. It was the same filing and tracking system that RHSP used at headquarters: clients who were pregnant in one stack, those who had missed appointments in another, those with detectable viral loads in another, and so on.

I knew the pharmacist needed to get back to work, but I allowed myself one reminiscence. There were once all these beds, I said. All these empty wooden bed frames. "Oh, yeah," the pharmacist replied, then walked me around to the back of the clinic where a rank of pale, blond, mattress-less frames sat under the eaves. "They're still here."

The Rakai project investigators had turned over the reins of the ART project to the next generation. Dr. Joseph Kagaayi, who'd been just out of medical school when I met him in 2005, was now the director of the field office. I was also interested in what the long-time researchers thought of the new emphasis on data. "I was very skeptical," RHSP cofounder Dr. David Serwadda told me one afternoon while we ate chicken salad sandwiches at his office at the Institute of Public Health. When he'd been told that the project would need to look at their data every week—as a recent "surge" had required—he'd thought, "How is this going to help us? How are we going to change this every week?" But he'd come around. "It has really made us focus our mind. . . . We are using data all the time. Not one month or six months but every week. That really has put us on our toes but it has also made us focus where we are not doing well much sooner than we would have otherwise. . . . Everybody's game is up." Serwadda also told me how much he relished the independence that the Rakai Project had secured in its earliest negotiations. "I credit Jonathan [Mermin]," he said. "He has been our best head so far. I realized much later that the way Uganda got its money is not the way every other country did."[40]

As I spoke with Dr. Serwadda, Abisagi Nampijja, and the others, I could almost see the numbers in the Data Pack scrolling between us, like the lines of binary code in *The Matrix*. The health professionals had the same satisfaction that activists had when we hacked through the thicket of abbreviations to locate a problem that we knew could be solved. In a report from the Office of the Inspector General, the overwhelming majority of PEPFAR staff surveyed said also that they appreciated the emphasis on data and the quarterly data reviews.[41]

Dr. Joshua Musinguzi, the head of Uganda's Ministry of Health AIDS Control Program (ACP), told me he appreciated the emphasis on data too. A veteran of the AIDS response, Musinguzi could reel off names and acronyms from programs of past decades; he could remember when, as a young doctor, he'd been asked to sit in on AIDS-focused government meetings when the ACP's then head, Dr. Elizabeth Madraa, had been away on business travel. In those meetings, he'd listened to Peter Mugyenyi—"very pragmatic"—who'd urged the government to start to scale up AIDS treatment with TASO and JCRC and the other nongovernmental programs that were ready to go. He'd seen the initial "cooperative agreement" between CDC and the Ministry of Health put in place by Jono Mermin—"excellent guy"—to help build surveillance and testing capacity. The same "cooperative agreement" was in place nearly twenty years later, and it had grown to encompass a range of other activities.

But to Musinguzi, the "turning point" had come in 2009, when PEPFAR had insisted that the country redo its country operational plan with an eye on geographic prioritization, ambitious targets, and better use of data. "We had to go back to the drawing board," he told me. "Since that time, there has been a big leap in terms of results that we have continued to achieve in subsequent periods."

At the time that we spoke, PEPFAR paid for more than 90 percent of the country's AIDS response. Musinguzi knew that and likely knew that I did too. He had ample reason to tell an American writer whom he'd met a handful of times over the years that he had no complaints with the new approach. But he was also trying to control an epidemic in a country where the president had long since turned his attention to other issues, including reportedly deploying threats, violence, intimidation of opposition candidates, and efforts at constitutional reform to secure more years in the State House. When I heard him say PEPFAR was an ally, I thought he meant it and wasn't just being polite.

A few days before, I'd had coffee with Amy Cunningham, who'd returned the year prior to serve as the country's PEPFAR coordinator. She told me she felt like all of the jobs she'd had in her life—from high school cheerleader to military journalist to USAID AIDS advisor—had prepared her for the role, and she'd embraced it with enthusiasm and focus. When she'd set her sights on getting the government of Uganda to increase its financial contributions to the AIDS fight, she'd leveraged every relationship she had and relied on the political capital and savvy of the minister of health, Dr. Jane Aceng, who'd run an AIDS treatment clinic in northern Uganda in the earliest days of PEPFAR. Aceng had a reputation for being close with the First Lady and having conservative religious views that worked against comprehensive sexual health and HIV prevention services for adolescent girls and young women, but she'd worked with Cunningham and other development partners to secure a $13 million commitment from the government for buying AIDS drugs—a doubling of its prior investment.

To Musinguzi, that money had flowed despite, and not because of, government commitment, and PEPFAR had played a key role. "The COP [country operational plan] process was really, really well done," he said. "Ministry of Finance is always having all these [competing] issues that they see as priorities. But the pressure [to invest] this time was so strong that it was almost this time like a precondition." Cunningham had urged the investment because she figured that PEPFAR funding wouldn't be around forever—but she'd used the program's clout and presence to secure the commitment.

No one I spoke to, including Musinguzi, seemed to think that the Ministry of Health should be running the AIDS treatment programs directly. In a decentralized health system, it was a coordinating body that made rules, issued guidelines and policies, and dispensed funding to the district level. He and Cunningham were working on setting up a regional technical support role, which also didn't exist at the government level. But as for overall government management, that was "for discussion for the future."[42]

In the meantime, PEPFAR Uganda was, like all other PEPFAR programs, moving towards "indigenization"—an awkward term that referred to shifting resources from the international NGOs to local, nationally registered and run groups. By 2021, 70 percent of all PEPFAR resources needed to go to "indigenous" groups. Overnight, JCRC, TASO, and RHSP—the "legacy partners" who'd once bedeviled PEPFAR headquarters with their historic entanglements and distinct cultures—became a tremendous asset and were asked to do more, not less, to take on additional districts, and, in the case of JCRC, to resume providing antiretrovirals at a large scale with PEPFAR dollars.

Musinguzi was optimistic about indigenization and positive about PEPFAR overall. But the program and the process looked distinctly different to government officials working in the districts. In Tororo, I visited the district health officer, the government official in charge of the network of clinics and hospitals serving Tororo District. I'd met Dr. David Okumo in 2005, when he'd held the same position. Then, he'd professed confusion about the plethora of donor-funded efforts in his ward, which in 2005 included ART clinics run by TASO, JCRC, and Uganda Cares (a project of AIDS Healthcare Foundation), as well as a government program with drugs from the Global Fund.

Fifteen years later, Okumo had mastered the cast of characters, including the different agencies that spent PEPFAR money. He was, as he explained, fed up. Okumo didn't mind that money was coming into the district and going to NGOs, but up until 2016, the CDC had managed the PEPFAR program, consistently asked him what his priorities were for the district, and helped fund them. USAID had taken over and stopped asking. He wanted PEPFAR to hold the implementing partners accountable, to "show proof they have engaged the actors they are going to work with [and] not for them to sit in Kampala and [say], 'This is what we are going to do.'" CDC had listened to him; USAID did not. "They have lost track. Their needs are totally different," he said in exasperation. He said he got no money from the national government for HIV and about $2,000 per quarter for everything else: sanitation, immunization, supplies, and more. When PEPFAR came in with a goal, it changed everything. He thought index testing was fine, but it was happening "at the expense of other programs." Things were shutting down, he said. "Everyone is out there looking for HIV-positives. Nobody wants to talk about anything else."[43]

In Uganda, the program seemed, if anything, more tightly bound to American strategy than it had fifteen years prior. But it also seemed far more focused. Mercy for mercy's sake had given way to an all-out effort to end epidemic levels of new infections. Birx's first actions—geographic prioritization, rebuilding the COP modules, instituting the quarterly data reviews and site visits—put an end to an ambivalence at the heart of the AIDS war as to whether the US government had, with its resources, bought the right to dictate strategy. America was paying to control AIDS, not to learn what policymakers preferred.

To some extent, PEPFAR took steps to address some of these structural and social issues that elevated risk of HIV and made it difficult to start and stay on treatment. Birx and Achrekar teamed up with the American ambassador to Malawi to forge a collaborative plan with the government and USAID to construct secondary schools so that every Malawian adolescent girl had a class to attend during the period in her life when she was at highest risk of HIV. To do this, they'd obtained a commitment from the Malawian government and non-PEPFAR funds from USAID. In 2020, the country operational plan guidance—the annual strategy directive to the field—included sections on how to help local groups serving men who have sex with men, transgender people, and sex workers find grants and generate their own income, as well as on the role of debt relief in freeing up countries' own finances. The narrow slice of priorities for PEPFAR defined by the program's first head, Randall Tobias, had expanded. But the coordination of American aid agencies working on AIDS hadn't actually improved.

Birx and the Malawi team had leveraged non-PEPFAR funding for the work, but that was on their own initiative. There was no cohesive approach that linked a country's PEPFAR resources with, say, its Millennium Challenge Corporation (MCC) grant or other US-AID projects. In Malawi, while PEPFAR orchestrated the building of schools, a $350.7 million MCC "compact" paid for work on the power sector, infrastructure, and environmental stewardship. Electrifying the country, improving infrastructure, and managing resources would all indisputably benefit Malawians—eventually. At the close of the compact, the MCC and its government collaborators projected a twenty-year time frame for realizing benefits. In the short term, it was the private sector engaged in the power-sector work that almost certainly saw the most immediate benefit.[44]

Developing an American approach to aid and trade that was neither hypocritical—offering less in aid than was extracted in trade—nor fragmented according to different strategic objectives and time frames was a monumental task. So were the costs, whether measured in persistent pandemics or planetary destruction. "Thereby hangs a tale whose implications we could not and did not see at the time," Ngugi wa Thiong'o had written of the missed opportunity for newly independent nations to fully dismantle colonialism. As the tale of postcolonial capitalism had shown, the implications were grave indeed.

In Kampala, Thiong'o's verdant dreamscape had long since been replaced by traffic-clogged streets and mega-malls with water features and faux marble floors. The city's landscape had been remade in part to provide cappuccinos, hotel rooms, and prefurnished flats to the globe-trotting global health establishment and businesspeople—many from China—seeking land and economic partnership. A monument to convenience, the new urban sprawl was bad for the environment—and for public health. When trees and forests disappeared, sediment from denuded hillsides flowed into Lake Victoria, along with factory waste and fertilizer from agribusiness. Sociologist Sanyu Mojola linked the declining fish population in Lake Victoria to rising HIV risk in its fishing communities—as they traveled farther and competed for fewer fish, men found new sexual partners at the lake-side villages where they sold their catch.[45]

To truly tackle AIDS, or any other pandemic, one had to address the destruction of the climate, the violence of extractive capitalism, and the enduring fear of and urge to control the female body. I'd learned this lesson in the earliest years of working on HIV. For a time, after the drugs had come to sub-Saharan Africa, I'd waited for the revolution. Then I'd worried about whether and how the AIDS fight would survive. When the concept of treatment as prevention reinvigorated the "investment case" for AIDS, I watched as funding failed to keep pace with the rhetoric of ending AIDS. Now the talk was of epidemic "control," a word that evoked the exercise of power, self-restraint and denial, and ongoing effort all at once. Could a primarily biomedical response lead to a viral détente—one in which this pandemic waned, even as the conditions that would allow the next one to emerge remained the same?

— —

WHEN I RETURNED HOME from Uganda in 2018, I started asking people working in the field whether the science- and evidence-base for the program's targets justified the hands-on management approach that Birx and her team took with programs in the field. I knew that she assigned targets that, if met, would lead to "epidemic control" and that the DC headquarters team pushed for those targets even when country teams pushed back. As a report from the Office of the Inspector General (OIG) documented, she and her team refused at times, to reduce the targets when country teams or partners said they were simply unfeasible.[46] I wanted to understand the trade-offs between pushing for the numbers required to control the epidemic even when they were impossible and the risk involved in settling for less. The answer came back: it was a laser focus—and it burned.

"When you take a situation and you withdraw power from the parties that are meant to be your partners, then you are directing the show, and that means that you've not even doubled your job. You've multiplied it beyond any comprehension because you're now responsible for managing a situation where people don't necessarily have a belief in the goals any longer," one American public health expert, with years of PEPFAR work under his belt, said to me in 2019. He was starting to see data in the form of Americans voting with their feet. "I know a number of people who are leaving the program now . . . I see people saying they don't even want to get anywhere near a PEPFAR country or budget line."

Many people linked the program's identity directly back to Deborah Birx. The same OIG report collected sixty-eight PEPFAR staffers' views on the leadership provided by the ambassador and her team. Nearly two-thirds were negative, with the report plucking out three adjectives—"dictatorial," "directive," and "autocratic"—that would become an epithet for Birx in the months to come. People did not like to be told what to do—especially when "OGAC issues threats" or when the directive was "programmatically harmful."

"For the last three or four years they aren't decisions driven by Washington. They are decisions driven by one incredibly powerful individual, who sometimes does not like to be confused by facts and reality, much less what countries think is in their own best interest," an ex-PEPFAR staffer told me, saying he had "survivors' guilt" over not being involved with the program anymore.

Not everyone found Birx's power insurmountable. Deborah Malac, the US ambassador to Uganda when I visited in 2019, had worked with PEPFAR for years and had been ambassador to Liberia during the Ebola virus crisis. When I sat down with her at the embassy on Ggaba Road, she told me that her experiences had left her interested in public health and PEPFAR in ways that set her apart from her colleagues. "My willingness to push back on OGAC is a bit unique," she said. "I think sometimes they tend to take that direction from OGAC at face value." She and Birx shared the same goal of achieving epidemic control, but that didn't mean she'd agreed with the means to the end. She added, "Debbi Birx knows that she can't just order us around."[47]

When I asked Birx's predecessor, Ambassador Eric Goosby, about the decision to drive hard for "90-90-90" targets and other milestones on the path to epidemic control, he said, "Debbi's drive saved more lives." A program that placed more of a premium on, say, building local ownership might not have reached as many people with the medications.

Goosby did have concerns, just not ones he could say outweighed the decisions Birx had made. He had issues with a disease-specific program that seventeen years later still had not shifted power and decision making from Washington, DC, to the countries and that still had a stringent focus on a single virus. Middle and upper management were still American, often white. The geographic, racial, and cultural disconnect between payers, providers, and clients worked against local problem solving and accountability, which Goosby described as "a self-correcting feedback loop that's created by having allocations made by people accessible and available to people [receiving] the services."

Goosby had a problem with the fact that PEPFAR had moved farther away from redistributing its power. Even as the program shifted its emphasis to making grants to "indigenous partners"— TASO, JCRC, the Rakai Project—those partners still received their targets from the groups that managed them. To cede ownership of planning processes, one should also cede control of the resources and test the possibility that there are other forms of power besides that of the US government—that a country that did not run its programs well would be held accountable by its citizens, health workers, and technocrats working for change within the system. By the time Birx assumed control of PEPFAR, it was abundantly clear that the United States would not cede such power and that this was the trade-off for continued resources.

"We just have to be really real that decisions about PEPFAR funding are 100 percent made by people in Washington, DC," Matthew Kavanagh said.[48] It was the price of American involvement. "There is no world in which the US gives the level that would be needed to the Global Fund, and therefore if we're actually going to get anywhere near what we need to do on HIV, [PEPFAR is] the only vehicle through which this level of sustained investment ever is going to happen."

I'd gone to talk to Birx and Angeli Achrekar in the PEPFAR office on G Street too. Birx, her hair up in a banana clip, seemed tired, hugging herself as we spoke. A clock in her office was set to chime every fifteen minutes to help her keep track of her time. She knew that an investigation of her management style was underway. USAID raised issues about her every year. Once, Achrekar said, they'd accidentally emailed her the complaints they were drafting about them. "We know what people say about us. If we let it get to us, we wouldn't be able to get out of bed in the morning," she said.

"The one good thing about me, the one nice thing people say, is that I have good data, I use data well," Birx said. "We always tell the truth. If we don't know something, we say we don't know." I noticed how much lower her voice was when she wasn't speaking in front of a crowd.

I wondered aloud if anything in Birx's family life had given her this will to persevere. I knew her grandparents had owned a country store, that with two brilliant brothers, she hadn't even been considered the smartest one in the family. I knew she had a strong faith, that her parents—who now lived with her—were both active in an amateur radio group that had once broadcast proselytizing messages to missionaries overseas and persisted to this day. This time, she didn't have any personal stories. "Just hard work," she said matter-of-factly. "You just work hard."

But then the mood changed, and her voice filled with the helium thrill I'd heard the night I called her from my Brooklyn railroad flat in December 2003. "I remember the State of the Union," she said. "I still think it's the most incredible thing. We have six billion dollars, nobody has six billion dollars."

"A year," Achrekar breathed. Birx leaned back in her chair.

"We ask ourselves this all the time: Is it really worth it? Are those 75,000 people really worth it?"—she'd told a story about a PEPFAR staffer pushing back against her targets. They were, those people were worth it. That was why she stayed, why she hadn't left long ago. When Birx lifted her face toward the daylight, it was filled with lines.

— —

ON MY 2018 TRIP to Uganda, I hadn't tried to find Simon. During our last encounter, five years prior, I'd decided that my own curiosity about his life was less important than his well-being. I'd come to that meeting in 2013 with hopes of understanding him better than I had in the past. I had a translator with me for the first time in years. I was there with my husband and both our sons, then three years old and four months old. We'd met on the grounds of a local church where Simon was friendly with the reverend. While Liam took our older son to play, my translator Jane and I took seats on a bench beside Simon, close by a large pot and a cooking fire.

"I'm so happy to see you," I told him. "It's been so long, and I have so many questions I'd like to ask. Is that okay?"

In reply he took out a small piece of paper, covered end to end, with no margins, with his text, and said a few lines in Lutooro. "The question I am writing is here," Jane relayed. "You tell me the answer. A good answer."

He'd answered my question with his own. I was not sure that he understood, but I handed my four-month-old to the translator and looked at the letter. It was a list of things that Simon wanted me to buy for him: pork, beef, chicken, beans, milk, the dried milk called Nido, rice, a lantern, a chair, a table, a mattress, a flashlight, a helicopter, a Pajero, a house, a cell phone of a very specific make and model, another car, and many more things. He'd run out of room on the page, which was perhaps four by six inches, squeezing his name in below the last line at the end.

I struggled not to thrust the letter back into Simon's hands or to crumple it up. I was frightened by the apparent madness of the text, which combined details of make and model and gigabytes of cell phone memory with a child's list of furnishings. I was distressed by the idea that Simon thought that happiness lay in these things and that I—the good consumer that I was—wondered for a moment if, after receiving every last item on the sheet of paper, he might smile as I remembered. I knew the answer was no. He had never had enough of anything; nothing would ever be enough.

I also felt a twisting disappointment at having yet another relationship in Uganda turn transactional. I'd been asked, over the years, for everything from the water bottle in my hand to an American husband. I'd been called to help find drugs for a man with cryptococcal meningitis—I'd found them; he'd still died—and asked to buy a refrigerator and an entire inventory worth of food for an HIV-positive woman from the Focus on Women conference who'd wanted to open a store. I'd been asked for so many things so many times that I had often said no before I'd even heard the full request. Cissy and Sandra were alive because I'd helped them twelve years prior. If they'd asked me for assistance now, I might have refused them too.

A woman who worked at the church came by and told us it would soon be time for lunch. Jane murmured to the baby. "Put you in the big pot, roll you and roll you and roll you. You want to see the big pot? I'll put you there."

"Are you working?" I asked Simon. My voice was rough and tense. I had a cold; my infant son wasn't sleeping through the night. He wasn't doing much, he explained, as he had two years prior; he said he was in pain, had a fever, felt sick all the time. "It seems like we must solve the problem of how to make it easier for you to work," I said. I told him that there was so much in the letter, that I'd found it was better to help someone find a job so they had steady income. If he did that, then we could see if he needed any extra help from me. He said he wanted to work, but he was weak. I said we needed to figure that out. What did the clinic say about how he felt, I asked. "Their words are the same," the translator relayed.

I tried to change the subject then. "I want to talk about work, but can I ask you some questions about when you were little?" I'd thought over the years of all the things I wished I could know about him. He was not the only one who'd come with a list of desired things. I began to ask my questions. His answers were brief, halting. His mother had been a teacher; he'd sometimes fallen asleep in the back of her classroom. He had been young when his parents died; he had been sad. He could not remember a favorite day or time in his life. I asked if he remembered when we had met. He said he had no recollection.

After a time, Liam came and called us to lunch. When we had arranged ourselves around heaping plates of mashed, boiled banana, bitter greens, and rice, I fussed over the baby, who had a wheezing cough, at one end of the table. Simon and Jane sat at the other end. After a long and silent meal, Simon began to speak. It was a torrent of words—more than I had heard him say since the day, three years prior, when he'd argued with Hajjarah so vociferously about wanting to go to school.

"Supposing you are to meet somebody, and then a table is set for you and then someone else messes it up," Jane eventually relayed. "How would you feel?"

"I'd feel bad," I said. "I'd feel mad. I'd feel like I didn't trust the person anymore." I wanted to know what he meant.

"It's just an example, one anyone can use."

"But what do you mean?" I pressed.

"You can find a table set. If you just go ahead and start eating without knowing why the table was prepared then you are in the wrong. You have to ask whose table it is and why it was prepared," Jane said.

"What brought it into his head?" I asked.

"It's just a picture."

But usually, I ventured, a story like that has a message, something the person is trying to say. "He's giving an example of somebody who can come, you have prepared your table, and then somebody comes and destroys it, messes it up." Jane had listened to Simon speak for some time. "Anyone can use it."

We went back and forth like that, jousting over what he meant, until finally Simon explained that I was the one who had asked him to be at the church grounds at a specific time. He had come, prepared, with his letter. After I had read it, I told him that we should talk about how to find him work, how it would be great for him to have a way to make his own money. But that had not been an answer. I had not said yes or no, only that I did not like the question. He had prepared carefully. I had not listened.

I could have apologized then, perhaps picking an item or two off the list, perhaps even opening my notebook and drawing as we had so long ago. But I didn't. Instead I lectured him, tight voiced, prim and unyielding. He had to work. I'd help if he worked. I didn't know why he couldn't work. Later, I could hardly bear to listen to the recording to transcribe it. I sounded Calvinist, ferocious, and unkind. I was speaking to myself as much as Simon, telling myself that I had to keep on writing, reporting, parenting, showing up for my job even though on many days all I wanted to do was sleep, alone, for an entire year. That was no excuse. The only grace I showed that day was realizing that I could not keep coming back to look for this young man, could not sit through another encounter in which we raised and then crushed each other's expectations.

I said good-bye to Simon for the last time in 2013. The following year, at Birx's invitation—extended to AVAC and other US-based advocacy groups—I entered Dataland, where the great heap of failures that accounted for Simon's disappointment with life would be dissected and quantified in the form of the Monitoring, Evaluation, and Reporting (MER) indicators that broke the work of fighting AIDS into strings of abbreviations—"Tx_Curr" for the number of people on treatment, "Htx_Pos" for new diagnoses.

With limits on my travel away from home, those trips to the PEP-FAR planning meetings became a time to reconvene with friends I used to visit in Uganda. At first, Lillian Mworeko hadn't been so sure she wanted to get involved. "My world was telling stories [about] women, and [now] you are telling me I have to look into figures." She thought, "That is not my world; my world is different from that." But she didn't like how the presentations sometimes ended without anyone raising a question, and so she'd set herself the task of mastering the funder's language. "We reached a level where it was very clear...if we [were] to get anything good out of the processes, we needed to be better than they [PEPFAR] expected." Always a quick study, she paid close attention when Brian Honermann, a bearded, rock-climbing activist lawyer who'd built a database to help activists decipher PEPFAR data, came to town. She'd learn PEPFAR's way of looking at the world, but she wouldn't abandon her own. "You do your statistics, your figures, your country maps but...help me understand so that I can tell a story," she remembers thinking.[49]

Birx herself expected nothing less than full fluency. She began most meetings with slide decks like the one I'd seen that day in Frankfurt. They were voluminous, often approaching one hundred screens of text and images, including population pyramids that broke down a country's HIV epidemic by gender, age band, the percentages of people with HIV in each category who did and did not know their status, and "cascades" of MER indicators showing who did and did not have AIDS drugs and did or did not have detectable levels of virus in their blood.

Seldom content to show one country's data, Birx presented three or four different case studies, breaking down where things had gone well and where they had not. She worried constantly about children like Simon—who had low rates of testing, linkage, and retention—and about adolescents who existed in an in-between world and needed specific, holistic forms of care. She seemed to worry, too, about maintaining a sense of urgency in her audience.

Birx gave her slide decks out like a hostess gives out fruitcakes, and I'd often pore over them trying to discern messages hidden in the idiosyncratic font sizes and colors that showed her handiwork as clear as fingerprints. Almost all of them ended with a slide that contained two images: a red-packed earth graveyard and a bench filled with buxom Black African women and their babies. The slide would always have the current figures for the numbers of AIDS deaths and babies born with HIV that week. The title was always a variation on a theme. It would read, "Our work is far from done," sometimes with the next line "How can we do better?" Or "Our work is far from done BUT possible." But in the slide deck Birx used on January 6, 2017, a little more than two months after the election of Donald J.

Trump, there was no subtitle, no riff at all. "Our work is far from done," the last slide's title read, and that was all.

— —

By 2016, KATY TALENTO had done a stint in a convent and almost taken religious orders, then reemerged, gotten married, and reentered the political world of American public health as a member of the Trump-Pence transition team, contributing to an internal memo that warned against giving the Global Fund too much money and setting out plans for walking back the Obama administration's firm commitments to expanding contraception and women's health coverage as part of foreign aid.

She also fielded calls about which, if any, Obama appointees should stay on. "People were lobbying us on two people. One was the head of the [National Institutes of Health (NIH), Francis Collins] and one was Debbi Birx. And I'm like, Why would they keep her? Anyone who funds Planned Parenthood is off the list," Talento recalled. The people on the other end of the phone pressed her. "No, Katy, really, she's really great."[50] Talento did take a second look and was won over by the woman she'd admiringly call "shrewd, winsome" and a master of the "simple public health math" focused on testing and treatment that Talento valued above all.[51]

Talento's phone was ringing because, when Birx had decided she wanted to stay on, she'd reportedly mobilized another campaign, getting the right people to speak up for her good name. Under Obama, this had been a largely left-leaning contingent. But Birx had a similarly sizeable and impassioned conservative corps behind her. They loved her for how she'd used data to turn the program into a target-hitting machine. Shepherd Smith, the influential Evangelical Christian AIDS advocate, thought that between the government's approach and challenges in tracking funding, PEPFAR had been "on autopilot" before Birx came on board, in spite of Ambassadors Mark Dybul and Eric Goosby's best efforts. "I don't think the program would even be potentially around now. It was that bad," Smith said.[52]

The Smiths rallied support everywhere they could. George W. Bush speechwriter and PEPFAR creator Mike Gerson would say that Ivanka Trump and Mike Pence lobbied the new president on Birx's behalf.[53] The messages got through. In late 2016, the transition team issued a survey about PEPFAR's utility during the transition weeks, with questions like "Is PEPFAR worth the massive investment when there are so many security concerns in Africa? Is PEPFAR becoming a massive, international entitlement program?"[54] But on January 19, the White House announced that both Birx and NIH head Francis Collins had been asked to stay on until their replacements could be found. Collins, like Birx, was a Christian with a strong track record of leadership and results who'd mustered Republican support along the way—several senators signed a letter in December 2016 urging the incoming president to keep the founder of the Human Genome Project in his post.

On Trump's first day in office, Birx's strategy for working with the administration became even clearer. As every Republican president did, Trump reinstated the Mexico City Policy that prohibited recipients of US foreign aid from speaking about, referring for, or providing abortion with any funding, American or otherwise. In every prior administration, the MCP had applied only to American foreign aid for family planning, about $600 million per year. Trump announced that the MCP would now apply to all US foreign aid for health, including PEPFAR. A total of more than $9 billion would now be subject to the so-called global gag.

Groups working on sexual and reproductive health and rights gasped—and gagged. The expansion was so vast and deleterious, some people wondered if Trump even knew what he was doing. But Birx, when asked, said it wouldn't be a problem. PEPFAR was "a more mature program," unlike in 2013, when the Bush administration had chosen not to apply the MCP to the fledgling initiative. There were many partners; if one opted out, she'd find another who could fill in. She had good data, "granular" data, as she loved to say. She'd use it to see whether there was any impact. She said, too, that if the funding for PEPFAR got reduced, she'd be able to manage that too. The granular details would allow her to save money on nonessential costs; she'd keep the program running no matter what.[55]

Birx's public gamble appeared to be to accept the administration's rhetoric and policies in order to keep her hands on the wheel of the program, which she insisted would remain unchanged, just like herself. It frustrated her to no end that people thought she'd begun to act differently in order to keep her job. She chafed at gossip that she'd started to wear a larger crucifix around her neck to garner Christian conservative support, an observation I reported to her. She didn't need me to tell her that observers thought she was exhibiting "chameleonlike" behavior. All of this was, to her, another example of how people discounted women's intelligence.

"What scares me the most for my daughters, for the next generation after us, is that we still can't believe that a woman can be competent, that she actually could know what she's doing and have a strategy," she said to me one day in December 2018. It was just after World AIDS Day, and she, Achrekar, and I had met for an interview at a restaurant by the Rockefeller Center skating rink. She still had her pancake makeup on from an appearance on *Good Morning America*. They were as relaxed as I'd seen them since the election.

A few days prior to our conversation, Mike Pence had called PEPFAR "inarguably one of the most successful investments in healthcare and humanitarian aid in American history."[56] In September, President Trump had signed the PEPFAR Extension Act of 2018, reauthorizing PEPFAR for another five years and $48 million.[57] He'd done so even as he derided foreign aid, African countries, the State Department, and America's role as a global citizen.

Pence was a dyed-in-the-wool conservative who'd been negligently slow to authorize syringe exchange when an opioid-related HIV outbreak surged in Indiana while he was governor. With swift action on syringe exchange, the epidemic would have been "entirely preventable," but he'd hemmed and hawed over whether the service violated antidrug policy, extending years of lethal debate within America about whether or not to follow the clear public health evidence supporting harm reduction and syringe exchange as part of a comprehensive, rights-based approach to working with people who use drugs.[58]

But one did not have to believe in evidence or resolve hypocritical positions on professed compassion and antiscience stances to support PEPFAR, and Pence had always been a believer. As far back as 2003, during the initial lawmaking, he'd risen in the House of Representatives to sing its praises, albeit while peddling the mendacious party line that the Global Fund was a payola scheme for abortionists. If he cared for the wrong reasons, he still cared—and Pence was undoubtedly a help in getting PEPFAR five more years of funding in the midst of Trump's assault on American foreign aid.

Birx knew that no one would thank her for positioning the program to get funding for another five years. "What I hear all the time is, 'She sold her soul to Republicans.' And I'm like, 'Oh yeah, honey, you don't know,'" she said that day at Rockefeller Center. She and Achrekar said they worked tirelessly to protect the program's essence—and its funding—in a volatile political environment. "It's the small little needle that we're threading every single day," Birx said. "It is every single day," Achrekar murmured, their contrapuntal dialogue in full swing. "It's so discounting, it's so dismissive," Birx went on.

Every day that they stood in the breach, the two were accused of being sellouts. I knew by then that clinics had closed rather than accept the expanded Mexico City Policy, and other programs were so worried about losing their funding that they'd stopped talking about or offering contraception—which they were still legally able to do. In a handful of documented instances, women had died of complications from unsafe abortions or unplanned pregnancies, unable to receive care from clinics that had once been there to serve them.[59] Every day brought new questions about whether the ends justified the means.

To Birx, those questions were evidence of the world's vendetta against her and other strong women. "People will use everything that I do to demean what I've accomplished. And I don't know why, but it's gonna continue to happen," she said at Rockefeller Center. She looked at me. "It would be good if you figured that out."

"Oh, you want *me* to figure that out?" My voice squeaked. Earlier, she and Achrekar had chuckled over the people who met with them without researching them first. They always made it a point to know whom they were talking to. We talked about how society underestimated women, how it discounted Birx, how it dismissed female intellect and turned demanding women into difficult people. We'd circled around these topics for more than an hour while the skaters on the Rockefeller Center rink slid past like fish in an aquarium. I thought I was asking questions dispassionately; now I wasn't so sure. I'd turned to Birx for different things over the years: permission to believe in PEPFAR in 2003, clues about how to be a woman in the world. I thought I'd been discrete, now I wondered if she'd noticed, and wanted to be sure I understood what it meant to be her ally at a moment when she was losing some of the activist confidence that had carried her into her position in the first place.

It wasn't just the position on the expanded Mexico City Policy that had activists worried. After Trump's election, "I felt like [she] and Angeli went into their bubble," Paul Zeitz said. "They didn't see the whole picture because they were trying to fit in [with the new administration] and protect the program overall. I don't think it was about ego. It was like she hadn't done what she came to do and she could navigate these choppy waters and there was high risk of someone worse coming in."[60]

To some extent, it worked. As the Trump administration put children in cages, split up families, sought to undo the patchy public health safety net of the Affordable Care Act, and eviscerated the morale and personnel roles of the State Department, Birx and Achrekar continued to lead a program that kept its funding and mandate. The DREAMS program, which focused on adolescent girls and young women, continued to pay for gathering spaces where girls and the leaders in their communities were taught to value young female lives as worthy of education, independent income, and choice. Many girls learned about their bodies and the options for preventing pregnancy and acquisition of HIV; in 2020, PEPFAR presented evidence that new HIV infections in adolescent girls and young women had dropped by more than 25 percent in nearly all the places where the program operated. In some geographies, by PEPFAR's calculations, it had dropped even more.[61] In 2019, after significant delays PEPFAR also launched a $100 million program focused on gay men, transgender men and women, sex workers, and people who inject drugs—the Key Populations Investment Fund—even as Trump "gutted" domestic and international commitments to LGBT rights.[62]

Where there were complaints, there was also caution and discretion: If Birx left, who would be put in charge? If she was not there to lead the program, and if a new Trump appointee took over, would there be any program left to lead?

Even as activists grappled with these questions, they also kept on working in Dataland, traveling annually to the PEPFAR planning meetings in those strange no-place South African hotels where a country became a conference room with its name on a sheet of paper taped to a door. I loved sitting in those rooms as much as I loved sitting in clinics, and for many of the same reasons. Tedious or frustrating hours went by, but if I waited long enough, I would witness an individual, through the sheer force of will, changing the system, manifesting a world.

In 2018, Tony Fauci told me that the activists were talking in "vagaries" when PEPFAR was launched. I admired him tremendously and valued his contributions and candor. In 2020, I repeated that phrase to him and asked if I'd understood his analysis correctly.

"The activist role was much less of an issue with regard to PEPFAR," he said. "That's just because the most vocal and the most effective was, you know, the ACT UP crowd." He named a number of indispensable activists. They were all white men. They'd been my mentors and changed the world. But they were not the only heroes.

In the PEPFAR planning rooms, I watched Maureen Milanga brace her hand on the table before she spoke, like a sprinter taking her mark, while in the room next door, my indefatigable friend and colleague Maureen Luba flipped pages in her native Malawi's data and plans, pointing out discrepancies and advancing demands with patient stubbornness that dispensed with her country's proclaimed collegiality. "No more 'Malawi-nice,'" she'd say. In the Uganda room, a government representative had once demanded that Margaret Happy come and stand at the front of the room to apologize for claiming, correctly, that there were major stockouts. Ken Mwehonge had stood with her. No one took the heat alone.

Felix Mwanza wouldn't come back after the year he won the treatment slots. There was, he said, "bad blood" between him and the PEPFAR team. But new Zambian advocates arrived and took up the work of pushing for greater ambition.

Finding Lillian Mworeko in the hall, she'd raise a hand and slap it into mine. "My dear, these people," she'd say, and burst out laughing. These people didn't stand a chance against her, as long as they let her in the room. And that was why, in spite of everything, I loved Dataland. For one or two weeks every year, it was home to the most powerful and effective activists I had ever seen.

You never knew who would turn up there either. In 2017, Prudence Mabele sliced through the crowd beside me during the coffee break. I knew of her, but I did not think we'd ever officially met. When we locked eyes, she broke into a giant, toothy grin. If she didn't know me, she seemed to know why I was there.

Four months later, Pru was gone. On July 10, 2017, she died of pneumonia, leaving a world of questions about how she had grown so depleted and why so few people talked openly about the enormous pressure of taking daily medications for decades to control HIV. Yvette Raphael tried to take over the Positive Women's Network. She went through the books Mabele had kept, found the budget lines for members' funeral funds, food parcels, support groups and counseling. She became the interim executive director even as she set up her own organization. She tried hard but eventually realized that the organization was enmeshed with her friend, perhaps by design. "Pru set it up not to survive without her," she said.[63] We'd started the call with our video on, but she turned it off as we spoke. "Pru was a perfectionist," she said. "She believed in her own hard work." She listed the people, including herself, including me, who took on more than they should and then tried to do it all themselves because no one could do it better.

Deborah Birx, who believed in her own hard work as much as anyone I had ever known, was at the annual in-person PEPFAR meeting in Johannesburg when she'd been summoned back to Washington, DC, to become the national coronavirus response coordinator at the end of February 2020. "We need her!" an activist messaged in dismay. Without her gimlet eye and willingness to stand her ground, negotiations with countries on key activist issues might be jeopardized. But she'd already departed for a world that the people she'd left behind could not yet apprehend. By the time they did, the illusion of control and order afforded by the data would be shattered— gone for good. In its place, only a question: What happened to an unfinished plague war when another one began?

CHAPTER 14

THE BEGINNING

I T'S LIKE WE ARE back to the beginning again," Lillian Mworeko said one day in June 2020, when the COVID-19 pandemic was well underway. In the earliest days of the AIDS epidemic, when there had been no drugs in the clinics and people with the virus had often been shunned by their families, women like Mworeko, Yvette Raphael, Milly Katana, and so many others had gone door to door, seeing who needed food, care, or support. They'd helped comrades survive and received the same comfort when they themselves faltered. That local web of community-based care had been eroded as funding went to pills and the clinics that provided them. Now the life and death impact of devaluing community-based work was abundantly clear.

With the COVID-19 lockdowns, people were back in their homes, often without food or income; gender-based violence was rising, as were unplanned pregnancy rates. No clinic-based service could help. Mworeko went to the Ugandan Ministry of Health and picked up a sticker that allowed her to drive her vehicle during lockdown. The virus that had once been a source of stigma now afforded stature. She packed her car with food and went to see women living with HIV. She was back at the beginning again.

Back at the beginning but also changed. Raphael, Mworeko, and others who lived with HIV and had lived through the years of untreated AIDS knew what was coming, even before the COVID-19 pandemic recapitulated AIDS with fearsome fidelity and accelerated velocity. Anyone could get the virus, and at first all sorts of people did. But within a month of the first closures in America, reports began flowing in. The virus spread disproportionately among those whom the state was most likely to neglect: Black, indigenous, and other people of color in the United States, the elderly, and low-wage frontline workers. HIV itself did not cause gender-based violence; nor did COVID-19. Yet beatings, rapes, and unplanned pregnancies surged amid COVID lockdowns, as predictable as fever and shortness of breath.

"Are you breathing?" Raphael, Mworeko, and I took turns asking that question in a WhatsApp chat. Sometimes Raphael posted pictures of the meals she'd prepared; Mworeko shared the chore chart she and her extended family devised. We laughed about how Mworeko—who did not like to cook—would cope with a weekly assignment of preparing breakfast. We tried to keep it light, but when a message did not arrive for too long, the question came: "Are you breathing?" We held vigils for each other as one of us, then the next, ran a fever, felt her chest tighten, or confessed she wasn't sleeping. Our families and incomes were intact, our fridges full. We knew we were lucky; we also knew that many people living close by and thousands of miles away were not. To work on "global AIDS" was to have a bodily sense of a pandemic's reach. The work of doing it for both AIDS and COVID-19 was exhausting.

"I want to go look at nothing but water for two days," Mworeko said to me in September 2020. It had been three months since she'd gotten the vehicle sticker. President Museveni had eased the lockdown, and the anticipated explosion of COVID cases in Africa had not yet occurred. Nevertheless, poor people were getting poorer, rates of HIV testing and new treatment initiations were dropping, and gains in childhood immunization, tuberculosis diagnosis, and preventive treatment were all being undone as health systems diverted attention and resources to the new pandemic. She made plans to go to Kalanagala, the lakeside district that had been home to some of the earliest cases of AIDS. I imagined her staring at the tarnished silver surface of the lake and nothing else, taking a break from seeing key gains unraveling. You should go, I urged.

My own eyes ached from hours spent scrolling the news on my phone. But even as I longed to take a break from reading, I kept on swiping through stories, clicking on maps, pinching out, zooming in. Every day, I checked the colors on the map: my county in New York City, then the country, then the world. For much of the second half of 2020, the global maps of COVID-19 prevalence showed sub-Saharan Africa as largely pale, while other parts of the world—and all of the United States—turned ever-deeper shades of red.

Many things were missing from those COVID-19 maps. In November 2020, the United Nations Children's Fund (UNICEF) reported "steep declines in facility-based care such as childbirth services, immunizations, treatment of children with severe malnutrition and healthcare for sick children," with especially acute effects in South Asia, the Middle East, and countries in Latin America. UNICEF forecast up to 10,000 additional childhood deaths due to wasting or malnutrition each month and projected that these preventable fatalities would occur primarily in sub-Saharan Africa and South Asia.[1] The United Nations Population Fund (UNFPA) projected millions of unplanned pregnancies and documented the surge in gender-based violence.[2] Two-thirds of countries surveyed by the World Health Organization reported disruptions in family-planning and contraceptive services between mid-May and early July 2020.[3] In March 2020, the world's largest condom manufacturer was briefly forced to close, then reopened at half capacity.[4] The maps did not track rates of condom-less sex in men who have sex with men or transgender women. Nor did the COVID-19 maps show disruptions in services for people who use drugs, including drops in visits to methadone-maintenance treatment programs—an essential element of harm reduction.[5]

Almost as soon as the COVID pandemic took on global proportions, both PEPFAR and the Global Fund took steps to ensure that countries could use their resources to respond to the new pandemic—while continuing to work on the other diseases. The Global Fund put hundreds of millions of dollars into a COVID-19 Response Mechanism.[6] PEPFAR used its granular data to track and address service and supply disruptions and issued guidance to the field. Where it could, the program rapidly shifted to multi-month dispensing of antiretroviral refills available at community locations close to people's homes.[7] Giving people three- or six-month supplies of medications in churches, schoolyards, or town squares helped decongest clinics, a boon to the health system and to people living with HIV. According to PEPFAR's own analysis, these shifts helped the program rebound from drops in HIV testing and treatment initiation in the first months after COVID.[8] PEPFAR's "Data Dashboard" also tracked an uptick in people starting pre-exposure prophylaxis (PrEP).[9] The program's flexibility helped stave off initial crisis-level declines in testing and treatment. But holding steady had never been the plan. The work to achieve epidemic control depended on continuing to prevent new infections, and to continue expanding treatment rolls as COVID rates climbed.

The week in March 2020 that UNAIDS shut down its offices and turned to teleworking, I called Dr. Winnie Byanyima, the Ugandan feminist who'd headed Oxfam International before becoming the agency's new head in 2019, and asked her how the world could possibly address COVID-19, HIV, escalating gender-based violence, and disruptions in reproductive health services at the same time. "It's really challenging to governments that have been designed by men and continue to be run and led by men," she replied. "The challenge is that it's about being able to work at many levels at the same time."[10] She said she knew that women in the markets and villages knew what they needed; politicians just had to listen.

Months later, in December 2020, UNAIDS released a new set of targets, looking beyond the "90-90-90" goals and designed to address ongoing failures to prevent new infections in adolescent girls, young women, LGBT individuals, and drug users. Byanyima and her team had put together a set of aims that broke the siloes she'd spoken about. UNAIDS said that epidemic control depended on testing, treatment, and virologic suppression—as it always had—but it also required ensuring that 95 percent of women of reproductive age had "their sexual and reproductive health services needs met" and that 95 percent of people at risk of HIV infection used "appropriate, prioritized, person-centred and effective combination prevention approaches."[11]

The new vision was exciting and inspiring—and it would be profoundly challenging to deliver. Within days of the UNAIDS report release, the monthly status report of the Global Fund to Fight AIDS, Tuberculosis, and Malaria found that 16 percent of countries surveyed had "high" or "very high" rates of HIV service disruption.[12] Unlike PEPFAR, which tracked its specific programs, the Fund surveyed governments. The reported disruptions were a decline from previous reports, but each day of disruption left a backlog of people in need of diagnosis, treatment, and care, not only for HIV but for tuberculosis, malaria, and other endemic diseases.

The segments of society most likely to suffer as a result of these disruptions were also those most vulnerable to COVID-19: poor, marginalized Black and brown people and wage-based and frontline workers. In other ways, the two pandemics were quite different. The hugely ambitious and highly coordinated attempt to make and manufacture a vaccine was unlike any mobilization that had ever occurred in research on AIDS or other diseases. Yet familiar fault lines emerged too. Wealthy nations prepurchased vaccine doses for their own citizens at rates that far outpaced their contribution to funds for low-income countries.[13] Concerns about intellectual property, patents, and global access emerged—just as they had with antiretrovirals. When the first vaccines were licensed, America's distribution efforts often seemed disastrously ill planned. But at least the country had doses to distribute; low-income countries, including those in Africa where rates of COVID were creeping up, would be expected to wait up to a year.[14] "Revolt is the word. Has it reached you?" Mworeko wrote to me one day on the thread we shared with Raphael. "The vaccine or the revolution?" I asked. Raphael answered first. "Both."

— —

WHEN NEW YORK SHUT its schools, I rearranged my day so that I could be my younger son's teaching aide. Our family life, which had once been marked by comings and goings, was now defined by the appearance of dirt, the announcement of appetites. I went days without leaving the house for more than a few minutes, just as I had when the children had been newborns. Time seemed to loop backward and to move herky-jerky fast.

When President Yoweri Museveni declared a lockdown, I thought of Maama Apollo, her daughter Olivia, and Apollo in their house in the slum. Informal workers like Maama Apollo risked fines or beatings for walking the streets selling clothing. With the schools closed, Olivia was home all the time, along with her brother, who was now a teenager. I worried about what would happen to their bodies without food, without a way to earn money, without permission to move. "What do they need?" I asked Cissy. "What do you need?" She worried about herself, her children, her mother in the village many kilometers away. I sent her money, and we pieced together plans for survival, just as we had at the beginning of our friendship when I'd given her a few hundred dollars at a time to purchase antiretroviral drugs. I emailed the reverend who'd been Simon's steadfast benefactor and asked him how Simon was faring. He was well, the reverend replied. He was happiest when he was working in the garden, only sometimes coming to him with requests that the reverend buy him a plane. I was happier than I should have been to get this news. In the past I'd wished for Simon to find peace, reliable strength, and perhaps a partner and a family. Now I was overjoyed that nothing had changed.

One of the strangest losses—not the greatest but among the most surreal—was Dr. Deborah Birx. I'd last seen her in January 2020, when I'd gone to her home to interview her husband, Paige Reffe, for this book. She'd made me toast and offered me jam, then padded off in loose-fitting fleece pants to try to put together a briefing on the issues that would arise if China or other countries started using an HIV medication to treat the coronavirus that I was hardly paying any attention to. Reffe, who'd been an advance man for President Bill Clinton, knew how to tell a story—and he told me plenty. But all his tales, in one way or another, were about how much he loved his wife. He loved how she'd impressed their contractors by noticing what high-quality two-by-fours they were using and how she'd refused to get married to him until their children from previous marriages had had their own weddings. "It was *their* time," she'd told him. She'd been right, he said, just as she'd been right to go ahead and purchase the high-top tables, flatware, and china needed for multiple events.[15] It was cheaper than renting them, and anyway, Birx put on even the largest parties on her own. She and Angeli Achrekar did all the cooking for the annual Christmas party that I'd attended a month before—that was where I'd met Reffe.

Like most people I'd spoken to who counted Birx as an intimate, Reffe loved her because of, not despite, her ferocious attention to every last detail in her world, her dauntingly boundless energy, and her belief that she needed to do many things herself. Though she was not yet the Coronavirus Task Force coordinator, she was heading to the White House that afternoon for a briefing. The next time I saw her, she was on my television screen.

After Birx became the White House coronavirus response coordinator on February 27, 2020, she appeared to do precisely what she'd done with PEPFAR. She demanded data, insisting that the information, when she got it, would provide the answers. I listened to her talk at the White House briefings and heard her say things she'd said many times before in the context of AIDS—how she needed the data to understand where infections were happening and why. "Using data" had a sort of vagueness to it in a world where just about everything used data in one way or another and anyone with a smartphone was billed for how much they used per month. Birx had precious little time to explain what it was that she did with data and why she thought it was important—but as the briefings went on and the epidemic engulfed the United States with unforgiving speed, it became clear, too, that the data were not enough.

The obstacles appeared daily, hourly, nightly—the president meting out new forms of humiliation to a physician who was also a colonel, an oath-sworn healer with faith in the chain of command. During a televised briefing in which the president suggested drinking bleach, she clasped her hands and looked at her feet. Birx served at the pleasure of the vice president; if she launched a direct critique, she risked losing her job. She also believed deeply in the chain of command that had defined her military career. She would only speak—as she did in the bleach briefing—when she was called on.

The same did not hold true for Dr. Anthony Fauci, who emerged as both advisor and critic as the months wore on. In contrast with Fauci's caustic commentary, Birx's combination of silence and affirmation of the president's leadership played terribly with the general public—and with many of those who knew her best in the AIDS world. "Dr. Birx, what the hell are you doing? What happened to you? Your AIDS colleagues are ashamed," veteran activist and Yale epidemiologist Gregg Gonsalves tweeted when she was a month into the job.[16]

As the head of PEPFAR, Birx had brought along many in the activist world by recruiting us to look at the same information she had. Now she tried in vain to explain segmentation, tracking the virus, and putting resources where the outbreaks were. She used her gee-whiz hand gestures, turned her palms on their sides, made a brick of air, and held it before her slides. She won few converts. In her slide decks on HIV, the numbers supported her strategy. With COVID-19, the numbers continued to climb. American testing was a debacle, treatment an exercise in improvisation. The president hawked unsafe, unproven remedies, disparaged masks, and hosted massive, maskless rallies.

Birx worked within and at the pleasure of a White House that was, on a daily basis, telling lies about unproven treatments and taking actions, like leaving the World Health Organization and undermining the authority of the Centers for Disease Control and Prevention (CDC), that undermined all hope of a cohesive, effective

American response. She could not distance herself from it without walking away completely. I was aghast, often in despair, but seldom confused about her calculus. She'd played an outsized role in reshaping PEPFAR and, by extension, the course of epidemics in some communities, if not countries, around the world. I imagined that she thought that she could do it again. Birx's close friend Sarah Schlesinger, a physician and scientist at Rockefeller University, agreed. "She is somebody who has done things that have been impossible. She's a zealot," Schlesinger said. She meant it favorably—even as she noted the peril that came with this sense of conviction and competence. "She's Daniel in the lion's den."[17]

Schlesinger, who'd worked alongside the Nobel Prize–winning researcher Ralph Steinman for many years, said that Birx was one of the smartest people she'd ever met. Yet when it came to COVID-19, assessments of her pedigree were often offset by critiques that suggested she was missing crucial and obvious pieces of information about her new viral foe. "Birx is, wrongly, analogizing from AIDS," AIDS activist Gonsalves tweeted after reports that she was looking at counties in terms of level of risk.[18] "HIV is a slowly spreading virus through sex etc. This is a highly-contagious respiratory virus. Ugh." ("I'm pretty sure she knows that," came one tart reply.) A CDC official told a *Science* reporter, "She couldn't understand why that wasn't happening in the United States" with COVID-19. According to the CDC sources, Birx didn't seem to see the difference between a slow-moving HIV outbreak and a raging respiratory pandemic. "[CDC Principal Deputy Director] Anne Schuchat had to say, 'Debbi, this is not HIV.' Birx got unhappy with that."[19]

The *Science* article dissected Birx's role shifting data collection from the CDC to the Department of Health and Human Services, honing in on the use of TeleTracking, an untested, for-profit company that received the contract to build a data management system for the pandemic through an opaque, accelerated process that prompted at least one congressional investigation.[20] CDC employees provided the reporter with details that allowed him to paint the scene in sharp, familiar strokes. Through her deputy, PEPFAR's chief epidemiologist Irum Zaidi, Birx reportedly issued an ultimatum: the CDC had to do better with its data, or she'd pull the plug. People wept and raged at the "arbitrary" decision.

Zaidi is a second-generation CDC staffer; her father worked there too. She has dimples so deep they might hold cherry pits and, like Achrekar, is deeply connected to Birx in ways that bridge the domestic and the professional. A few months before the epidemic started, Zaidi, donned a gingham apron at the end of Birx's annual Christmas party to help wash dishes; when Birx took the role at the White House, Zaidi tried to help, even as she continued her day job at PEPFAR.

She told me that shifting data collection from CDC to HHS was a last resort. She'd approached her CDC colleagues, some of whom she'd worked with for years, and suggested that now was the time to modernize the data collection systems—offering the experience with PEPFAR's shift to DATIM as an example. It was time to move to a collection system that reflected all patients across the country, without relying on modeling to fill in gaps; the system needed to be easily adaptable during a pandemic, in part to ensure equitable distribution of therapeutics, vaccines, and other supplies. She said that after an initial positive response, there hadn't been any movement; in the aftermath, she and Birx undertook the controversial shift to centralize data collection at HHS, with hospitals feeding information via TeleTracking or their own systems, into a repository called "HHS Protect," developed by Palantir, a company cofounded by a major Trump supporter. Tales of tears and ties to Trump notwithstanding, the shift to the HHS-based system paid off. By early 2021, Alexis Madrigal, a cofounder of independent Covid Data Tracking project wrote, "The current, HHS-run system works—unlike so much else in the response." It was, he said, "The best available data about the pandemic."[21]

By the time this assessment came through, it was, in many ways, too late to serve as a corrective to the assessment that Birx and Zaidi had acted in accord with a president who seemed intent on eviscerating the CDC's power and prestige. But while the toxic, mendacious White House could in no way claim to be doing a better job than the CDC, the CDC itself had made grievous missteps many times in the epidemic, including botching the swift development and release of a test early on when containment efforts might have been possible.[22]

Birx's experience lay in managing the US-funded response to a global pandemic. But in some respects, the American federal government had more influence over foreign countries than it did with its own states. Jono Mermin explained this to me when I'd gone to see him and Becky Bunnell in Atlanta in May 2020. Mermin was now director of the National Center for HIV/AIDS, Viral Hepatitis, STD, and TB Prevention at the CDC; Bunnell was director of the Office of Science. He told me how he'd run into Birx at a meeting and told her he was interested in learning more about PEPFAR's data systems, "partially because that clinic level of information seems almost impossible to get in the United States," he said. "Why is that the case? I think there's some structural reasons. If you fund the entire program, you can fund information systems . . . [T]he US has much more of a fragmented health-care system."[23] At the time that Mermin and I spoke, external donors paid for 90 percent of Uganda's AIDS response, with America accounting for 99.8 percent of that funding—as it had for the last three years.[24] There were other countries, like South Africa, where the ratio of domestic to US financing favored the national government. But overall, the US contribution to AIDS in PEPFAR countries in proportion to local contributions was larger than federal contributions to state health budgets.

Many key decisions, from mask ordinances to social distancing guidelines, sat with the states, where decisions about these and other critical actions were often guided by political affiliation, not public health wisdom. The mere fact that the White House was holding briefings was evidence of the same lethal dysfunction that made a ravaging American pandemic all but inevitable. The CDC's own epidemic handbook stated that public health responses needed to be apolitical, led by professionals with training in communicating complex, balanced messages that the public could act on and understand. But Donald Trump seized the spotlight and would not let it go.

With each passing day, the limitations of Birx's new role showed. America's longest plague war had been waged with what was, ultimately, a mighty budget and an empowered, ambassador-level leader at the helm.

The same person in her native country, lacking the muscle of funding and most of her ability to impel others to act, was left with little other than her formidable intelligence, her iron-clad belief in working within the chain of command, and perhaps her most unpredictable weapon: her own instinct about when to beguile, berate, or demand action.

I thought these things as I watched the TV clips where Birx wrapped urgent epidemiological advice in grandmotherly tones, remained silent while the president lied, and then gave interviews praising his scientific acumen. Then I stopped watching, not because I did not want to see her but because I did not like who I became as I toggled between the briefing and the Twitter storm that erupted, often before she was done speaking. Many of my own criticisms and concerns died out, half formed, when I saw them amplified and laid out in excoriating terms on social media. The choice between being part of broad-reaching critique and giving Birx the benefit of the doubt was a new version of a familiar self-imposed referendum on my character.

From the outset of my work on AIDS, I attached myself to individuals, their stories, and their lives. During the time that I had ridden the subway with Cissy to a doctor in the Bronx, I'd resented the AIDS activists who critiqued President George W. Bush's new global AIDS initiative. I'd allowed my love for Cissy, and my excitement about the program that might help women, to become a righteous defensiveness. How could spending all of that money be bad? I resented how my fellow activists attacked Bush, because I wanted there to be an end to the nightmare of untreated AIDS. I did not understand then that a massive gain can also be a monumental loss and that there are no simple, happy endings to pandemics and never will be until the structures that cause them are dismantled and rebuilt. Lethal public health emergencies only come to an end when a pathogen is viewed in isolation and not as a mutating form—malleable and adaptable. Tuberculosis replaces HIV; police brutality swaps in for syphilis. Without substantial, radical change, COVID-19 would become something else that also revealed, in daily death tolls, the stark realities of health inequities.

Now I understood those things—but I still could not stop finding heroes where I was not supposed to. George W. Bush had changed my life; Deborah Birx had too. They'd taken actions on AIDS that made me ask questions and move forward out of a strange and dismal time; those actions had, on a global scale, alleviated untold suffering. It had not been only them, never only them. Each had also done things that caused them to be labeled as irredeemable. Bush had his military wars, his ideologically based approaches to AIDS. It was a wholly different scale, but Birx now had her thankless tour of duty as the coronavirus response coordinator. When I set myself the task of writing a history of PEPFAR, I hoped that, after a full accounting of the story, I would finally find a balance between my intellect and my unruly sympathies. But when I tuned in to Birx's briefings, I felt like I was back at the beginning again.

When I next began to pay attention to her, though, I thought perhaps I'd made a mistake—not by indulging in my sympathetic assessment of Birx, but in doubting it. In the summer months, Birx left the White House for an extended period, reportedly fed up with the pontification of Dr. Scott Atlas, a radiologist who'd assumed an outsized role on the task force, espousing views on the pandemic so contrary to public health best practices that Stanford University, where he'd had an appointment, issued a statement distancing itself from his views.[25] Previously, she'd flown on Air Force Two with Vice President Mike Pence. Toward the end of the summer, she called her friend Dr. Sarah Schlesinger and told her she'd driven thousands of miles in a rental car, often with Irum Zaidi at her side.[26] They drove all through the fall, steering past campaign signs spiked into median strips, more pro-Trump the further south she drove. She took meetings with university presidents, state and public health officials, and governors when they would sit down with her. "Wear masks," she urged, and reportedly roved the aisles of grocery stores checking on supplies of masks and gloves. It was easy to see this as a move to distance herself from the Trump administration and its ignominious final days, but taking on unglamorous, grueling work that needed to be done was precisely what she'd always done her entire life. She was the only federal official working on COVID-19 to take simple, effective public health measures across the country. "I'm always the same person," she'd once said to me—as though one could walk into the belly of the beast and remain unchanged.

For a time, Birx was everywhere in the media. Then she began to fade from view. In December 2020, President-elect Joe Biden announced that Dr. Tony Fauci would be the chief medical advisor for the COVID-19 response. When asked whether Birx would remain involved, a member of Biden's pandemic task force—which also included Eric Goosby and Ezekiel Emanuel—said, "It's complicated."[27]

In the end, a story about her family sealed her fate. Birx lived in two houses—the one she shared with Reffe, where she'd once fed me toast, and a house in Potomac that had room for her elderly parents, her daughter and son-in-law, and their two children. Before COVID-19, she'd shuttled between the two, cooking meals for the week and freezing them in the multigenerational home, putting up eight or ten or twelve Christmas trees with a theme meant to please her grandchildren. After warning the nation not to travel for Thanksgiving, she and the family that spread across those two homes gathered at a third one. The media thought she'd gone too far, leaping on the number of houses and generations involved. She put on a mask, called an obscure news outlet, and told them she'd be happy to be of service to the next administration but that she was retiring.

— —

As COVID-19 UNFOLDED, THE general media started to take an interest in AIDS too. Was this pandemic like that one? In which ways, and for whom? US-focused stories highlighted the similarities in racial disparities, ethnic slurs, and blaming. A few contrasted the government's lethal inaction on AIDS with the rapid global mobilization to find a COVID-19 vaccine. But PEPFAR, the most sustained, well-endowed American effort to end a plague ever in the country's history, received scant mention or was left out entirely—even in stories about how America could do better, this time, at preparing for a pandemic response.

It had been nearly two decades since global HIV was a health-security issue and just over a decade since the Barack Obama administration's brief experiment with a global health initiative that tied global AIDS and primary health care to American safety from future pandemics. In response to existential threats—a cessation of funding, donor fatigue—the AIDS world had secured sustained support by promising control of a single pandemic. In spite of eminent scientists' pleading, the AIDS response had not been used to inform post-Ebola global preparedness work. The program was perceived as a Bush legacy, a monument to mercy—and not a source of lessons about dealing with emergencies that did not end on schedule, pandemics that did not simply go away. Yet the lessons abounded. PEPFAR used and shared data to fight a pandemic in ways that no other initiative did. It created a fragile union of government agencies and acted on scientific evidence as it became available, to the extent that finite resources allowed. It was conceivable to think of "PEPFAR-ing" other problems, particularly those where a specific strategy with a measurable impact, like a drug or vaccine, could help address an issue.

To do so, though, America had to see it as a national asset; not a work of mercy but a source of self-preservation in a world where a pandemic anywhere threatened us all. For better or for worse, PEP-FAR was the best American pandemic response in the twenty-first century, and that meant a great deal. PEPFAR was far from perfect, but its insights about how to sustain a long haul were invaluable. Pandemics were not going away, Fauci and a colleague warned. "We remain at risk for the foreseeable future."[28]

Perhaps the most important lesson was that ordinary people—for that was all that activists were—had never ceased to pay attention. People made incandescent, brilliant, and fearless out of fear and rage had stepped into the breach time and again to prevent a global retreat from never-ending AIDS and refused to be turned away from decision-making tables because they lacked the right degrees. Even after Bush had, with his largesse, purchased the story rights to their revolution, they'd continued to work within the system, inside the decision-making rooms. There would have been no comparable, continuous AIDS response without them—and there would almost certainly be no cessation to any plague that ran along the fault lines of inequality without comparable civilian engagement, leadership, and activism. The lesson was double-edged. Activists' success in sustaining the AIDS response was a victory; the fact that they'd had to fight in the first place was a failure of the first degree. Humanity is always its own greatest threat.

PEPFAR didn't belong at the center of a broader pandemic preparedness response, but it could help guide a reconfigured American approach to global health and development. "Its success is illustrative but not a structural example," Dr. Kenneth Bernard said when I asked him. Bernard had served Bill Clinton as the first health-focused member of the National Security Council. George W. Bush eliminated his position, then hired him back, and Bernard had helped to write a proposal for what would be called Project BioShield—the $6 billion biodefense program that Bush had announced in the 2003 State of the Union mere minutes after he'd launched his war on AIDS.[29]

Bernard thought PEPFAR could be mined for lessons for the coronavirus epidemic, but that the program was flourishing where it was. It wasn't broke, don't try to fix it, he told me. Besides, it couldn't be used as the cornerstone for an expanded effort. A larger, elevated American global health effort couldn't live entirely at the State Department, as PEPFAR did. Nor could it be housed at the Department of Health and Human Services (HHS). In either location it would be "too buried," Bernard opined. He favored instituting a health-security position on the National Security Council (NSC), with a portfolio that encompassed biological epidemics and biodefense. A program like PEPFAR would fall in the purview of this security-focused position, changing it from a work of mercy to one of truly global protection. Bernard's former boss, Senator Bill Frist, thought this could work, "but only if [the NSC] understands they should work closely with and listen to the HHS assistant secretary for preparedness and response."[30]

In January, when President Biden unveiled his National Security Council, it included senior director positions for "development, global health and humanitarian response" and for "global health security and biodefense," filled by Linda Etim and Beth Cameron, respectively—both veterans of the Obama administration with significant experience in their fields. The pairing marked the first time in American history that there had been two health roles at the NSC level. With Samantha Power, Obama's ambassador to the United Nations, at the head of the US Agency for International Development, there was no shortage of political clout, expertise, and ideas.

To build a cohesive, effective global health security response, the Biden Administration's team needed to deal with COVID-19 and with challenges that predated the pandemic by decades. Success depended in no small part on the ability to circumvent turf wars and false dichotomies between altruism and self-interest, outbreaks and ongoing epidemics, and put funding and political will toward an agenda based on the reality that most emergencies did not so much end as change. "Once diseases no longer threaten those living in the wealthiest countries, they are reclassified as development or humanitarian issues, rather than being considered as global health security threats. That reclassification means they attract a fraction of the resources," warned Peter Sands, executive director of the Global Fund.[31]

A global health–security agenda that downgraded endemic epidemics, like HIV, and funneled money into emerging pathogens might secure some countries, but it would not secure the global nation. A full embrace of the notion of "human security," as an alternative to the concept of "national security," could prevent this outcome. First popularized by the Nobel Prize–winning economist Amartya Sen and others, "human security" was part of a mid-1990s effort to reconfigure notions of threat and safety in a globalized, post–Cold War world.

The notion of "human security" lends itself to expansive lyrical formulations, like "freedom from fear and freedom from want" and "creating political, social, environmental, economic, military and cultural systems that together give people the building blocks of survival, livelihood and dignity."[32] In the two decades since its emergence, human security has spawned a UN index, a bevy of reports, and a predictable array of counter-critiques: that it is too all-encompassing to implement, that it means everything and therefore nothing.[33] But health, with its focus on the borders of the body and the well-being of inner terrain, is uniquely well suited for an intentional extension of this definition into programs that track, monitor, and respond to the physical symptoms of global inequity as they manifest in the bodies of the world's citizens.

A notion of human security had for years animated the AIDS activist movement, which refused to settle for pills alone and persisted in demanding housing, human rights, and sexual and reproductive freedoms. The people I knew best in this movement took the work of ensuring security as their own personal responsibility—even as they urged the state to assume its own essential role. In October 2020, Milly Katana's voice came crackling out of my computer's speakers. "Emily!" she exclaimed. "I'm really worried." The community structures that had helped people before the government had stepped in were all eroded; she knew that nothing would continue without them. She told me how, before COVID-19, she'd been visiting a community program in a northern district and, at the end of the meeting, noticed an attendee who appeared too weak to leave. She'd asked who could take him home, and no one had offered to help, so she'd driven him herself. In the old days, she said, in the days before treatment, people looked out for each other. That was what you did in pandemic time.

"My phone's a mess," Yvette Raphael said to me one day. She was approaching the twentieth anniversary of her HIV diagnosis and wanted to use it to raise funds for counseling for women who'd been raped and experienced sexual violence. She wanted something more to offer young women than her response as "Auntie" to their text messages written in the anguished aftermath of assault. She wanted a legion of women with resources to give one another strength to report, denounce, and some day defeat rape. Any honest, human-centered health security agenda would want this too.

—— ——

"This can never last," James Mugeni, my HBAC guide, had said to me in 2005, and in a way he'd been right. HBAC was a research study, not a program; it had been destined to come to an end. Many of the programs that offered mobile clinics or other forms of home-based care had been scaled back, often as part of efforts to cut costs and match program models to those in the government system. The pendulum swung back and forth. The "90-90-90" treatment goals had brought a new emphasis on community-based approaches to find people, link them to care, and deliver HIV medication. At the very outset of the epidemic, when treatment first arrived, people living with HIV had said that they held the expertise needed to design programs that would work over the long term. Fifteen years on, the world was still only half listening.

In May 2019, I visited Jono Mermin and Becky Bunnell in Atlanta. Over beers and an enormous platter of sushi, Mermin popped open his laptop and read me a list of points he thought it was important to make about PEPFAR in Uganda—how it had married research with implementation, relied on local partners, moved fast, and sought at every turn to understand what the 95 percent of Ugandans who did not have access to antiretrovirals needed to go on with their lives. "Go find the clients," Bunnell urged me. "See what they say."

My reporting was coming to an end. I did not need to make another trip to Tororo to complete the book. But I was not ready to be finished, and I hadn't spoken to clients in years, so I emailed Dr. Rebecca Amongi and then traveled out to see Tororo one more time. I told her I wanted to meet clients, and when I arrived, she assembled a group to talk to me—a pharmacist who was just a few years older than PEPFAR itself, a nurse counselor who could remember the time before there had been any AIDS drugs at all, and a man and a woman who were "expert clients"—people living with HIV whose lives had been saved by HBAC, who now helped other people cope with their diagnosis and the burden of taking pills daily, for life.

We sat in a circle, and the expert clients told their stories, familiar to me as fables. These were the tales from the first days of AIDS. "The counselors called us to a certain small awareness [meeting] and then they told us these people are going to start you on ART," the man said. "So we came to the CDC center there, and they removed our bloods, and we were given proper counseling, then started on ART. I went on improving, and now I have my grandson," the man said. He had been thirty-five when he started the medications. "I was dying then," he said. "Now I am sixty-two years old." He'd been on those medications the entire time. Years later, he marveled at what had seemed to him like HBAC's luxuriant kindness. "When you fell sick, they collect[ed] you with a vehicle; when you were admitted [to the hospital], they paid for everything," he said. They'd even provided lunch. An ambulance service and free hospital stays with food included were essential, basic elements of a functioning, equitable health system. The man remembered them as luxuries that had gone when the project ended. "If HBAC could be brought back, we would be very happy," he said.

The woman, Rose, said that her husband had died while she was pregnant. Her father had remained stalwart, by her side. She'd summoned up her courage to begin telling people that she had HIV and then found that she was good at providing educational testimonials. The HBAC team had taken notice and asked her to help educate other people with HIV. She started on antiretrovirals and began doing trainings. "I was glittering," she said of finding her calling.

When she finished talking, I ventured that some years before I had gone to a woman's house in Tororo and heard a story about how she had fought for a cow that was her rightful inheritance. That woman was also named Rose, I said. She smiled wide and clapped her hands. It was her! We embraced, even as she confessed that she had no memory of my visit. So many people had come through in that time. It was an extraordinary story, I told Dr. Amongi. She'd gotten the cow, then given it back. The point had been to prove that she could do it. Now Rose shook her head. That hadn't been the case at all. She'd kept the cow and sold it, she explained. She'd used the money to build a house adjacent to her father's land. I wondered if I'd written the story down wrong, or if James Mugeni, who'd translated that day, had tried to make it more dramatic, perhaps not realizing, as a man, that this woman's survival was an act of grand defiance that needed no embellishment.

When Bunnell told me to find the clients, I thought of the woman with the cow but assumed that it would take enormous effort to locate her. In my comings and goings from Uganda, I had lost sight of the fact that most people there, and in most other parts of the world, lived and died in the same place and knew each other well. A question or two might have led me to Rose, had she not appeared in the office that day. Years earlier, I had said that I wanted to understand how free AIDS drugs would change the world and set out to find evidence of massive transformation. Over the years, as I'd gone back to see Sister Natalya, Cissy, and Maama Apollo, I'd come to value most that they were there each time I was able to return. The fight to control the epidemic was complex, costly, political—and incomplete. To find the energy to continue, one had to celebrate not only what had changed but what had remained. In Tororo, this was individuals like Rose and a lingering sense of having been part of something beautiful, if only for a time. Contrary to Mugeni's prediction, something had endured. The research project had long since vanished but not the sense of being valued, listened to, and loved. That had remained.

— —

IN MARCH 2020, NEARLY sixteen years after Cissy had left my railroad flat with a year's worth of medication and some relief from the pain that had brought her to my futon, she returned to the Brooklyn apartment that I shared with Liam and my two sons. She came with her warmest winter coat, her heavy bag; she slept, as she always did, beneath the blankets and towels that I gave her, the coat spread out on top.

In all the years that we'd spent together, we had never done a formal interview. I had taken notes at the Bronx clinic and in her home. But we had never faced each other with a recorder between us so that I could hear the story of her life as she wanted it to be told.

We did two oral histories during that visit. In the first one, she told me about how she'd grown up in a place that sounded like paradise. At her grandfather and grandmother's home, they'd eaten only what they grew. Everything they needed was right there. There had been fruits, vegetables, chicken, beef, her brothers, and her uncles. Her lips formed the shape of a tender kiss when she said "protected." "I wish I could go back to being young," she said. Of her grandparents, she said, simply, "They showed us what love was."

We did our second conversation on March 6, 2020, in my kitchen. I lit a candle and did an audio tag. I asked her to tell me about her husband. "What was he like?" I prodded her. She thought for a moment, her lips folded in on themselves. She was careful when the recorder ran. When she finally spoke, she smiled just a bit. "He taught me to wear pants." On one of his business trips, he'd brought back a brightly patterned pair of trousers, the first she'd ever owned.

After we had spoken for some time, I asked her what is always my final question. Was there anyone she wanted to bring into the story she'd told, anything unspoken that felt important?

"I don't know whether this can be in your story, but I really—I don't know how to appreciate people," she replied. "I don't know how to thank people, but from the bottom of my heart I thank all the people who supported me." There was her brother Mike, who had "gone the extra mile," she said. "And then my children. They have been there, through thick and thin, they have really walked with me." There was the doctor who had seen her in the Bronx, her boss, and Dr. Addy, who had let her stay away for as long as she needed to heal. Her father who had given her education, and "Emily. I had never seen her but when someone comes to support you, to love you—" She paused. She spoke as though I wasn't there, as though people who had never met either of us were listening and needed to understand.[34]

As we ended the interview, I thanked her too. I had lived nearly two decades with the feeling of her grip on my arm, keeping me steady, urging me on. She smiled, but her face was strained in a way that I had not seen since she'd tuned the channel to the Christian station in my railroad flat in 2003. Before I started recording, I'd told her that she did not need to worry. I'd told her she could fly home early, that she would be just fine. There were not that many cases of the novel coronavirus in New York City, and there wouldn't be. She had nodded and looked right through me. Old trauma, I'd thought. I still hadn't finished learning how to listen. Some weeks later, when the schools had been shut and I had not left the house for more than five minutes for weeks, I transcribed our interview and heard what I had missed—and she surely had not. Sirens had been screaming, on and off, the whole time.

AUTHOR'S NOTE

THIS IS A WORK of journalism whose subject is also the professional and personal context of my adult life. In seeking to navigate this reporting, I have applied principles of transparency, consent, and collaboration in ways that I describe below.

I moved to Uganda in 2004 with the intention of researching a book on the introduction of AIDS treatment in the country and the region. All of the reporting from this time in these pages took place with people to whom I had explained this. Many of the quotations cited come from recorded interviews. When I was visiting clinics, and in some instances conducting interviews, I took notes in real time and made additional typewritten field notes within twenty-four hours. I have relied on the notebooks and field notes, as well as audio recordings and conversations with other people present at the time, to depict events and interactions. When I indicate someone's thoughts at the time or exchanges for which I was not present, I have used content from interviews as cited. I have interviewed many people in this book many times over the years. Almost all of those individuals are named in the narrative; in a few instances, in addition to the steps described below, I have omitted or changed the names of Ugandan health professionals, either because they are actively working or because I could not secure permission for interviews from 2004–2005.

AUTHOR'S NOTE

Where there is chronological separation, the notes indicate the timing of the interviews in relation to scenes described.

From 2004 to 2005, I did my reporting with the support of a Fulbright grant. Thank you to my sponsor, Dr. Moses Kamya, and the staff of the US Embassy at the time. During my time in Uganda, I visited a range of health facilities and ART programs. In each instance, I obtained permission to visit those clinics from relevant authorities, including the hospital administrator at the hospital where the Joint Clinical Research Center (JCRC) clinic was located, the leadership of JCRC, the Rakai Health Sciences Program, The AIDS Support Organisation, US agency and PEPFAR staff in country, and, in 2018 and 2019, the USAID staff in Washington, DC.

From 2005 onward, I worked on this book while also working in the field as a staff member at AVAC. In a handful of instances, I have provided descriptions of physical locations or non-data-related elements of PowerPoint presentations; however, I have not used any dialogue or data that I had access to in the context of my work at AVAC. I have, instead, relied on interviews with others who were present at the time and on information that was either supplied to me by informants or, in the majority of instances, is available in the public domain.

Between 2006 and 2017, I made several trips to Uganda, Kenya, and South Africa as an AVAC employee. I benefited immensely from a job that afforded me the opportunity to return to East and Southern Africa several times a year. As noted in the text, I conducted interviews and did reporting during days added on to these trips. I did the same on shorter trips to Washington, DC. I covered all of the costs associated with those reporting days. I was solely responsible for financing all reporting in Uganda and the region from 2004 to 2006 and in 2018 and 2019. AVAC is an ethical employer and seeks to accommodate working parents. For trips made from 2010 to 2011, AVAC purchased a ticket for my son to travel with me. When he was under the age of two and did not require his own airplane seat, AVAC covered the cost of airfare for his nanny.

AUTHOR'S NOTE

AVAC has received funding from the Bill & Melinda Gates Foundation and USAID under the auspices of PEPFAR. I have, since 2017, managed a Bill & Melinda Gates Foundation–funded transnational advocacy coalition focused on ensuring that civil society guides and leads the HIV response. Several of the activists interviewed in this book have received grants or fellowships from AVAC to do this and other work. I have managed, and continue to manage, some of those grants. I conducted interviews with individuals who collaborate with and/or receive funding from AVAC while on sabbatical from the organization, during a period in which all of my management responsibilities had been assumed by my generous, accommodating colleagues. This step gave both the interviewees and me some separation from the day-to-day work of collaborative activism. However, this symbolic shift in personal configurations did not alter the broader, structural context in which the conversations occurred or the power dynamics inherent in an activist movement that continues to be funded by grants to groups in the Global North, who then pass the funds on to the Global South. We addressed those dynamics in the interviews and in the collaborative review process as I developed the manuscript. To have omitted these leaders' voices because I was also working with and, in some instances, funding them was an erasure I could not abide. In these pages, they speak for themselves in actions and words.

AVAC's leadership, board, and funders were aware that I was working on this book. They did not review this manuscript, save for this author's note. All of the views presented in these pages are my own.

It is a privilege and a responsibility to write the stories of people who are fellow travelers in this field, many of whom are friends, comrades, and chosen family. Milly Katana, Chamunorwa Mashoko, Maureen Milanga, Felix Mwanza, Lillian Mworeko, Kenneth Mwehonge, and Yvette Raphael all reviewed the portions of the text in which they are quoted. I offered these and other sources copies of their audio files and transcripts, and I discussed the quotes that I wanted to use as well as the context in which they would appear before publication. Kate Sorensen gave me her permission to share facts about her life and my version of our time together. Where I have indicated someone's HIV status or sexual orientation, he or she has also disclosed it and is living openly in the world.

In several other instances, sources agreed to speak with me on background and with the condition that I review quotes and context with them prior to attribution. I honored these agreements. I was not asked to make any changes that were factually different from what I had written.

I met the people who, in this book, are known as Maama Apollo, Taata, Apollo, Peace, Olivia, and Stella in 2005. I am lucky that they allowed me to enter their lives. Between 2005 and 2007, I visited them approximately twenty times, with each visit lasting at least an hour and frequently much longer. On many of those visits, we discussed why I was there and what I was hoping to learn. I often brought a bag of rice, beans, or silver fish with me when I came.

Maama Apollo, the sole breadwinner of her family, earned her money as a hawker. When she was with me, she was not working, and, as I explained to them then, I valued their time. In 2007, I made what I considered a more formal break from my journalistic approach, as described in this book. I connected Maama Apollo with an income-generation program. I did not provide her with any money to make the phone calls or obtain the transport to that program. I did not provide the family any financial support at all until 2018, when I began paying school fees for Maama Apollo's daughter, who is called Olivia in this story. I did so because I was more interested in helping her to avoid HIV and find a way in the world that allowed her some level of financial security than in being an objective observer. While I brought food and, on one occasion, a bundle of used clothes for Maama Apollo to sell, I did not give them any money during the years that I was most immersed in their lives. I was, however, paying school fees while I was completing the manuscript. I am very grateful to Cissy, who lent her skills as a counselor and expert in community engagement in ethical research to a process of sharing the content in the book with Maama Apollo and her family and describing the risks and benefits associated with sharing their story. We emphasized that decisions about whether to include any or all of the content I intended to use in the book would not affect the support I was providing. Maama Apollo was concerned that no pictures of her family be used and that names and identifying details be changed, as they have been. With those assurances, she consented to my sharing her story.

I have taken great care to change details that might allow Maama Apollo, Taata, Apollo, Peace, Stella, or Olivia to be identified. I have done the same for some of the staff members at the JCRC clinic where I met the young man I call Simon in this book and for Simon himself. In the eight-year period when I knew Simon and visited with him regularly, I did not provide any financial assistance. I paid for three lunches that we shared. While the core elements of his story are accurate, the identifying details have all been changed to preserve his privacy and confidentiality. While I am in touch with his benefactor, he and I have not been in contact since 2013. Based on my experience of reconnecting at that time, I felt that the process of reestablishing contact remotely for the sole purpose of affirming that I could tell his story could cause psychological distress that outweighed the benefits I would get by claiming he had given me permission. I have sought, through a thoroughly anonymized account, to show the incalculable human costs of the ongoing failure to diagnosis and treat children living with HIV and to ensure that they, like all children, grow up in loving, supportive, self-determining communities that have control of the land they live on and access to the resources they need to build programs that support mind, body, and soul.

The woman called Cissy in this book is a part of my family and one of my closest friends. She has, since the day that we met, taught me how to live and listen ethically and with compassion. Many years ago, I approached Adrian Nicole LeBlanc on a dais at the Nieman Conference on Narrative Journalism and asked her what to do if I thought I was going to write about a friend. "Tell them," she said, and so I did, on a D train in 2003 while we were traveling to a clinic in the Bronx. "I might want to write about you someday," I said, and took out my steno notebook. I am grateful to LeBlanc for her simple, sound advice and to Cissy for agreeing not once but over and over again to share her story. I began paying for Cissy's antiretroviral treatment before I knew that I would write about her. She shared my home and resources during an extreme health crisis. Over the years, when the condition for which she sought treatment in 2003 has returned, I have helped her to find doctors in America and paid for medications. When COVID-19 began, I also began to offer her and her family financial support for living expenses. These decisions may compromise journalistic objectivity, but they uphold an ethics of humanity that is far more valuable to me. Cissy read several versions of this book and provided written comments on the text. We had detailed conversations about the risks and benefits of having her story told. Cissy has, over the years, sought to be a health provider first and to keep her life as a woman with HIV private. She is concerned for her children and her grandchildren—a reflection of the stigma that still makes life profoundly difficult for so many people living with HIV. I explained to her that, of all the people in the book, she would be the one who was easiest to identify and that I knew this concerned her. She replied that it was important that people know what life was really like for women like her. I have done my utmost to do that story justice.

ACKNOWLEDGMENTS

Tнis воок вegins and ends with thanks to the African women living with HIV who have shared their stories and comradeship with me for many years and whose work has changed the lives of countless girls, women, and people living with or at risk of HIV. Cissy, Milly Katana, Dr. Lydia Mungherera, Lillian Mworeko, Yvette Raphael, Martha Tholanah, and Jacque Wambui are just a few of those women doing this work today. I was fortunate to know Faith Akiki, Nokulunga Mazibuko, and Prudence Mabele. They, and so many other fighters, left too soon. *You multiply.* Heartfelt thanks too to Richard Lusimbo, Kenneth Mwehonge, Chamunorwa Mashoko, Felix Mwanza, and all of the activist allies whose voices animate this story and remain in the struggle to this day.

Uganda's physicians, researchers, and frontline nurses and pharmacists began welcoming me into their lives in 2000, and they have been extraordinarily generous ever since. Thank you to Dr. Alex Coutinho, Dr. Addy Kekitiinwa, Dr. Sabrina Bakeera, Dr. Bernard Etukoit, Dr. Rebecca Amongi, Dr. Peter Mugyenyi, Dr. Betty Nsangi, Dr. David Serwadda, Dr. Nelson Sewankambo, Professor Fred Wabwire-Mangen, and Sister Angela Rweyora. Dr. Elizabeth Namagala, Dr. Elizabeth Madraa, Dr. Joshua Musinguzi, Dr. David Apuuli, and the late Professor John Rwomushana provided essential and tireless leadership in the

ACKNOWLEDGMENTS

national fight. To others whom I have not mentioned by name, the days I spent watching you work are some of the richest of my life.

I am indebted to the many people whom I interviewed, often more than once, and peppered with follow-up queries. All of those conversations informed this work, and I am grateful to those named and many others who provided insights, analysis, correspondence, and archival material that informed this account. A few people have been answering my questions for more than fifteen years, including Dr. Jono Mermin and Dr. Becky Bunnell, Dr. Chris Beyrer, Dr. Deborah Birx, Amy Cunningham, Dr. Paul Zeitz, Jen Kates, Chris Collins, and Ambassador Jimmy Kolker. Dr. Seth Berkley gave me my first chance to go to Uganda and provided support years later. Thank you.

One day in 2004, I walked down from my flat on Makerere Campus and climbed into a taxi driven by a kind, astute, profoundly hardworking man. He and I spent sixteen years driving around Uganda, discussing our families, politics, health, HIV, and life. Out of an abundance of caution, I will not use his given name. Taata Erick, thank you for the ride.

Thank you to Jamila Headley, Richard Jeffreys, Karyn Kaplan, Kim Nichols, Gregg Gonsalves, Mark Harrington, Amanda Lugg, Michael Marco, Mark Milano, Eustacia Smith, Daniel Wolfe, and Uncle Mike for the fight and the fun. From the moment they entered my life, JD Davids, Paul Davis, Rachel Cohen, Matthew Kavanagh, Sharonann Lynch, and Asia Russell have challenged me to get it right. Over years of working in this field and on this book—down to the hours before it was completed—they shared documents, edits, analysis, and insights on how to make the impossible possible.

I conducted nearly two hundred formal interviews for this book between 2017 and 2020. I am grateful to each person who shared their story and perspective. Many individuals fielded numerous questions in conversations and correspondences that spanned years, if not decades.

Thank you to each and every one of my colleagues at AVAC for your smarts, passion, and belief in community. Mitchell Warren offered friendship, encouragement, and flexibility for which I will always be grateful. Thank you to Manju Chatani-Gada, Kevin Fisher, and Deirdre Grant for being on the long haul, and to my team, including Amanda Banda, Micheal Ighodaro, and Terry Mukuka. Justine MacWilliam arrived with mad skills and the steadiest of hands at a crucial moment. I met Jeane Baron, Cindra Feuer, Stacey Hannah, Angelo Kaggwa-Katumba, Erin Kiernon, and Maureen Luba before they joined AVAC and am grateful to them as colleagues and friends.

The late Louise DeSalvo taught me how to have a writing life, which is to say, she taught me how to be alive. This book would not exist without her. Deep thanks to my classmates at the Hunter College MFA program and to my other teachers of writing, including Anne-christine d'Adesky, Kip Zegers, Jennifer Huebner, Kathryn Harrison, Maggie Holley, Patrica Kahn, Eileen Myles, and Laurie Weeks.

Lisa Freedman, Beth Gould, Sangamithra Iyer, Adrienne Jones, Jennifer Lutton: *Salon rules. Arms up.* The What Would an HIV Doula Do Collective challenged, held, and expanded me and this project. Theodore (Ted) Kerr and Alex Juhasz provided critical feedback. Early readers Brian Honermann and Meg Halverson provided encouragement and gently caught critical omissions.

A double round of gimlets and a litter of kittens' worth of gratitude to my agent, Kent D. Wolf, who trawled the fine print of *Best American Essays* and then coaxed the story that needed to be told into being. Benjamin Adams is the most patient, deft editor I could have hoped for. Great thanks too to the team at Hachette Book Group, including Melissa Raymond, Melissa Veronesi, and Jen Kelland.

Avram Finkelstein and Amy Scholder led me to David Groff, whose gentle, steady hand helped me to step back, start fresh, and stay the course. Sean Strub led me to Martin Duberman, whose bracing questions about and belief in this project were an elixir of hope and possibility. Marty and Eli Zal: thank you both.

Jason Baumann, Melanie Locay, and the archival staff at the New York Public Library (NYPL) were profoundly generous throughout my time as the Martin Duberman Visiting Scholar at the New York Public Library. Thank you to the NYPL for that much-needed support and magical time. The Vermont Studio Center offered quiet, company, and

ACKNOWLEDGMENTS

mountains when I needed them most. Deep thanks to Neil Carlson, Erin Carney, and the Brooklyn Creative League community.

Marguerite Bass, Carolyn Flaherty, Dr. Ann Jones, Mallory Jones, and Mary, Sol, Allan, and Ralph Pred provided love, guidance, and nurturing to me while they were alive, as did Alberta Kornegay. It is my tremendous loss not to have met my father-in-law, the great writer Joe Flaherty. I wrote with all of their spirits in mind and in hopes of making them proud.

Thank you to my parents, Lane Bass and Suzanne Pred Bass, for unwavering support, boundless love, and the lesson that one should travel often and, when home, welcome every human with warmth, genuine curiosity, and excellent meals. My sister, Becky Bass, never fails to make me up my game.

Thank you to Jeannine Johnson Flaherty and Siobhan, Eddie, and Maeve Haber for being family.

Mark Breda, Gizmo and Ilonka Brew, Keith Chervenak, Jan DeBont, Sabrina Egan, Ray Harvey, Leslie Nielsen, Steve Reynolds, and Ali Taylor dwell in the lake house of my soul.

Zoe Goldberg, Margaret Horlick, and Johanna Pinzler are friends so valuable I have no words. Becky Karush: *exactly*. Benjamin Birch changed our lives and the lives of our children. Chloe Shane, thank you for being on 8th Street when we needed you.

Sebastian and Clyde fill my world with joy, laughter, and hope for the future. For those who have read this far, they would like you to know how much time I was gone while writing this. Coming home to you is my greatest joy; being your mother (and your messenger) is the glorious delight of my life.

On the night that we met, Liam Flaherty's pickup line was a riff on a V. S. Naipaul quotation about memory and the past. Naipaul writes, "In the beginning it is like trampling on a garden. In the end you are just walking on ground." For nearly two decades now, it has been my great good fortune to walk the world with him as guide, fellow traveler, coparent, and partner in crime. My heart's dearest companion was also this book's staunchest ally. Liam: there is no one in the world with whom I could have taken this walk but you.

NOTES

Prologue

1. "President George W. Bush's Inaugural Address," George Bush White House Archives, January 20, 2001, https://georgewbush-whitehouse .archives.gov/news/inaugural-address.html.
2. "President Bush's 2003 State of the Union Address," *Washington Post*, January 28, 2003, www.washingtonpost.com/wp-srv/onpolitics/transcripts/bush text_012803.html.
3. Harold Varmus, "Making PEPFAR: A Triumph of Medical Diplomacy," *Science & Diplomacy* 2, no. 4 (December 2013), www.sciencediplomacy.org /sites/default/files/making_pepfar_science__diplomacy.pdf.
4. Dylan Matthews, "George W. Bush Was a Much Better President Than Liberals Like to Admit," *Vox*, July 8, 2015, www.vox.com/2015/7/8/8894019 /george-w-bush-pepfar.

Chapter 1: The Inside-Outside Game

1. Anne-christine d'Adesky, *The Pox Lover: An Activist's Decade in New York and Paris* (Madison: University of Wisconsin Press, 2017).
2. David France, *How to Survive a Plague: The Story of How Activists and Scientists Tamed AIDS* (New York: Vintage, 2017).
3. Chris Collins, phone interview with the author, April 29, 2019.
4. Eric Sawyer, "Remarks at the Opening Ceremony," XI International Conference on AIDS, Vancouver, Canada, July 7, 1996. https://actupny.org /Vancouver/sawyerspeech.html.

5. Eric Sawyer, interview by Sarah Schulman, New York City, March 10, 2004, ACT UP Oral History Project Interview #049: early personal history: 1–3; ACT UP response to housing advocates: 19.

6. Centers for Disease Control and Prevention (CDC), "30 Years of AIDS in African American Communities: A Timeline," CDC, 2011, www.cdc .gov/nchhstp/newsroom/docs/timeline-30years-hiv-african-american -community-508.pdf.

7. CDC, "30 Years of AIDS."

8. David Brown, "AIDS Death Rate Down 47% in 1997," *Washington Post*, October 8, 1998, www.washingtonpost.com/archive/politics/1998/10/08/aids -death-rate-in-97-down-47/6ca3a56d-2015-42fa-b4f4-0ffe2aa22d12.

9. W. D. King et al., "Racial, Gender, and Geographic Disparities of Antiret-roviral Treatment Among US Medicaid Enrolees in 1998," *Journal of Epidemiology and Community Health*, 62, no. 9 (September 30, 1998), https://doi .org/10.1136/jech.2005.045567; "Update: Trends in AIDS Incidence—United States, 1996," Centers for Disease Control and Prevention, September 19, 1997, https://wonder.cdc.gov/wonder/help/AIDS/MMWR-09-19-1997 .html#00002692.htm.

10. Michelle Esther O'Brian, interview with JD Davids, New York City Trans Oral History Project Interview #19, March 11, 2017, 11. Available at https://s3.amazonaws.com/oral-history/transcripts/NYC+TOHP+ Transcript+019+JD+Davids.pdf.

11. Both quotations from James in this section are from John S. James, "GATT and the GAP: How to Save Lives," posted on E-drug list by Richard Laing, November 17, 1998, http://lists.healthnet.org/archive/html/e-drug/1998-11 /msg00059.html.

12. Carlton Hogan, "Give 'Em Hell, Hogan: Pointers and Prerogatives from and for the Unrepentant Problem Patient," *TAGline*, December 2003, www.treatmentactiongroup.org/resources/tagline/tagline-2003/give-em -hell-hogan.

13. JD Davids and Karen L. Lyons, "An Assay Is a Test or How to Talk to Real People," *The Body*, March 1, 1997, www.thebody.com/article/assay -test-or-talk-real-people.

14. Leslie Feinberg, "Jail House Rocks! Matthew Shepard Lives," in *From ACT UP to the WTO: Urban Protest and Community Building in the Era of Globalization*, ed. Benjamin Shepard and Ronald Hayduk (New York: Verso, 2002). Feinberg describes the protest as a moment of post-Stonewall triumph. Sarah Schulman, in *The Gentrification of the Mind: Witness to a Lost Generation* (Berkeley: University of California Press, 2013), describes a "transitional crowd" with many seasoned activists going through well-practiced motions.

15. For more on many of these New York City–based developments and the broader context of 1990s antigentrification and antiglobalization activism, see Benjamin Shepard and Ronald Hayduk, eds., *From ACT UP to the WTO: Urban Protest and Community Building in the Era of Globalization* (New York: Verso, 2002).

16. For a summary of the events at CROI, see Tim Horn, "Tracing the Origin of the AIDS Pandemic," Physicians' Research Network, September 2005, www.prn.org/images/pdfs/58_hahn_beatrice.pdf. For the original publication of Hahn and her colleagues' findings, see F. Gao et al., "Origin of HIV-1 in the Chimpanzee *Pan troglodytes troglodytes*," *Nature* 397 (February 4, 1999): 436–441. doi:10.1038/17130.

17. Rainforest Action Network, "World Bank Approves 'Nightmare' African Oil and Pipeline Project," June 6, 2000, Internet Archive, https://web.archive.org/web/20000525135446/http://www.ran.org/ran_campaigns/africa/index.html.

18. JD Davids, text message to the author, October 31, 2020.

19. James Gallagher, "AIDS: Origin of Pandemic Was 1920s Kinshasa," *BBC News*, October 2, 2014, www.bbc.com/news/health-29442642.

20. Jacques Pepin, *The Origins of AIDS* (Cambridge: Cambridge University Press, 2012).

21. For more about Kuromiya's remarkable life and his work as a pioneer of internet freedom, see Cait McKinney, "Crisis Infrastructures: AIDS Activism Meets Internet Regulation," in *AIDS and the Distribution of Crises*, ed. Jih-Fei Cheng, Alexandra Juhasz, and Nishant Shahani (Durham, NC: Duke University Press, 2020).

22. Dan Royles, "Don't We Die Too? The Political Culture of African-American AIDS Activism" (PhD diss., Temple University, 2014).

23. Asia Russell, phone interview with the author, November 10, 2020.

24. John Riley, interview by Sarah Schulman, New York City, January 2, 2013, ACT UP Oral History Project Interview #151, 39–40, www.actuporalhistory.org/interviews/images/riley.pdf.

25. Susan Reverby, *Co-conspirator for Justice: The Revolutionary Life of Dr. Alan Berkman* (Chapel Hill: University of North Carolina Press, 2020), 243.

26. Reverby, *Co-conspirator for Justice*, 247.

27. Reverby, *Co-conspirator for Justice*, 260.

28. Jonathan M. Mann, "Statement at an Informal Briefing on AIDS to the 42nd Session of the United Nations General Assembly," National Library of Medicine, National Institutes of Health, October 20, 1987, https://apps.nlm.nih.gov/againsttheodds/pdfs/OB0855.pdf.

29. Reverby, *Co-conspirator for Justice*, 260.

30. Reverby, *Co-conspirator for Justice*, 256.

31. David W. Dunlap, "From AIDS Conference, Talk of Life, Not Death (Published 1996)," *New York Times*, July 15, 1996, www.nytimes.com/1996/07/15/us/from-aids-conference-talk-of-life-not-death.html.

32. Sharonann Lynch, text message to the author, October 27, 2020.

33. Sharonann Lynch, interview with the author, New Jersey, May 14, 2019.

34. Susannah Markandya, "Timeline of Trade Disputes Involving Thailand and Access to Medicines," *CPTech*, July 23, 2001, www.cptech.org/ip/health/c/thailand/thailand.html.

35. Raymond A. Smith and Patricia Siplon, *Drugs into Bodies: Global AIDS Treatment Activism* (Westport, CT: Praeger, 2006).

36. Sharonann Lynch, email to the author, September 8, 2020.

37. Mark Milano, "Zapping for Drugs," *AIDS Community Research Initiative of America (ACRIA) Update* 15, no 4 (2006).

38. Katharine Q. Seelye, "Embracing Clinton at Arm's Length, Gore Formally Begins Run for President," *New York Times*, June 17, 1999, www.nytimes.com/1999/06/17/us/embracing-clinton-at-arm-s-length-gore-formally-begins-run-for-president.html.

39. "AIDS Action Council and Compulsory Licensing," email from Rachel Maddow to aidsact@critpath.org, July 6, 1999. See page 13 in pdf document at https://catalog.archives.gov/OpaAPI/media/24325773/content/presidential-libraries/foia/2006-0003-F/ag-t-20015426-20060003f-004-006-2015.pdf.

40. "Africa AIDS Plan," email from Richard Socarides to multiple recipients, June 30, 1999. See pages 1–2 in pdf document at https://catalog.archives.gov/OpaAPI/media/24325773/content/presidential-libraries/foia/2006-0003-F/ag-t-20015426-20060003f-004-006-2015.pdf.

41. By 1999, two studies had found that a "short course" of roughly four weeks of the antiretroviral AZT during the last trimester of pregnancy, plus additional doses during labor, halved the rate of transmission to infants during labor and delivery. Previous research had established the benefit of starting AZT at fourteen weeks' gestation, but this long-duration regimen was deemed unfeasible for low-resource settings. The term "mother-to-child transmission" places pregnant and lactating women as bearing sole responsibility for transmitting HIV to newborns. This construction, which removes the male partner, reinforces stigma centered on cis-gendered women, who often receive HIV tests in the context of antenatal care and are blamed for bringing HIV into the family when they share their diagnosis. "Vertical transmission" or "parent-to-child transmission" are the terms preferred by women living with HIV and their allies. In this book, I use "prevention of mother-to-child transmission" and its variations when it is in the context of an official program name or a discussion where the source used that language.

42. Sandra Thurman and Cornelius Baker, interview with the author, Washington, DC, January 21, 2020; "Candidate Gore Zaps," ACT UP, https://act upny.org/actions/gorezaps.html.

43. The letter in question is Exhibit 13 in this case study, which provides a detailed background on other key events described in this chapter. William Fisher and Cyrill Rigamonti, "The South Africa AIDS Controversy: A Case Study in Patent Law and Policy," Harvard Law School, February 10, 2005, https://cyber.harvard.edu/people/tfisher/South%20Africa.pdf.

44. "Greed 2000: Medical Apartheid Worldwide," ACT UP flier from the archive of Paul Davis.

45. Neil Lewis, "U.S. Industry to Drop AIDS Drug Lawsuit Against South Africa," *New York Times*, September 10, 1999, www.nytimes.com/1999/09/10 /world/us-industry-to-drop-aids-drug-lawsuit-against-south-africa.html.

46. "US–South Africa Understanding on Intellectual Property," Office of the US Trade Representative, September 17, 1999, Internet Archive, https://web.archive .org/web/20010925231605/http://192.239.92.165/releases/1999/09/99-76.html.

47. Barton Gellman, "DEATH WATCH: The Global Response to AIDS in Africa," *Washington Post*, July 5, 2000.

48. Samuel Hale Butterfield, *U.S. Development Aid—an Historic First: Achievements and Failures in the Twentieth Century* (Westport, CT: Praeger, 2004).

49. Irvin D. Coker, interview by W. Haven North, July 29, 1998, Association for Diplomatic Studies and Training, Foreign Affairs Oral History Project.

50. Steven Radelet, "Bush and Foreign Aid," *Foreign Affairs* 8, no. 5 (September/ October 2003), 108.

51. John Norris, "USAID: A History of Foreign Aid—the Clashes of the 1990s," *Devex*, July 13, 2014, www.devex.com/news/the-clashes-of-the-1990s-83341.

52. Barton Gellman, "AIDS Is Declared Threat to Security," *Washington Post,* April 30, 2000, www.washingtonpost.com/archive/politics/2000/04/30/aids -is-declared-threat-to-security/c5e976e4-3fe8-411b-9734-ca44f3130b41.

53. Kenneth W. Bernard, "Health and National Security: A Contemporary Collision of Cultures," *Biosecurity and Bioterrorism: Biodefense Strategy, Practice and Science* 11, no. 2 (November 2, 2013). doi: 10.1089/bsp.2013.8522.

54. For an in-depth account of Clinton-era efforts to mobilize funding for global HIV through the National Security Council and the Office of National AIDS Policy, see Greg Behrman, *The Invisible People: How the U.S. Has Slept Through the Global AIDS Pandemic, the Greatest Humanitarian Catastrophe of Our Time* (New York: Free Press, 2004).

55. UNAIDS, *AIDS Epidemic Update: 2000* (Geneva: UNAIDS, 2000), 17, https://data.unaids.org/publications/irc-pub05/aidsepidemicreport2000 _en.pdf.

56. For a detailed account of the history and impact of South African AIDS denialism, see Didier Fassin, *When Bodies Remember: Experience and Politics of AIDS in South Africa* (Berkeley: University of California Press, 2007).

57. "Global Manifesto," ACT UP, July 9, 2000, https://actupny.org/reports /durban-access.html.

58. "The Durban Declaration," *Nature* 406 (2000): 15–16. doi: 10.1038/35017662.

59. Kim Nichols, interview with the author, New York City, April 30, 2019.

60. Alexandra Juhasz, "Forgetting ACT UP," *Quarterly Journal of Speech* 98, no. 1 (January 2012): 69.

61. Dan Royles, "Black Gay History and the Fight Against AIDS," *Black Perspectives*, December 23, 2017.

62. Juhasz, "Forgetting ACT UP," 69.

63. The "Africa" folders and tagged content in the New York Public Library archives for Gay Men's Health Crisis and ACT UP for the 1980s and 1990s primarily contain peer-reviewed scientific articles, media stories, and the occasional first-person account, including one by a participant in a US government delegation to examine "AIDS in Africa" and another from Robert Rygor, a white, gay ACT UP New York member who attended an AIDS conference in Côte d'Ivoire. In the context of untreated AIDS in America and of issues closer to hand like the stigmatization and quarantine of Haitians, AIDS in Africa was more a subject for study than a site for sustained solidarity-based action.

64. Amanda Lugg, interview with the author, New York City, April 24, 2019.

65. Yvette Raphael, phone interview with the author, October 10, 2020.

66. Jeanette Chabalala, "Maimane Pays Tribute to Aids Activist Lucky Mazibuko," *News24*, April 20, 2019, www.news24.com/news24/SouthAfrica/News /maimane-pays-tribute-to-aids-activist-lucky-mazibuko-20190420; "Treatment Free for All," *Guardian*, November 23, 2003, www.theguardian.com /world/2003/nov/23/aids.theobserver4.

67. Raphael interview, October 10, 2020.

68. For an early history of Uganda's AIDS response, see Uganda AIDS Commission, *The Story of AIDS in Uganda—and Banana Trees Provided the Shade* (Kampala: Uganda AIDS Commission, 2001). For a history of the Joint Clinical Research Center and the country's epidemic in the late 1980s and 1990s, see Peter Mugyenyi, *Genocide by Denial: How Profiteering from HIV/AIDS Killed Millions* (Kampala: Fountain Publishers, 2008).

69. Mugyenyi, *Genocide by Denial*, 7

70. Mugyenyi, *Genocide by Denial*.

71. Dr. Peter Mugyenyi, interview with the author, Kampala, June 20, 2019.

72. Mugyenyi, *Genocide by Denial*.

CHAPTER 2: THE HARD THINGS

1. Paul Davis, phone interview with the author, May 29, 2020. All quotes are from this interview unless otherwise indicated.

2. Copies of the letters, responses, and a range of media articles and other primary documents related to Cipla can be found at CPTech's "Cipla" webpage: www.cptech.org/ip/health/cipla.

3. Letter from G. G. Bereton, Head of Patents, Global Intellectual Property Department, Glaxo Wellcome, to Director and Mr. Amar Lulla, Cipla, Ltd., November 20, 2000, www.cptech.org/ip/health/africa/glaxocipla11202000.html.

4. Ellen 't Hoen et al., "Driving a Decade of Change: HIV/AIDS, Patents and Access to Medicines for All," *Journal of the International AIDS Society* 14 (March 27, 2011). doi:10.1186/1758-2652-14-15.

5. Davis interview, May 29, 2020.

6. "Jubilee 2000," Advocacy International, www.advocacyinternational.co.uk /featured-project/jubilee-2000.

7. "Re: Bulk Procurement," email from Dr. Thuthula Balfour to Paul Davis, January 24, 2001.

8. Health GAP, "Global Bulk Drug Procurement and Distribution System: Discussion Document Regarding Efficient Large-Scale Programs Delivering Drugs to People in Impoverished Countries," March 28, 2001 (in the author's possession).

9. Davis interview, May 29, 2020; email from Asia Russell, June 3, 2020.

10. Derek Hodel, *At the Crossroads: A Study of Federal HIV/AIDS Advocacy* (New York: Ford Foundation, 2004).

11. "Re: Bulk Procurement Language," email from Michael Riggs to Paul Davis, March 21, 2001.

12. Jeffrey Sachs, "AIDS, Drugs and Africa: Industrialized Nations and Pharmaceutical Companies Have a Responsibility to Tackle Disease in the Continent," *Financial Times*, February 13, 2001, www.jeffsachs.org/news paper-articles/gjrdp3tpa6pz8rh86z9hnxy63bb2lf.

13. Jeffrey Sachs, "A Global Fund for the Fight Against HIV/AIDS," *Washington Post*, April 7, 2001, www.washingtonpost.com/archive/opinions/2001/04 /07/a-global-fund-for-the-fight-against-aids/6df48270-67f7-4b8b-956b -9a9e0ac71bc4.

14. Individual members of the faculty of Harvard University, "Consensus Statement on Antiretroviral Treatment for AIDS in Poor Countries," April 4, 2001, Internet Archive, https://web.archive.org/web/20011125192218/http:// www.hsph.harvard.edu/hai/overview/news_events/events/consensus_aids _therapy.pdf.

15. Carol Bellamy, "How to Distribute AIDS Drugs," *New York Times*, March 26, 2001.

16. "Bulk Procurement and Distribution System," email from Paul Davis to treatment-access@hivnet.ch, April 19, 2001, Internet Archive, https://web.archive.org/web/20010627230601/http://www.hivnet.ch:8000/topics/treatment-access/viewR?983.

17. United Nations, "Secretary-General Proposes Global Fund for Fight Against HIV/AIDS and Other Infectious Diseases at African Leaders Summit," United Nations Office of the Secretary-General, April 26, 2001, www.un.org/press/en/2001/SGSM7779R1.doc.htm.

18. Matthew Kavanagh, interview with the author, Washington, DC, March 7, 2018.

19. David E. Sanger, "Bush Plans to Stress Effects of Economics on Security," *New York Times*, January 16, 2001, www.nytimes.com/2001/01/16/world/bush-plans-to-stress-effects-of-economics-on-security.html.

20. Lindsey would keep his position for less than two years, losing it weeks after projecting astronomical costs for the proposed Iraq War. See Bob Davis, "Bush Economic Aide Says the Cost of Iraq War May Top $100 Billion," *Wall Street Journal*, September 16, 2002, www.wsj.com/articles/SB103212813421806655; Edmund Andrews, "Bush, in Shake-Up of Cabinet, Ousts Treasury Leader," *New York Times*, December 7, 2002, www.nytimes.com/2002/12/07/us/upheaval-treasury-treasury-secretary-bush-shake-up-cabinet-ousts-treasury-leader.html.

21. Sanger, "Bush Plans to Stress Effects of Economics on Security."

22. Harold Varmus, "Making PEPFAR: A Triumph of Medical Diplomacy," *Science & Diplomacy* 2, no. 4 (December 2013), www.sciencediplomacy.org/article/2013/making-pepfar.

23. Jay Lefkowitz, "AIDS and the President: An Inside Account," *Commentary*, January 2009, www.commentarymagazine.com/articles/jay-lefkowitz/aids-and-the-president-an-inside-account.

24. John Donnelly, "The President's Emergency Plan for AIDS Relief: How George W. Bush and Aides Came to 'Think Big' on Battling HIV," *Health Affairs* 31, no. 7 (July 1, 2012): 1389–1396. doi: 10.1377/hlthaff.2012.0408.

25. Carol Lancaster, *George Bush's Foreign Aid: Transformation or Chaos?* (Washington, DC: Center for Global Development, 2008).

26. Lancaster, *George Bush's Foreign Aid*.

27. Kenneth Bernard, phone interview with the author, October 30, 2020.

28. For a detailed history of the late-1990s militarization of the police response to protest and the "R2K" protests and legal defense, see Kris Hermes, *Crashing the Party: Legacies and Lessons from the RNC 2000* (Oakland, CA: PM Press, 2015).

29. Walter Benjamin, *Illuminations* (New York: Schocken Books, 1968), 257.

30. "United Nations Millennium Declaration," September 8, 2000, Internet Archive, https://web.archive.org/web/20010405070654/https://www.un.org/millennium/declaration/ares552e.htm.

31. Development Assistance Committee, "History of the 0.7% ODA Target," *DAC Journal* 3, no. 4 (2002): III-3–III-11, revised March 2016.

32. Isaac Shapiro, "As a Share of the Economy and the Budget, U.S. Development and Humanitarian Aid Would Drop to Post-WWII Lows in 2002," Center on Budget and Policy Priorities, June 18, 2001, www.cbpp.org /archiveSite/6-18-01bud.pdf.

33. George W. Bush, *Decision Points* (New York: Crown Publishing, 2011): "handout": location 329; "G8 tradition" and "guilty": location 330 in e-pub edition.

34. Bush, *Decision Points*, e-pub location 331.

35. Condoleezza Rice, *No Higher Honor: A Memoir of My Years in Washington* (New York: Crown Publishing, 2011), 142.

36. Gary Edson, interview with the author, Washington, DC, January, 21, 2020.

37. Bush, *Decision Points*, e-pub location 317.

38. "President Announces Proposal for Global Fund to Fight HIV/AIDS, Malaria and Tuberculosis," press release, US Department of State, May 11, 2001, https://2001-2009.state.gov/p/af/rls/74806.htm.

39. "USA: Action Alert / Failing the Test on Global AIDS," Health GAP, May 10, 2001.

40. "Critical Issues Surrounding an International Fund for HIV/AIDS and Other Infectious Diseases," Health GAP, May 15, 2001.

41. "Declaration of Commitment on HIV/AIDS: United Nations General Assembly Special Session on HIV/AIDS, 25–27 June 2001," UNAIDS, June 2001, www.unaids.org/sites/default/files/sub_landing/files/aidsdeclaration_en_0.pdf.

42. Donald G. McNeil, "US at Odds with Europe over Rules on World Drug Pricing," *New York Times*, July 20, 2001, www.nytimes.com/2001/07/20 /world/us-at-odds-with-europe-over-rules-on-world-drug-pricing.html.

43. Asia Russell, email to the author, July 6, 2020.

44. "Statement by Kofi Annan on the Global Fight Against AIDS," G7 Information Centre, July 20, 2001, www.g7.utoronto.ca/summit/2001genoa/annan.html.

Chapter 3: Fight Like a Woman

1. Milly Katana, phone interview with the author, June 25, 2020.

2. Milly Katana, personal communication with the author, Kampala, December 2001.

3. Laura Guay et al., "Intrapartum and Neonatal Single-Dose Nevirapine Compared with Zidovudine for Prevention of Mother-to-Child Transmission of HIV-1 in Kampala, Uganda: HIVNET 012 Randomised Trial," *The Lancet* 354, no. 9181 (September 4, 1999). doi: 10.1016/S0140-6736(99)80008-7.

4. Amy Kapcyzynski and Jonathan Berger, "The Story of the TAC Case: The Potential and Limits of Socio-Economic Rights Litigation in South Africa,"

in *Human Rights Advocacy Stories*, ed. Deena R. Hurwitz and Margaret L. Satterthwaite (New York: Foundation Press, 2008).

5. Remarks by President Yoweri K. Museveni, 9th International Conference on AIDS and STIs in Africa, Kampala, Uganda, December 10, 1995, https://web.archive.org/web/20040511170431/http://www.museveni.co.ug/reader.php?process=speeches&speechSpec=5.

6. Uganda AIDS Commission, *The Story of AIDS in Uganda—and Banana Trees Provided the Shade* (Kampala: Uganda AIDS Commission, 2001).

7. These two sources document the facts here and provide a deeper exploration of President Museveni's active cultivation of personal and professional ties with Western donors: Jonathan Fisher, "International Perceptions and African Agency: Uganda and Its Donors 1986–2010" (PhD diss., Oxford University, 2011); Helen Epstein, *Another Fine Mess: America, Uganda, and the War on Terror* (New York: Columbia Global Reports, 2017).

8. G. Asiimwe-Okiror et al., "Change in Sexual Behaviour and Decline in HIV Infection Among Young Pregnant Women in Urban Uganda," *AIDS* (London, England) 11, no. 14 (1997): 1757–1763. doi:10.1097/00002030-1997 14000-00013.

9. Asiimwe-Okiror et al., "Change in Sexual Behaviour."

10. UNAIDS, *A Measure of Success in Uganda: The Value of Monitoring Both HIV Prevalence and Sexual Behaviour* (Geneva: UNAIDS, 1998), www.un aids.org/sites/default/files/media_asset/value_monitoring_uganda_en_0 .pdf.

11. Ellen Hauser, "Ugandan Relations with Western Donors in the 1990s: What Impact on Democratisation?," *Journal of Modern African Studies* 37, no. 4 (1999): 621–641.

12. Ian Fisher, "AIDS Permeates Uganda Politics Too," *New York Times*, March 12, 2001, www.nytimes.com/2001/03/12/world/aids-permeates-uganda-politics -too.html.

13. Human Rights Watch, "Uprooted and Forgotten: Impunity and Human Rights Abuses in Northern Uganda," *Human Rights Watch* 17, no 12A (September 2005), www.hrw.org/reports/2005/uganda0905/uganda0905.pdf and Margaret E. McGuinness, "Territory of the Congo: The ICJ Finds Uganda Acted Unlawfully and Orders Reparations," *ASIL Insights* 10, no. 1 (January 9, 2006), www.asil.org/insights/volume/10/issue/1/case-concerning -armed-activities-territory-congo-icj-finds-uganda-acted. Joseph Tumushabe, *The Politics of HIV/AIDS in Uganda* (Geneva: United Nations Research Institute for Social Development, 2006).

14. Cissy, interview with the author, Brooklyn, New York, March 4, 2020.

15. Quotations are from an interview Cissy and I conducted in New York City on March 4, 2020. The narrative of her life reflects stories she told me many times; she reviewed the versions presented here.

16. Lillian Mworeko, interview with the author, Ssenge, Uganda, June 21, 2019.

17. Mworeko interview, June 21, 2019.

18. Ann T. Rossetti, dir., *Pills, Profits, Protest: Chronicle of the Global AIDS Movement* (New York: Outcast Films, 2005).

CHAPTER 4: THE WORK OF MERCY

1. Unless otherwise noted, Edson quotations and content throughout this chapter are from Gary Edson, interview with the author, Washington, DC, January, 21, 2020.

2. Condoleezza Rice, *No Higher Honor: A Memoir of My Years in Washington* (New York: Crown Publishing, 2011), 142.

3. I am indebted in this analysis to an unpublished 2007 paper by Jen Kates, prepared in the course of graduate work, titled "The President's Emergency Plan for AIDS Relief (PEPFAR): An Examination of a New Budgetary Initiative for Global AIDS."

4. Jonathan Fisher, "International Perceptions and African Agency: Uganda and Its Donors 1986–2010" (PhD diss., Oxford University, 2011).

5. Jamie Drummond, phone interview with the author, November 9, 2018.

6. "President Proposes $5 Billion Plan to Help Developing Nations," White House, March 14, 2002, https://georgewbush-whitehouse.archives.gov/news/releases/2002/03/20020314-7.html.

7. "President Proposes $5 Billion Plan to Help Developing Nations."

8. Jamie Drummond, phone interview with the author, November 9, 2018.

9. Dr. Anthony Fauci, phone interview with the author, January 16, 2018.

10. Allen Moore, phone interview with the author, October 29, 2020.

11. Kenneth Bernard, phone interview with the author, October 30, 2020.

12. Jesse Helms, "We Cannot Turn Away," *Washington Post*, March 24, 2002, www.washingtonpost.com/archive/opinions/2002/03/24/we-cannot-turn-away/9daf68e2-2bd5-4be3-a863-a88b7bd45210.

13. Allen Moore, email to the author, December 13, 2020.

14. Allen Moore, phone interview with the author, October 29, 2020.

15. Washington Post Editorial Board, "Sen. Frist Backs Down," *Washington Post*, June 12, 2002, www.washingtonpost.com/archive/opinions/2002/06/12/sen-frist-backs-down/7a1ab174-24fd-4d71-8a93-41e6209d5357.

16. Josh Bolten, interview by Russell Riley and Barbara Perry, January 15–16, 2013, Miller Center Presidential Oral History Project.

17. US Congress, House Committee on International Relations, *The United States' War on AIDS*, 107th Cong., 1st sess., June 7, 2001, Internet Archive, https://web.archive.org/web/20011130163016/http://www.house.gov/international_relations/72978.pdf, 10–11.

18. US Congress, House Committee on International Relations, *The United States' War on AIDS*, 28.

19. Andrew Natsios, phone interview with the author, April 12, 2019.

20. A detailed account of pre-PEPFAR legislative activity can be found in Derek Hodel, *At the Crossroads: A Study of Federal HIV/AIDS Advocacy* (New York: Ford Foundation, 2004).

21. US Congress, Senate Committee on Health Education Labor and Pension, "Capacity to Care in a World Living with AIDS," 107th Cong., 2nd sess., April 11, 2002, Internet Archive, https://web.archive.org/web/20081208165619/http://frwebgate.access.gpo.gov/cgi-bin/getdoc.cgi?db name=107_senate_hearings&docid=78-812, 5–10.

22. US Congress, Senate, *United States Leadership Against HIV/AIDS, Tuberculosis, and Malaria Act of 2002*, S2525, 107th Cong., 2nd sess., introduced in Senate on May 15, 2002, www.congress.gov/107/bills/s2525/BILLS-107s 2525rs.pdf.

23. Health GAP, "Health GAP on Kerry/Frist AIDS Bill: Important Step, More Needed for Global Fund in 2004," Health GAP, May 15, 2002, https://archive.commondreams.org/news2002/0515-16.htm.

24. Fauci interview, January 16, 2018.

25. Bolten interview, 2013.

26. *Minister of Health v. Treatment Action Campaign (TAC)* (2002) 5 SA 721 (CC), www.escr-net.org/caselaw/2006/minister-health-v-treatment-action -campaign-tac-2002-5-sa-721-cc.

27. Asia Russell, phone interview with the author, November 10, 2020.

28. Mark Dybul, interview by Russell Riley, December 6, 2016, Miller Center Presidential Oral History Project, https://millercenter.org/node/52296.

29. Dr. Peter Mugyenyi, interview with the author, Kampala, June 20, 2019.

30. Dr. Eric Goosby, phone interview with the author, January 18, 2018.

31. Fauci interview, January 16, 2018.

32. Gary Edson, phone interview with the author, December 2, 2020.

33. John Donnelly, "The President's Emergency Plan for AIDS Relief: How George W. Bush and Aides Came to 'Think Big' on Battling HIV," *Health Affairs* 31, no. 7 (July 1, 2012): 1389–1396. doi: 10.1377/hlthaff.2012.0408.

34. Congressional aide quotation and description of jurisdictional disputes are from Derek Hodel, *At the Crossroads: A Study of Federal HIV/AIDS Advocacy* (New York: Ford Foundation, 2004).

35. *The National Security Strategy of the United States of America* (Washington, DC: White House, 2002), https://2009-2017.state.gov/documents/organization /63562.pdf.

36. "The Bush Doctrine," Frontpage Symposium, October 7, 2002, Carnegie Endowment for International Peace, https://carnegieendowment.org/2002 /10/07/bush-doctrine-pub-1088.

37. "Saving Families and Communities: A Proposal for a US Presidential Global AIDS Initiative," Health GAP, https://web.archive.org/web/200301 09155502/http://www.healthgap.org/PAI.html.

38. "Congressional Black Caucus Leaders Demand That President Bush Provide Greater Resources for HIV/AIDS Epidemic," Barbara Lee: Congresswoman for the 13th District of California, https://lee.house.gov/news/press-releases/congressional-black-caucus-leaders-demand-that-president-bush-provide-greater-resources-for-hiv/aids-epidemic.

39. Jay Lefkowitz, phone interview with the author, December 1, 2020.

40. Charles Fishman, *One Giant Leap: The Impossible Mission That Flew Us to the Moon* (New York: Simon & Schuster, 2019).

CHAPTER 5: THE COST OF VICTORY

1. Sandra Thurman and Cornelius Baker, interview with the author, Washington, DC, January 21, 2020.

2. Shepherd and Anita Smith, phone interview with the author, April 8, 2019.

3. Senator Bill Frist, phone interview with the author, September 14, 2020.

4. Unless otherwise noted, Lefkowitz quotations and content throughout this chapter are from Jay Lefkowitz, interview with the author, New York City, January 27, 2020.

5. Allen Moore, phone interview with the author, October 29, 2020.

6. Jay Lefkowitz, phone interview with the author, December 2, 2020.

7. KHN, "Frist Withdraws Support for Senate 'AIDS Bill' Passed Last Year; Instead Supports White House Draft of Bill," *KHN Morning Briefing*, February 14, 2003, https://khn.org/morning-breakout/dr00016062.

8. Thurman and Baker interview, January 21, 2020.

9. Dr. Pearl-Alice Marsh, phone interview with the author, August 1, 2019.

10. Sheryl Gay Stolberg, "The World: A Calling to Heal; Getting Religion on AIDS," *New York Times*, February 2, 2003, www.nytimes.com/2003/02/02/weekinreview/the-world-a-calling-to-heal-getting-religion-on-aids.html.

11. "FW: More from Austin Ruse on the HIV/AIDS Initiative," email from Susan Cohen to Heather Boonstra, February 5, 2003 (in the author's possession).

12. For extensive background and links to other sources on the MCP, see "The Mexico City Policy: An Explainer," Kaiser Family Foundation Fact Sheet, November 4, 2020, www.kff.org/global-health-policy/fact-sheet/mexico-city-policy-explainer.

13. There is a long history of women's-health-focused medical organizations endorsing a definition of comprehensive health that includes abortion. For one recent example, see Eve Espey, Amanda Dennis, and Uta Landy, "The Importance of Access to Comprehensive Reproductive Health Care,

Including Abortion: A Statement from Women's Health Professional Organizations," *American Journal of Obstetrics and Gynecology* 220, no. 1 (January 2019): 67–70.

14. Adrienne Germain, interview by Rebecca Sharpless, June 19–20, September 25, 2003, Population and Reproductive Health Oral History Project, Sophia Smith Collection.

15. Michelle Goldberg, *The Means of Reproduction: Sex, Power, and the Future of the World* (New York: Penguin Books, 2009).

16. "Bush Bars UNFPA Funding, Bucking Recommendation of Its Own Investigators," Guttmacher Institute, September 22, 2004, www.guttmacher.org/gpr/2002/10/bush-bars-unfpa-funding-bucking-recommendation-its-own-investigators.

17. "Access to Condoms and HIV/AIDS Information: II. The United States' 'War on Condoms,'" Human Rights Watch, www.hrw.org/legacy/backgrounder/hivaids/condoms1204/2.htm.

18. Jocelyn Kaiser, "Studies of Gay Men, Prostitutes Come Under Scrutiny," *Science* 300, no. 5618 (April 18, 2003): 403. doi: 10.1126/science.300.5618.403.

19. Rumors and concerns that the White House would apply the Mexico City Policy to PEPFAR continued to appear in the press and in correspondence with public officials after February 10, 2003; Lefkowitz attributes this to individuals outside the White House seeking information from sources who were not privy to the decision; his account that the decision was made early is confirmed by Mark Dybul. Mark Dybul, interview by Russell Riley, December 6, 2016, Miller Center Presidential Oral History Project, https://millercenter.org/node/52296.

20. Not all people who get pregnant, breastfeed, or seek to prevent pregnancies identify as women. Not all people who identify as women are born or live in bodies that can bear children. Rigid definitions of sex, gender identity, and gender expression cause individual pain and work against effective health programming. With full acknowledgment of this reality, in this chapter and throughout the book, where the subject is cisgender women and girls from East and Southern Africa, I use the term "women."

21. Stephanie Bi and Tobin Klusty, "Forced Sterilization of HIV-Positive Women: A Global Ethics and Policy Failure," *American Medical Association Journal of Ethics Policy Forum* 17, no. 10 (October 2015). doi: 10.1001/journalofethics.2015.17.10.pfor2-1510.

22. Peter Yeo, phone interview with the author, October 4, 2019; Sam Stratman, phone interview with the author, June 11, 2019.

23. Marsh interview, August 1, 2019.

24. Pearl-Alice Marsh, *But Not Jim Crow: Family Memories of African American Loggers of Maxville, Oregon* (Wallowa, OR: African American Loggers Memory Project, 2019).

25. Pearl-Alice Marsh, "Grassroots Statecraft and Citizens' Challenges to U.S. National Security Policy," chap. 5 of *On Security*, ed. Ronnie D. Lipschutz (New York: Columbia University Press, 1998).

26. Heather Boonstra, phone interview with the author, September 30, 2019.

27. Adrienne Germain, phone interview with the author, August 26, 2019.

28. "Congresswoman Barbara Lee and Congressional Black Caucus Address President Bush's Global HIV/AIDS Proposal Given in State of the Union," Barbara Lee: Congresswoman for the 13th District of California, https://lee .house.gov/news/press-releases/congresswoman-barbara-lee-and-congressional -black-caucus-address-president-bushs-global-hiv/aids-proposal-given -in-state-of-the-union.

29. "Congresswoman Barbara Lee Declares President Bush's FY 04 Plan the Worst Budget in Decades; Bush's Proposal Sends Country Back into Deep Deficits While Cutting Taxes for Wealthy," Barbara Lee: Congress-woman for the 13th District of California, https://lee.house.gov/news/press -releases/congresswoman-barbara-lee-declares-president-bushs-fy-04-plan -the-worst-budget-in-decades-bushs-proposal-sends-country-back-into -deep-deficits-while-cutting-taxes-for-wealthy; "Global AIDS Alliance: Press Releases," May 2, 2003, Internet Archive, https://web.archive.org/web /20030502235045/http://www.globalaidsalliance.org/press040203.html.

30. After envelopes containing anthrax were delivered to members of Congress and media houses, Tommy Thompson, head of the Department of Health and Human Services, threatened to change US law so that the country could access cheaper, generic versions of ciprofloxacin, the antibiotic used as treatment. The cost and availability of Bayer's brand-name version were obstacles to amassing a national stockpile. Bayer ultimately offered a price reduction, but the hypocrisy of America seeking to invoke the trade-related intellectual property provisions it had opposed in the context of AIDS medications did not go unnoticed. For more on this, see Thomas F. Mullin, "Aids, Anthrax, and Compulsory Licensing: Has the United States Learned Anything? A Comment on Recent Decisions on the International Intellec-tual Property Rights of Pharmaceutical Patents," *ILSA Journal of Interna-tional and Comparative Law* 9 (2002): 185–209.

31. Katy French Talento, phone interview with the author, August 12, 2019.

32. Katy French Talento, "Ladies: Is Birth Control the Mother of All Med-ical Malpractice?," *Federalist*, January 5, 2015, https://thefederalist.com /2015/01/05/ladies-is-birth-control-the-mother-of-all-medical-mal practice.

33. Talento's views on sex education and "flirting classes" are well captured in this report (see p. 42), which she helped prepare: US Senate Subcommittee on Federal Financial Management, Government Information and Interna-tional Security, Minority Office, *CDC Off Center: A Review of How an*

Agency Tasked with Fighting and Preventing Disease Has Spent Hundreds of Millions of Tax Dollars for Failed Prevention Efforts, International Junkets and Lavish Facilities, but Cannot Demonstrate It Is Controlling Disease (Washington DC: US Senate, 2007).

34. See, for example, the statement that teaching "sexual communication skills" is effective with "sexually experienced adolescents" in APA Council of Representatives, "Resolution in Favor of Empirically Supported Sex Education and HIV Prevention Programs for Adolescents," American Psychological Association, February 20, 2005, www.apa.org/about/policy/adolescents. The Committee on Adolescent Health of the American College of Obstetricians and Gynecologists (ACOG) notes that "comprehensive sexuality education should begin in early childhood and continue through a person's lifespan" and that programs should focus not only on reproductive development but on "forms of sexual expression, healthy sexual and nonsexual relationships, gender identity and sexual orientation and questioning, communication, recognizing and preventing sexual violence, consent, and decision making." Committee on Adolescent Health Care, "Comprehensive Sexuality Education," Committee Opinion No. 678, November 2016, ACOG, www.acog.org/clinical/clinical-guidance/committee-opinion/arti cles/2016/11/comprehensive-sexuality-education.

35. Michael Fleshman, "Women: The Face of AIDS in Africa," *United Nations Africa Renewal*, October 2004, www.un.org/africarenewal/magazine /october-2004/women-face-aids-africa.

36. "FW: Rep. Pitts and Pro-Life Caucus Concerns on Hyde Bill," email from Susan Cohen to Heather Boonstra, March 26, 2003 (in the author's possession).

37. George W. Bush Presidential Library, Domestic Policy Council Collection, Jay Lefkowitz Subject Files, [AIDS: Correspondence] Folder.

38. Shepherd and Anita Smith, interview with the author, Sterling, Virginia, May 16, 2019.

39. Ann M. Moore et al., "Coerced First Sex Among Adolescent Girls in Sub-Saharan Africa: Prevalence and Context," *African Journal of Reproductive Health* 11, no. 3 (May 5, 2008).

40. Shelley Clark, "Early Marriage and HIV Risks in Sub-Saharan Africa," *Studies in Family Planning* 35, no. 3 (September 1, 2004): 149–160. doi: 10.1111/j.1728-4465.2004.00019.x.

41. Dybul interview, 2016.

42. Derek Hodel, *At the Crossroads: A Study of Federal HIV/AIDS Advocacy* (New York: Ford Foundation, 2004).

43. "H. Rept. 108-60—UNITED STATES LEADERSHIP AGAINST HIV/ AIDS, TUBERCULOSIS, AND MALARIA ACT OF 2003," legislation,

2003/2004, Congress.gov, www.congress.gov/congressional-report/108th
-congress/house-report/60/1.

44. Janet Museveni to Senator Richard Lugar, April 2, 2003, Domestic Policy
Council Collection, Jay Lefkowitz Subject File, AIDS: [Comments and
Material Related to H.R.1298-United States Leadership Against HIV/
AIDS, Tuberculosis and Malaria Act of 2003], George W. Bush Presidential
Library.

45. Helen Epstein, *Another Fine Mess: America, Uganda, and the War on Terror*
(New York: Columbia Global Reports, 2017).

46. George W. Bush Presidential Library, Domestic Policy Council Collection,
Jay Lefkowitz Subject Files, [AIDS: Correspondence] Folder.

47. Henry J. Hyde, "Actions—H.R.1298—108th Congress (2003–2004):
United States Leadership Against HIV/AIDS, Tuberculosis, and Malaria
Act of 2003," May 27, 2003, 2003/2004, Congress.gov, www.congress.gov
/bill/108th-congress/house-bill/1298/all-actions.

48. "Bush Makes Historic Speech Aboard Warship—May 1, 2003," CNN.com,
www.cnn.com/2003/US/05/01/bush.transcript.

49. Frist interview, September 14, 2020.

50. Jay Lefkowitz, phone interview with the author, December 2, 2020.

51. Jay Lefkowitz, phone interview with the author, December 2, 2020.

52. Zena Stein, "HIV Prevention: The Need for Methods Women Can Use,"
American Journal of Public Health 80, no. 4 (April 1990).

53. All quotations are from the *Congressional Record—Senate*, May 15, 2003,
www.congress.gov/crec/2003/05/15/CREC-2003-05-15-pt2-PgS6475.pdf.
Alexander's remarks appear on S6497, Leahy's on S6477, Clinton's on
S6484, and Kennedy's on S6478.

54. "The US and the Global Fund to Fight AIDS, Tuberculosis, and Malaria," Kaiser Family Foundation Fact Sheet, November 26, 2019, www.kff
.org/global-health-policy/fact-sheet/the-u-s-the-global-fund-to-fight-aids
-tuberculosis-and-malaria.

55. Hyde, "Actions—H.R.1298—108th Congress (2003–2004)."

56. Letter from Representatives Nancy Pelosi and Henry Waxman to Joe
O'Neill, May 23, 2003, George W. Bush Presidential Library, Domestic Policy Council, pp. 61–62.

57. Marsh interview, August 1, 2019.

58. PL 108-25, the law that enacted PEPFAR in 2003, allowed for "assistance
that can help avoid substance abuse and intravenous drug use that can lead
to HIV infection." At the time that the law was signed, and for almost all
of the next seventeen years, a federal law banned use of federal funding for
domestic American syringe exchanges. This ban arguably did not apply to
foreign aid. USAID, in non-PEPFAR-related activities, worked with Open

Society Institute and other partners to support harm-reduction services for people who use drugs. While USAID would not use federal funds to purchase sterile injecting equipment, USAID did push back against a 2005 congressional effort to limit US funding for harm-reduction activities and to investigate whether federal funds had been used to purchase syringes overseas. (USAID, Response to Congressional Inquiries Regarding Health Activities in Central Asia: Briefing Book, February 16, 2005, in the author's possession.) Within the PEPFAR context, harm-reduction advocates would find the program far more conservative.

59. Dybul interview, 2016.
60. Dr. Deborah Birx, interview with the author, Washington, DC, March 7, 2018.

CHAPTER 6: STRETCHING THE WEEK

1. November 24th March on White House Coalition, "2003 Year in Review: HIV/AIDS US Policy Briefing Paper" (in the author's possession). The coalition that authored this paper comprised a range of activist groups, including Health GAP, the American Foundation for AIDS Research, the Center for Health and Gender Equity, Housing Works, and several others.
2. Dr. Deborah Birx, phone interview with the author, December 12, 2003.
3. Roland A. Erlandson, "Era Ends as Sparks Family Says Goodbye. Leaving: At 92, Sherman Sparks and His Wife, Helen, 88, Are Calling It Quits at the Landmark Store They Ran for Seven Decades," *Baltimore Sun*, June 28, 1996, www.baltimoresun.com/news/bs-xpm-1996-06-28-1996180069-story .html.
4. Susan Reverby, *Co-conspirator for Justice: The Revolutionary Life of Dr. Alan Berkman* (Chapel Hill: University of North Carolina Press, 2020).
5. PEPFAR launched in 2003 with an initial list of fourteen "focus countries": Botswana, Côte d'Ivoire, Ethiopia, Haiti, Kenya, Mozambique, Namibia, Nigeria, Rwanda, South Africa, Tanzania, Uganda, Vietnam, and Zambia ("The U.S. President's Emergency Plan for AIDS Relief," KFF Global Health Policy Fact Sheet, Kaiser Family Foundation, May 27, 2020, www .kff.org/global-health-policy/fact-sheet/the-u-s-presidents-emergency-plan -for-aids-relief-pepfar/#:~:text=Of%20these%2025%20countries%2C%201 4,Uganda%2C%20Vietnam%2C%20and%20Zambia). Additional countries and regionally focused programs were added over time. For a full list of programs as of 2020, see "Where We Work—PEPFAR," The United States President's Emergency Plan for AIDS Relief, US Department of State, www.state.gov/where-we-work-pepfar.
6. Dr. Eugene McCray, phone interview with the author, January 17, 2018.

7. Andrew Natsios, phone interview with the author, April 12, 2019.

8. Dr. Donna Kabatesi, interview with the author, Kampala, June 17, 2019.

9. Amir Attaran, "Adherence to HAART: Africans Take Medicines More Faithfully Than North Americans," *PLOS Medicine* 4, no. 2 (February 2007). doi: 10.1371/journal.pmed.0040083.

10. Dr. Sten Vermund, phone interview with the author, January 23, 2018.

11. Dr. Deborah Birx, interview with the author, Washington, DC, March 7, 2018.

12. Birx interview, March 7, 2018.

13. Mark Dybul, interview by Russell Riley, December 6, 2016, Miller Center Presidential Oral History Project, https://millercenter.org/node/52296.

14. Natsios interview, April 12, 2019.

15. Michele Moloney-Kitts, phone interview with the author, December 4, 2018.

16. Dybul interview, 2016.

17. David Stanton, phone interview with the author, August 10, 2018.

18. Stanton interview, 2018.

19. Dybul interview, 2016.

20. Kathy Marconi, phone interview with the author, July 24, 2019.

21. 108 *Congressional Record*, July 17, 2003, S9549 "Exhibit 1, Letter from Dr. Joseph O'Neill to Senate Majority Leader Bill Frist," in *Congressional Record*, www.congress.gov/crec/2003/07/17/CREC-2003-07-17-senate.pdf; "'Dr Doo Little' Goes to Africa," OneWorld.net, September 9, 2003, Internet Archive, https://web.archive.org/web/20030909113110/http:/www.oneworld.net/article/view/66291.

22. "President Bush Names Randall Tobias to Be Global AIDS Coordinator," White House, July 2, 2003, https://georgewbush-whitehouse.archives.gov/news/releases/2003/07/images/20030702-3_aids-070203-d-pm-515h.html.

23. Randall Tobias and Todd Tobias, *Put the Moose on the Table: Lessons in Leadership from a CEO's Journey Through Business and Life* (Bloomington: Indiana University Press, 2003).

24. Donald G. McNeil Jr., "From Eli Lilly to Front Line in AIDS War," *New York Times*, July 29, 2003.

25. Randall Tobias, phone interview with the author, May 15, 2019.

26. Treatment Action Campaign, "TAC Welcomes Cabinet Adoption of HIV Treatment Plan—'Hope for Millions.'" November 20, 2003, Internet Archive, https://web.archive.org/web/20031129042448/http://tac.org.za. One month prior, in October 2003, TAC notched another significant victory in a case brought against GlaxoSmithKline and Boehringer Ingelheim in the country's Competition Commission. In the "Hazel Tau" suit, one of its complainants accused the drug companies of excessive pricing. The

Competition Commission determined that the drug companies had "abused their dominant positions" in the antiretroviral market and referred it to the Competition Tribunal, affirming the need for affordable, generic versions of patented medications and the licenses to produce them. "Competition Commission Finds Pharmaceutical Firms in Contravention of the Competition Act," Competition Commission of South Africa, October 16, 2003, www.cptech.org/ip/health/sa/cc10162003.html.

27. Health GAP, "GFATM: HGAP on Round 3 Results, OCT 03," March 1, 2004, Internet Archive, https://web.archive.org/web/20040301153913 /http://www.healthgap.org/press_releases/03/101603_HGAP_PR_GFATM _round3.html.

28. Health GAP, "World AIDS Day Protest White House, Nov 03," November 20, 2003, Internet Archive, https://web.archive.org/web/20040118084115 /http://www.healthgap.org/press_releases/03/112003_HGAP_PR_WAD _protest.html.

29. Dr. Phyllis Kanki, phone interview with the author, April 12, 2018; Dr. Richard Marlink, phone interview with the author, May 5, 2018.

30. For timing of PEPFAR funding disbursals, see Tobias testimony in Subcommittee of African Affairs of the Committee on Foreign Affairs of the United States Senate, *Fighting HIV/AIDS in Africa: A Progress Report*, April 7, 2004.

31. Margrethe Juncker and Father Joseph Archetti, *Reach Out Mbuya Annual Report* (Kampala: Reach Out Mbuya, 2004), www.reachoutmbuya.org /reports/Annual%20Report%202004.pdf.

32. President's Emergency Plan for AIDS Relief, *Engendering Bold Leadership: First Annual Report to Congress on PEPFAR* (Washington, DC: Office of the Global AIDS Coordinator, 2005), https://2009-2017.state.gov/s/gac /rl/c14961.htm; President's Emergency Plan for AIDS Relief, *Action Today, a Foundation for Tomorrow: Second Annual Report to Congress on PEPFAR* (Washington, DC: Office of the Global AIDS Coordinator, 2006), https://2009-2017.state.gov/s/gac/rl/c16742.htm.

33. A. Jahn et al., "Scaling-Up Antiretroviral Therapy in Malawi," *Bulletin of the World Health Organization* 94 (2016): 772–776. doi: http://dx.doi .org/10.2471/BLT.15.166074; E. E. Zijlstra and J. J. G. van Oosterhout, "The Introduction of Antiretroviral Therapy in Malawi," *Nederlands Tijdschrift voor Geneeskunde* 150, no. 50 (December 16, 2006): 2774–2778.

34. "Fund Signs US$36.3 Million Grant to Support Uganda's Ongoing Fight Against HIV/AIDS," Global Fund to Fight AIDS, Tuberculosis and Malaria, 2003. Disbursement delays for Global Fund treatment were part of regular conversation when I was reporting in Uganda in 2004; they are mentioned in the country's FY2005 Country Operational Plan.

35. Dr. Francois Venter, phone interview with the author, October 12, 2020.

36. Dr. Yogan Pillay, phone interview with the author, October 19, 2020.

37. "South Africa Fails to Accept $41 Million from Global Fund," i-base, June 1, 2003, https://i-base.info/htb/11255.

38. Helen Epstein, *Another Fine Mess: America, Uganda, and the War on Terror* (New York: Columbia Global Reports, 2017).

39. Subcommittee of African Affairs, *Fighting HIV/AIDS in Africa*.

40. "Conference on Fixed-Dose Combination Products: Scientific and Technical Issues Related to Safety, Quality and Effectiveness. Gaborone, Botswana. March 29–30, 2004," CPTech.org, www.cptech.org/ip/health/aids/fdc/botswana.html.

41. "U.S. Official Defends Policy on Generic AIDS Drugs; Business Coalition Says Policy Undermining Efforts to Fight Disease," *Kaiser Health News*, April 1, 2004, https://khn.org/morning-breakout/dr00022983.

42. Médecins Sans Frontières, "MSF Statement on Fixed Dose Combination Antiretrovirals," CPTech.org, March 3, 2004, www.cptech.org/ip/health/aids/fdc/msf03302004.html.

43. Donald G. McNeil Jr., "Views Mixed on U.S. Shift on Drugs for AIDS," *New York Times*, May 18, 2004.

44. Nazanin Ash, interview with the author, Washington, DC, November 26, 2018.

45. Sharonann Lynch, interview with the author, New Jersey, May 14, 2019.

Chapter 7: Small Heavens

1. Sir Gerald Portal, *The British Mission to Uganda in 1893* (London: Forgotten Books, 2016).

2. Ngugi wa Thiong'o, *Birth of a Dream Weaver* (New York: The New Press, 2020).

3. wa Thiong'o, *Birth of a Dream Weaver*.

4. "Wayne Bennett's *Uganda Argus* Scrapbook," The Bennett Collection: *Uganda Argus* Newspaper, Carleton University, https://carleton.ca/uganda-collection/the-bennett-collection-uganda-argus-newspaper.

5. Ambassador Horace G. Dawson, interview with Charles Stuart Kennedy, February 7, 1991, Association for Diplomatic Studies and Training, Foreign Affairs Oral History Project.

6. Ambassador Michael Pistor, interview with Charles Stuart Kennedy, June 6, 2001, Association for Diplomatic Studies and Training, Foreign Affairs Oral History Project.

7. Pistor interview and Ambassador Hendrik Van Oss, interview with Lillian Mullin, February 8, 1991, Association for Diplomatic Studies and Training, Foreign Affairs Oral History Project.

8. Rebecca Bunnell and Jonathan Mermin, video interview with the author, January 17, 2018.

9. Reuben Granich and Jonathan Mermin, *HIV, Health, and Your Community* (Berkeley, CA: Hesperian Foundation, 2001), www.unaids.org/sites/default/files/media_asset/jc0038_hiv_health_and_your_community_en_1.pdf.

10. Jonathan Mermin, interview with the author, Atlanta, Georgia, June 5, 2019.

11. Dr. Alex Coutinho, interview with the author, Kampala, Uganda, June 24, 2019.

12. Dr. Alex Coutinho, interview with the author, Kampala, Uganda, June 24, 2019.

13. Jono Mermin, email to the author, January 10, 2021.

14. For a history of this period, see Edward Hooper, *Slim: One Man's Journey Through the AIDS Zone of East Africa* (New York: Vintage, 1990).

15. Amy Cunningham, interview with the author, Kampala, Uganda, June 17, 2019.

16. Dr. Peter Mugyenyi, interview with the author, Kampala, Uganda, May 12, 2005.

17. Rob Cunnane, phone interview with the author, January 15, 2018.

18. Rebecca Bunnell, interview with the author, Kampala, Uganda, May 10, 2005.

19. Jonathan Mermin et al., "Effect of Co-trimoxazole Prophylaxis on Morbidity, Mortality, CD4-Cell Count, and Viral Load in HIV Infection in Rural Uganda," *The Lancet* 364, no. 9443 (October 16–22, 2004). doi: 10.1016/S0140-6736(04)17225-5.

20. Jonathan Mermin et al. "Developing an Evidence-Based, Preventive Care Package for Persons with HIV in Africa," Tropical Medicine and International Health 10, no. 10 (September 26, 2005). doi: 10.1111/j.1365-3156.2005.01488.x.

21. Nearly fifteen years after hearing that story for the first time, I heard it again, unprompted, from a different source who'd also been living in Kampala and working on PEPFAR at the time.

22. Alex Coutinho interview with the author, Kampala, Uganda, March 1, 2005.

23. Christian Pitter, interview with the author, Chevy Chase, Maryland, May 16, 2008.

24. Ambassador Jimmy Kolker, phone interview with the author, December 22, 2017.

25. Helen Epstein, *Another Fine Mess: America, Uganda, and the War on Terror* (New York: Columbia Global Reports, 2017).

CHAPTER 8: THE MEANING OF LIFE

1. Natural Environment Research Council, Institute of Geological Sciences, *50th Anniversary Geological Survey and Mines Department Uganda*, Overseas Geology and Mineral Resources 41 (London: Her Majesty's Stationery Office, 1973); S. J. Mathers, *The Industrial Mineral Resource Potential of Uganda* (London: British Geological Survey, 1994).

2. Cliff Lord, "Military Signalling in East Africa," *Military History Journal of the South African Military History Society* 12, no. 5 (June 2003), http://samilitaryhistory.org/vol125cl.html.

3. Ralph Clark, *Aid in Uganda: Programmes and Policies* (London: Overseas Development Institute, 1966), 59. "The Tororo school is very much a showpiece; it has involved about twice the normal construction costs in Uganda of £600 per place, and has also taken twice as long to build. Tororo's very magnificence could prove unfortunate for it is in such startling contrast to most secondary schools in Uganda that it may encourage an undue sense of privilege amongst staff and pupils who attend it."

4. Helen Wataba (head teacher, Tororo Girls Secondary School), interview with the author, Tororo, Uganda, May 25, 2018.

5. "Photo 22 of 23, E.V. Townsend: Tororo on Independence Day. October 9th 1962," *History in Progress Uganda* (blog), www.hipuganda.org/collection/e-v-townsend/graham-townsend-independence-day.

6. Charles Mohr, "Outward-Bound Asians Tell of Maltreatment by Uganda Soldiers," *New York Times*, September 30, 1972.

7. Ippolytos Andreas Kalofonos, "'All I Eat Is ARVs': The Paradox of AIDS Treatment Interventions in Central Mozambique," *Medical Anthropology Quarterly* 24, no. 3 (September 1, 2010): 363–380. doi: 10.1111/j.1548-1387.2010.01109.x.

8. Yvette Raphael, phone interview with the author, October 13, 2020.

9. "About Us," WE-ACTx, www.we-actx.org/about-us.

10. Anne-christine d'Adesky, phone interview with the author, September 23, 2020.

11. Lillian Mworeko, interview with the author, Ssenge, Uganda, June 21, 2019.

12. "Gays and Lesbians of Zimbabwe (GALZ) (1990–)," Blackpast.org, November 15, 2012, www.blackpast.org/global-african-history/gays-and-lesbians-zimbabwe-galz-1990.

13. "Martha Tholanah," Front Line Defenders, www.frontlinedefenders.org/en/profile/martha-tholanah.

14. Bonnie Goldman, "An Interview with Dorothy Onyango, Founder of Women Fighting AIDS in Kenya," *TheBodyPro*, August 18, 2006, www.thebodypro.com/article/interview-dorothy-onyango-founder-women-fighting-aids-kenya.

15. Felix Mwanza, phone interview with the author, April 28, 2020.

16. "About PATAM," Pan-African Treatment Access Movement (PATAM), January 23, 2004, Internet Archive, https://web.archive.org/web/20040123 003936/http://www.patam.org.

17. The shift that occurred in low-income countries as AIDS drugs arrived mirrored transformations in the AIDS epidemics in wealthy nations a few years prior. There, too, in the years before antiretroviral treatment, and in the face of willful state neglect, communities organized their own networks of care and activism, with little distinction between the two. "AIDS activists...understood their work in terms of political resistance rather than compassion," wrote American historian and sociologist Cindy Patton. As happened in the African context, when government funding and effective biomedical treatment finally arrived, this work got recast, the revolutionary impulse removed, and local efforts redefined as "good works." Badly needed assistance came at the cost of what Patton termed an "amnesia" about the early response. "It ends any society-wide commitment to redistributing wealth, instead allocating resources to who makes an appealing 'victim' rather than according to who has been 'victimized' by society." Cindy Patton, *Inventing AIDS* (Milton Park, UK: Routledge, 1991).

18. Such activist-delivered and activist-designed health-care interventions were not unique to HIV. Abortion rights advocates and harm reductionists in many countries organized to provide medical services governments wouldn't pay for and often also considered illegal. See Naomi Braine, "Autonomous Health Movements: Criminalization, De-medicalization, and Community-Based Direct Action," *Health and Human Rights Journal* 22, no. 2 (December 2020): 85–98.

19. Francois Venter, phone interview with the author, October 12, 2020.

20. Sharonann Lynch, interview with the author, New Jersey, May 14, 2019.

21. All of the names of the people in Taata's family and many of their identifying features have been changed.

22. All of my conversations with Taata and Maama Apollo took place with a translator who worked with me for many years and whose assistance was invaluable. I have not named her or my other longtime translator in order to eliminate any risk that might come from being associated with this project. All of the quotes from Taata and Maama Apollo reflect my translator's English interpretation.

23. "Global Fund Suspends Grants in Uganda," Global Fund, August 24, 2005, theglobalfund.org/en/news/2005-08-24-global-fund-suspends-grants-in-uganda.

24. The names and identifying details of Simon and the clinic staff and location have all been changed.

25. "About Us," Uganda Program for Human and Holistic Development (UPHOLD), http://uphold.jsi.com/About.htm.

26. Vinh-Kim Nguyen, *The Republic of Therapy: Triage and Sovereignty in West Africa's Time of AIDS* (Chapel Hill: Duke University Press, 2010).

27. "The Millennium Challenge Account: Does the Program Match the Vision?," Committee on International Relations, 2005, http://commdocs.house.gov /committees/intlrel/hfa20918.000/hfa20918_of.htm.

28. J. Brian Atwood, M. Peter McPherson, and Andrew Natsios, "Arrested Development Making Foreign Aid a More Effective Tool," *Foreign Affairs* 67 (November/December 2008).

29. Sarah Rose and Franck Wiebe, "MCC @ 10: Focus on Results: MCC's Model in Practice," *Center for Global Development MCC Monitor*, January 2015, 4.

30. Nazanin Ash, interview with the author, Washington, DC, November 26, 2018.

31. Rose and Wiebe, "MCC @ 10," 5.

32. Congressional Research Service, *Millennium Challenge Corporation: Overview and Issues* (Washington, DC: Congressional Research Service, 2019).

33. Bradley C. Parks and Caroline Davis, "When Do Governments Trade Domestic Reforms for External Rewards? Explaining Policy Responses to the Millennium Challenge Corporation's Eligibility Standards," *Governance* 32, no. 2 (April 1, 2019): 349–367. doi: 10.1111/gove.12376.

34. Emma Mawdsley, "The Millennium Challenge Account: Neo-liberalism, Poverty, and Security," *Review of International Political Economy* 14, no. 3 (May 2, 2008): 487–509. doi: 10.1080/09692290701395742.

35. Brook K. Baker, "Global Fund's Granting System: Laissez-Faire Granting System Is Delivering Planned Failure," Health GAP Background Paper, April 25, 2005, Internet Archive, https://web.archive.org/web/20060907073811 /http://www.healthgap.org/press_releases/05/042505_HGAP_BP_GFATM _disbursements_Baker.doc.

36. Mark Dybul, interview by Russell Riley, December 6, 2016, Miller Center Presidential Oral History Project, https://millercenter.org/node/52296.

37. Lancaster, *George Bush's Foreign Aid*.

CHAPTER 9: WHERE THE BODIES ARE BURIED

1. Scott Shane and Mark Mazzetti, "Interrogation Methods Are Criticized," *New York Times*, May 30, 2007.

2. Susan Saulny, "Some Hitherto Staunch G.O.P. Voters Souring on Iraq," *New York Times*, May 30, 2007.

3. Jonathan Stempel, "New Century Files for Chapter 11 Bankruptcy," *Reuters*, April 2, 2007.

4. Jeffrey Klausner et al., "Scale-Up and Continuation of Antiretroviral Therapy in South African Treatment Programs, 2005–2009," *Journal of Acquired Immune Deficiency Syndromes* 56, no. 3 (March 1, 2011). doi: 10.1097/QAI.0b013e3182067d99.

5. "Uganda Country Operational Plan, FY 2008," PEPFAR, www.state.gov/wp-content/uploads/2019/08/Uganda-5.pdf.

6. Jane Gruber von Kerenshazy et al., *USAID/South Africa PEPFAR Treatment Program: Final Evaluation* (Washington DC: USAID, 2011).

7. PEPFAR's treatment tallies count individuals with HIV who attended ART programs receiving direct support from the US government, such as payment for drugs and staff costs, as well as clients who attended clinics receiving technical assistance, such as staff training.

8. "President Bush Announces Five-Year, $30 Billion HIV/AIDS Plan," White House, May 30, 2007, https://georgewbush-whitehouse.archives.gov/news/releases/2007/05/20070530-6.html.

9. Joint United Nations Programme on HIV/AIDS and World Health Organization, *AIDS Epidemic Update* (Geneva: UNAIDS and World Health Organization, 2007). UNAIDS would, in the coming years, change its data-collection and quantification approach and revise this figure downward.

10. "Significant Growth in Access to HIV Treatment in 2006," World Health Organization, April 17, 2007, www.who.int/mediacentre/news/releases/2007/pr16/en; World Health Organization, *Antiretroviral Therapy for HIV Infection in Adults and Adolescents: Recommendations for a Public Health Approach* (Geneva: World Health Organization, Department of HIV/AIDS, 2006). The 2006 recommendations also stated that people with CD4 cell counts below 350 could be considered for ART initiation.

11. Mike Igoe, "Exclusive: Documents Reveal Largest USAID Health Project in Trouble," *Devex*, August 25, 2017, www.devex.com/news/sponsored/exclusive-documents-reveal-largest-usaid-health-project-in-trouble-90933.

12. "SCMS Milestones: Building the Ship While Sailing," SCMS 10 Year Report, http://scms10yearreview.pfscm.org.

13. Personal communication from PEPFAR staff and minutes from US-Ugandan coordination meetings in 2004–2005 (in the author's possession).

14. "The Next Phase of the Global Fight Against HIV/AIDS," House Committee on Foreign Relations, October 24, 2007, 8.

15. Author's notes, Rakai, November 17, 2005.

16. "The Next Phase of the Global Fight Against HIV/AIDS," 10.

17. Gregorio A. Millett and John L Peterson, "The Known Hidden Epidemic: HIV/AIDS Among Black Men Who Have Sex with Men in the United States," *American Journal of Preventive Medicine* 32, no. 4 Suppl. (2007): S31–S33. doi:10.1016/j.amepre.2006.12.028.

18. Kaiser Family Foundation, "Public Opinion on the HIV/AIDS Epidemic in the United States," 2006, Internet Archive, https://web.archive.org/web/20090723173203/https://www.kff.org/spotlight/hivus/upload/HIV_US_Epidemic_outline.pdf.

19. Both Adimora and Millett have published extensively; papers produced during this period include A. A. Adimora and V. J. Schoenbach, "Social Context, Sexual Networks, and Racial Disparities in Rates of Sexually Transmitted Infections," *Journal of Infectious Diseases* 191 Suppl. 1 (February 1, 2005): S115–S122. doi: 10.1086/425280. PMID: 15627221; A. A. Adimora, V. J. Schoenbach, and I. A. Doherty, "Concurrent Sexual Partnerships Among Men in the United States," *American Journal of Public Health* 97, no. 12 (December 2007): 2230–2237. doi: 10.2105/AJPH.2006.099069. Also see G. A. Millett et al., "Explaining Disparities in HIV Infection Among Black and White Men Who Have Sex with Men: A Meta-analysis of HIV Risk Behaviors," *AIDS* 21, no. 15 (October 1, 2007): 2083–2091. doi: 10.1097/QAD.0b013e3282e9a64b. PMID: 17885299.

20. "President Bush Announces Five-Year, $30 Billion HIV/AIDS Plan."

21. President's Emergency Plan for AIDS Relief, *The Power of Partnerships: The President's Emergency Plan for AIDS Relief—Third Annual Report to Congress* (Washington, DC: PEPFAR, 2007), www.state.gov/wp-content/uploads/2019/08/PEPFAR-2007-Annual-Report-to-Congress.pdf.

22. Global Fund, "Pledges and Contributions Report," Global Fund, December 11, 2020, https://www.theglobalfund.org/en/government.

23. "United States Government, Global Fund Collaborate to Treat 1.58 Million People Living with HIV/AIDS," Global Fund, June 1, 2007, www.theglobalfund.org/en/news/2007-06-01-united-states-government-global-fund-collaborate-to-treat-1-58-million-people-living-with-hiv-aids.

24. Brian McKeon, phone interview with the author, July 19, 2018.

25. "PEPFAR: An Assessment of Progress and Challenges," House Committee on Foreign Affairs, April 24, 2007, https://foreignaffairs.house.gov/2007/4/pepfar-assessment-progress-and-challenges.

26. Committee for the Evaluation of the President's Emergency Plan for AIDS Relief (PEPFAR) Implementation, *PEPFAR Implementation: Progress and Promise* (Washington, DC: National Academies Press, 2007), x–xii.

27. Committee for the Evaluation of PEPFAR Implementation, *PEPFAR Implementation*, 11.

28. Committee for the Evaluation of PEPFAR Implementation, *PEPFAR Implementation*, x.

29. Howard Berman, "Tom Lantos and Henry J. Hyde United States Global Leadership Against HIV/AIDS, Tuberculosis and Malaria Act of 2008—Report Accompanying HR5501," House Committee on Foreign Affairs, March 10, 2008, 2.

30. K. A. Thomson et al. "Increased Risk of Female HIV-1 Acquisition Through-out Pregnancy and Postpartum: A Prospective Per-Coital Act Analysis Among Women with HIV-1 Infected Partners," *Journal of Infectious Diseases* 218, no. 1 (June 5, 2018); K. Brittain et al. "Determinants of Suboptimal Adherence and Elevated HIV Viral Load in Pregnant Women Already on Antiretroviral Ther-apy When Entering Antenatal Care in Cape Town, South Africa," *AIDS Care* 30, no. 12 (July 16, 2018), www.tandfonline.com/doi/abs/10.1080/09540121 .2018.1503637?journalCode=caic20; K. Brittain et al. "Long-Term Effects of Unintended Pregnancy on Antiretroviral Therapy Outcomes Among South African Women Living with HIV," *AIDS* 33, no. 5 (April 1, 2019).

31. "Perspectives on the Next Phase of the Global Fight Against AIDS, Tuber-culosis and Malaria," Senate Committee on Foreign Relations, December 13, 2007, 29.

32. "PEPFAR Reauthorization: From Emergency to Sustainability," House Committee on Foreign Affairs, September 25, 2007, 11–12.

33. "PEPFAR Reauthorization," 71.

34. Janet Fleischman and Allen Moore, *International Family Planning: A Common-Ground Approach to an Expanded U.S. Role* (Washington, DC: Center for Strategic and International Studies Global Health Policy Center, 2009), 16.

35. "PEPFAR Reauthorization," 26–30.

36. Mark Dybul, interview by Russell Riley, December 6, 2016, Miller Center Presidential Oral History Project, https://millercenter.org/node/52296.

37. "The Next Phase of the Global Fight Against HIV/AIDS," 7.

38. Mark Dybul, interview by Russell Riley, December 6, 2016, Miller Center Presidential Oral History Project, https://millercenter.org/node/52296.

39. "The Next Phase of the Global Fight Against HIV/AIDS," 19.

40. Michele Moloney-Kitts, interview with the author, Cape Cod, Massachu-setts, August 28, 2019.

41. Janet Fleischman, *Voices from the Field: The Role of Integrated Reproductive Health and HIV/AIDS Programs in Strengthening U.S. Policy* (Washington, DC: Center for Strategic and International Studies, 2008).

42. Yvette Raphael, phone interview with the author, October 13, 2020.

43. Yvette Raphael, phone interview with the author, August 21, 2020.

44. Paul Davis and two other activists present recall these events; Biden aides told me they did not.

45. "PEPFAR Re-authorization Prevention Working Group Meeting Notes," January 11, 2007 (in the author's possession).

46. Dr. Pearl-Alice Marsh, phone interview with the author, August 1, 2019.

47. Serra Sippel, phone interview with the author, January 23, 2020; "Discus-sion Draft HR—'To Authorize Appropriations for Fiscal Years 2009

Through 2013 to Provide Assistance to Foreign Countries to Combat HIV/ AIDS, Tuberculosis, and Malaria, and for Other Purposes,'" January 18, 2008 (in the author's possession).

48. Jeffrey T. Bergner, Assistant Secretary, Legislative Affairs, "Letter to Tom Lantos, Chairman, Committee on Foreign Affairs, House of Representatives," February 7, 2008.

49. Yeo interview, October 4, 2019. (Dybul would later say that the Democrats delayed too long in making concessions and that they might have kept some of the language in had they compromised earlier.)

50. Heather Boonstra, phone interview with the author, September 30, 2019.

51. "Markup Before the Committee on Foreign Affairs, House of Representatives," 110th Cong., 2nd sess., Serial No. 110–158, February 27, 2008, 252.

52. Katy Talento, interview with the author, Washington, DC, October 15, 2019.

53. 110 Cong. Rec. S7814 Daily Edition, July 31, 2008 (Statement of Sen. Coburn).

54. 110 Cong. Rec. S1999 Daily Edition, March 12, 2008.

55. 110 Cong. Rec. S2149 Daily Edition, March 13, 2008 (Remarks of Sen. Kyl).

56. "Bear Stearns Collapses, Sold to J.P. Morgan Chase," History.com, March 16, 2008, www.history.com/this-day-in-history/bear-stearns-sold-to-j-p-morgan -chase.

57. Sarah Schulman, *The Gentrification of the Mind: Witness to a Lost Imagination* (Berkeley: University of California Press, 2013).

58. Kaytee Ray-Riek, phone interview with the author, December 6, 2019.

59. Paul Davis, phone interview with the author, January 18, 2019.

60. Michael Weinstein, phone interview with the author, December 6, 2019.

61. John Blandford, phone interview with the author, April 24, 2019.

62. Senator Joseph Biden, *Report: The Tom Lantos and Henry J. Hyde Global Leadership Against HIV/AIDS, Tuberculosis and Malaria Reauthorization Act of 2008*, US Senate, 110th Congress, April 15, 2008, 22, www.congress .gov/110/crpt/srpt325/CRPT-110srpt325.pdf.

63. The letter, "Letter to Republican Leader Mitch McConnell," March 31, 2008, was cosigned by seven senators, including Tom Coburn, Jim Bunning, Saxby Chambliss, Jim DeMint, Jeff Sessions, and David Vitter (in the author's possession).

64. Ray-Riek interview, December 6, 2019.

65. H. Grosskurth et al., "Impact of Improved Treatment of Sexually Transmitted Diseases on HIV Infection in Rural Tanzania: Randomised Controlled Trial," *The Lancet* 346, no. 8974 (August 26, 1995): 530–536. doi: 10.1016 /s0140-6736(95)91380-7. PMID: 7658778.

66. M. J. Wawer et al., "Control of Sexually Transmitted Diseases for AIDS Prevention in Uganda: A Randomised Community Trial. Rakai Project Study Group," *The Lancet* 353, no. 9152 (February 13, 1999): 525–535. doi: 10.1016/s0140-6736(98)06439-3.

67. 110 Cong. Rec. S6384 Daily Edition, July 16, 2008 (Statement of Sen. Dodd).

68. 110 Cong. Rec. S6839, Daily Edition, July 16, 2008 (Statement of Sen. Coburn).

CHAPTER 10: ARRESTED DEVELOPMENT

1. Colleen Denny and Ezekiel Emanuel, "US Health Aid beyond PEPFAR: The Mother & Child Campaign," *JAMA* 300 (December 1, 2008): 2048–2051. doi: 10.1001/jama.2008.556.

2. Ezekiel J. Emanuel et al., "What Makes Clinical Research in Developing Countries Ethical? The Benchmarks of Ethical Research," *Journal of Infectious Diseases* 189, no. 5 (March 1, 2004): 930–937. doi: 10.1086/381709.

3. Lin Liu, phone interview with the author, March 13, 2020.

4. "Statement by the President on Global Health Initiative," White House, May 5, 2009, https://obamawhitehouse.archives.gov/the-press-office/statement -president-global-health-initiative.

5. For a concise review of the Obama administration's H1N1 and Ebola virus response work, see the second section of this documentary series: "America's Pandemic," Part 2: "Guided by Science," *Washington Post*, October 27, 2020, https://www.washingtonpost.com/graphics/2020/national/administrations -pandemic-documentary.

6. "President Obama's Global Development Policy and the Global Health Initiative," Fact Sheet, White House, September 22, 2010.

7. Kaiser Health News, "Bush Releases FY 2009 Budget with Funding for Global Health Programs," *Kaiser Health News*, June 11, 2009, https://khn .org/morning-breakout/dr00050215; US Department of State and the Broadcasting Board of Governors Office of the Inspector General, *Review of the President's Emergency Plan for AIDS Relief (PEPFAR) at Select Embassies Overseas*, Report Number ISP-I-11-07 (Washington, DC: Department of State and OIG, 2010), www.stateoig.gov/system/files/154967.pdf; Health Gap, "Obama Proposes $6.6 bn Cut to Global AIDS Programs," Internet Archive, May 5, 2009, https://web.archive.org/web/20100628095928/http:// www.healthgap.org/press/obamafy10budget.htm.

8. Mike Pflanz, "Barack Obama 'Breaks Four Aid Pledges for Africa,'" *Telegraph*, May 18, 2009, www.telegraph.co.uk/news/worldnews/barackobama /5344290/Barack-Obama-breaks-four-aid-pledges-for-Africa.html.

9. Ezekiel Emanuel, phone interview with the author, January 30, 2019.

10. Sharonann Lynch, interview with the author, New Jersey, May 14, 2019.

11. John Blandford, phone interview with the author, April 24, 2019.

12. Jodi Jacobson, "Dybul Out: Thank You, Hillary!!!," *Rewire News Group*, January 22, 2009, https://rewirenewsgroup.com/article/2009/01/22/dybul -out-thank-you-hillary.

13. The President's Emergency Plan for AIDS Relief, "Country Operational Plan (COP) Guidance: Programmatic Considerations, FY2010, The President's Emergency Plan for AIDS Relief," PEPFAR, June 29, 2009, 17.

14. US Department of State and the Broadcasting Board of Governors, *Review of PEPFAR at Select Embassies Overseas*. Report No. ISP-I-11-07 (Washington, DC: Office of the Inspector General, December 2010), https://www .stateoig.gov/system/files/154967.pdf.

15. Mead Over, "Prevention Failure: The Ballooning Entitlement Burden of U.S. Global AIDS Treatment Spending and What to Do About It," Center for Global Development, April 2008.

16. Helping to Enhance the Livelihood of People Around the Globe, *Beyond Assistance: The HELP Commission Report on Foreign Assistance Reform*, Center for American Progress, December 7, 2007, www.americanprogress.org/wp -content/uploads/issues/2007/12/pdf/beyond_assistence.pdf.

17. Dr. Eric Goosby, phone interview with the author, January 18, 2018.

18. Eric Goosby, phone interview with the author, March 30, 2018.

19. Mark Landler, "G-8 Leaders Reaffirm Promises of Billions to Battle AIDS and Other Diseases," *New York Times*, June 9, 2007.

20. "US Congress Approves $900 Million Record Support for the Global Fund," *The Global Fund* (blog), March 11, 2009, www.theglobalfund.org/en /news/2009-03-11-us-congress-approves-usd-900-million-record-support -for-global-fund.

21. "Global Fund Facing Shortfall," *New Humanitarian*, February 6, 2009, www.thenewhumanitarian.org/news/2009/02/06/global-fund-facing -shortfall; "UN-Backed Fund Needs Additional $4 Billion to Fund AIDS, TB and Malaria Efforts," *UN News*, April 1, 2009, https://news.un.org/en /story/2009/04/295662.

22. Anso Thom, "Africa: Moves to Decrease Aids Funding Slammed," *allAfrica*, July 22, 2009, https://allafrica.com/stories/200907220200.html.

23. "Drug Shortages Reach Crisis Levels in South African Province," *Science Speaks: Global ID News*, April 22, 2009, https://sciencespeaksblog .org/2009/04/22/drug-shortages-reach-crisis-levels-in-south-african-pro vince.

24. The three original papers showing the impact of voluntary medical male circumcision are listed here; subsequent follow-up research has confirmed and increased estimates of the efficacy of the procedure: B. Auvert, D. Taljaard,

and E. Lagarde, "Randomized Controlled Intervention Trial of Male Circumcision for Reduction of HIV Infection Risk: The ANRS 1265 Trial," *PLOS Medicine* 2 (2005): e298, doi:10.1371/journal.pmed.0020298; R. H. Gray et al., "Male Circumcision for HIV Prevention in Men in Rakai, Uganda: A Randomised Trial," *The Lancet* 369 (2007): 657–666; R. Bailey, S. Moses, and C. Parker, "Male Circumcision for HIV Prevention in Young Men in Kisumu, Kenya: A Randomised Controlled Trial," *The Lancet* (2007): 643–656.

25. Eric Lugada et al., "Rapid Implementation of an Integrated Large-Scale HIV Counseling and Testing, Malaria, and Diarrhea Prevention Campaign in Rural Kenya," *PLOS ONE* 5, no. 8 (August 2010): e12435. doi: 10.1371/journal.pone.0012435.

26. "Uganda's All-You-Can-Eat Corruption Buffet," Wikileaks Public Library of US Diplomacy (Uganda Kampala, January 5, 2010), https://search.wikileaks.org/plusd/cables/10KAMPALA5_a.html.

27. "Population Growth: Uganda's Ticking Time Bomb," Wikileaks Public Library of US Diplomacy (Uganda Kampala, August 21, 2009), https://search.wikileaks.org/plusd/cables/09KAMPALA955_a.html; "Museveni Mixes Toxic Brew of Ethnicity and Oil in Western Uganda," Wikileaks Public Library of US Diplomacy (Uganda Kampala, August 19, 2009), https://search.wikileaks.org/plusd/cables/09KAMPALA946_a.html.

28. "Scenesetter for OGAC Ambassador Goosby September 26–30 Visit to Uganda," Wikileaks Public Library of US Diplomacy (Uganda Kampala, September 23, 2009), https://search.wikileaks.org/plusd/cables/09KAMPALA1098_a.html.

29. "Forensic Audit May Uncover Corruption at the Uganda Aids Commission," Wikileaks Public Library of US Diplomacy (Uganda Kampala, August 26, 2009), https://wikileaks.org/plusd/cables/09KAMPALA985_a.html. A subsequent independent audit of the Uganda AIDS Commission confirmed mismanagement, as described in Danida, Irish Aid, USAID. *Joint Evaluation of Support to the National Response to HIV/AIDS in Uganda 2007–2012* (Denmark: Ministry of Foreign Affairs, 2014).

30. "Forensic Audit May Uncover Corruption at the Uganda Aids Commission."

31. "Uganda: Scenesetter for Visit of Assistant Secretary Carson," Wikileaks Public Library of US Diplomacy (Uganda Kampala, October 19, 2009), https://wikileaks.org/plusd/cables/09KAMPALA1197_a.html.

32. David Wendt, "If You Drive, I'll Pay for Gas: Critical Developments in the Ownership and Financing of the National AIDS Response," Center for Global Development Commentary and Analysis, July 29, 2009, www.cgdev.org/blog/if-you-drive-i%E2%80%99ll-pay-gas-critical-developments-ownership-and-financing-national-hivaids.

33. Centers for Disease Control and Prevention, "Letter to ART Implementing Partners, Cc: Zainab Akol, Program Manager, AIDS Control Program, Ministry of Health," October 21, 2009 (in the author's possession). While the CDC version of the letter was the one leaked to the public, sources familiar with the issue say that the directive was program wide and that other agencies funding ART, including USAID Uganda, wrote similar letters.

34. "Uganda-UPDF," AMISOM, https://amisom-au.org/wp-content/cache/page _enhanced/amisom-au.org/uganda-updf/_index.html_gzip.

35. "Uganda: Assistant Secretary Carson's Meeting with President Museveni," Wikileaks Public Library of US Diplomacy (Uganda Kampala, November 4, 2009), https://search.wikileaks.org/plusd/cables/09KAMPALA1276_a .html.

36. Charles Holmes, phone interview with the author, April 8, 2019.

37. Amy Cunningham, interview with the author, Kampala, Uganda, June 17, 2019.

38. Peter Mugyenyi, interview with the author, Lubowa, Uganda, July 30, 2013.

39. Vivikka Molldrem et al., *Uganda Indigenous Partners' Programs Assessment* (Washington, DC: USAID, 2009).

40. The Mitchell Group, Inc., *End-of-Project Evaluation of the ACE Program* (Kampala: USAID-Uganda, 2009).

41. "SUSTAIN: Strengthening Uganda's Systems for Treating AIDS Nationally," URC, www.urc-chs.com/sites/default/files/UgandaSUSTAINBrochure 2013.pdf.

42. Citation omitted to preserve confidentiality (in the author's possession).

43. Citation omitted to preserve confidentiality (in the author's possession).

44. "Scenesetter for OGAC Ambassador Goosby September 26–30 Visit to Uganda."

45. Felecia Peterson, CDC IRB G administrator, "Closure of Protocol Study 3666, 'Uganda Home-Based AIDS Care Project,'" March 26, 2009 (in the author's possession).

46. The CDC granted my Freedom of Information Act request to review documents related to the review of HBAC, but as of early 2021—nearly a year after approval—had not provided them.

47. James Mugeni, interview with the author, Kampala, Uganda, July 30, 2013.

48. Rajiv Shah, phone interview with the author, June 13, 2020.

49. Lois Quam, phone interview with the author, February 15, 2019.

50. Deirdre Shesgreen, "Will Infectious Diseases Get Slighted in Foreign Assistance Overhaul?," *Science Speaks: HIV & TB News*, August 5, 2009, https:// sciencespeaks.wordpress.com/2009/08/05/will-infectious-diseases-get -slighted-in-foreign-assistance-overhaul; Editorial Board, "USAID: An

Agency Without Leader and Direction," *The Lancet* 374, no. 9689 (August 15, 2009): 502. doi: 10.1016/S0140-6736(09)61466-5.

51. Josh Rogin, "Obama's Development Reviews Still at Odds After High Level Meeting," *Foreign Policy: The Cable*, April 22, 2010.

52. Guest Writer, "Global Center Weighs In on House Foreign Policy Overhaul," *Science Speaks: Global ID News*, August 14, 2009, https://science speaksblog.org/2009/08/14/global-center-weighs-in-on-house-foreign -policy-overhaul.

53. Médecins Sans Frontières, *No Time to Quit: HIV/AIDS Treatment Gap Widening in Africa* (New York: Médecins Sans Frontières, 2010), www.msf.org /sites/msf.org/files/msf-no-time-to-quit-hiv-aids.pdf.

54. Donald G. McNeil Jr., "In Uganda, AIDS War Is Falling Apart," *New York Times*, May 10, 2010; Farah Stockman, "US Seeks to Rein in AIDS Program," *Boston Globe*, April 11, 2010.

55. Gorik Ooms et al., "The 'Diagonal' Approach to Global Fund Financing: A Cure for the Broader Malaise of Health Systems?," *Globalization and Health* 4, no. 1 (2008): 6. doi: 10.1186/1744-8603-4-6.

56. Gorik Ooms, "Health Development Versus Medical Relief: The Illusion Versus the Irrelevance of Sustainability," *PLOS Medicine* 3, no. 8 (August 15, 2006), https://doi.org/10.1371/journal.pmed.0030345.

57. Francois Venter, phone interview with the author, October 12, 2020.

58. Lois Quam, email to Hillary Clinton, WikiLeaks—Hillary Clinton Email Archive, https://wikileaks.org/clinton-emails/emailid/5240.

59. Cheryl Mills, email to Hillary Clinton, WikiLeaks—Hillary Clinton Email Archive, https://wikileaks.org/clinton-emails/emailid/33656.

60. Eric Goosby, phone interview with the author, September 9, 2020.

61. Raj Shah, phone interview with the author, June 11, 2020.

62. Congressional Research Service (CRS), *The Global Health Security Agenda (GHSA): 2020–2024* (Washington, DC: CRS, March 16, 2020).

63. Kevin De Cock and Wafaa El-Sadr, "A Tale of Two Viruses: HIV, Ebola, and Health Systems," *AIDS* 29, no. 9 (June 1, 2015): 989–991. doi: 10.1097/ QAD.0000000000000726.

64. Deborah Birx, "Making the World Safer from Health Threats," *DipNote: Global Health* (US Department of State blog), April 6, 2018, https:// medium.com/statedept/making-the-world-safer-from-health-threats-2a45 ef770901.

65. De Cock and El-Sadr, "A Tale of Two Viruses."

66. John Donnelly, "Obama Administration Closes Global Health Initiative Office," *PRI: The World*, July 3, 2012, www.pri.org/stories/2012-07-03 /obama-administration-closes-global-health-initiative-office.

67. Amanda Glassman, "The Office of Global Health Diplomacy: A Christmas Miracle or Lump of Coal?" *Center for Global Health Diplomacy* (blog),

December 17, 2012, www.cgdev.org/blog/office-global-health-diplomacy-christmas-miracle-or-lump-coal.

68. National Academies of Sciences, Engineering, and Medicine; Health and Medicine Division; Board on Global Health; Committee on Global Health and the Future Role of the United States, *Global Health and the Future Role of the United States* (Washington, DC: National Academies Press, May 15, 2017), chap. 9.

69. Kolker interview, December 29, 2017.

70. "The Global Health Initiative: The Next Phase of American Leadership in Global Health Around the World" (remarks by Secretary of State Hillary Rodham Clinton, August 16, 2010, School of Advanced International Studies, Washington, DC), available on the website of the American Institute in Taiwan at www.ait.org.tw/the-global-health-initiative-the-next-phase-of-american-leadership-in-health-around-the-world-remarks-by-hillary-rodham-clinton-secretary-of-state.

71. Gayle Smith, phone interview with the author, April 25, 2019.

72. "The U.S. President's Emergency Plan for AIDS Relief (PEPFAR)," Kaiser Family Foundation, May 27, 2020, www.kff.org/global-health-policy/fact-sheet/the-u-s-presidents-emergency-plan-for-aids-relief-pepfar.

Chapter 11: The End of AIDS

1. Medical anthropologists engage with pharmaceuticals as social and cultural phenomena and propose a "biographical approach" to understanding the ideas, values, practices, and cultures that emerge as drugs enter communities. See, for example, Sjaak van der Geest, Susan Reynolds Whyte, and Anita Hardon, "The Anthropology of Pharmaceuticals: A Biographical Approach," *Annual Review of Anthropology* 25 (1996): 153–178, http://www.jstor.org/stable/2155822.

2. Myron S. Cohen et al., "HIV Treatment as Prevention: How Scientific Discovery Occurred and Translated Rapidly into Policy for the Global Response," *Health Affairs* 31, no. 7 (July 1, 2012): 1439–1449. doi: 10.1377/hlthaff.2012.0250.

3. Global Fund to Fight AIDS, Tuberculosis and Malaria (GFATM), "Chair's Summary: Third Voluntary Replenishment (2011–2013), Pledging Conference, New York, USA, 4–5 October, 2010," Global Fund, 2010, www.theglobalfund.org/media/1439/replenishment_2010newyork_chairsummary_en.pdf; GFATM, "Chair's Summary: The Third Global Fund Replenishment (2011–2013) Preparatory Meeting, 24–25 March 2010," Global Fund, 2010, www.theglobalfund.org/media/1417/replenishment_2010haguechair_summary_en.pdf?u=637319004577470000.

4. John Blandford, phone interview with the author, January 12, 2020.

5. Charles Holmes, phone interview with the author, March 31, 2020.

6. Sean Strub, email to the Health GAP listserv, circa August 9, 2011. The text of this email is in the author's possession; over the course of my research, the domain for the Health GAP email list archive ceased to work on the web or in the Wayback Machine.

7. Jeffrey Gettleman, "David Kato, Gay Rights Activist, Is Killed in Uganda," *New York Times*, January 27, 2011.

8. "Uganda: Homophobe Extremists and Homosexual Scapegoats," Wikileaks Public Library of US Diplomacy (Uganda Kampala, December 24, 2009), https://search.wikileaks.org/plusd/cables/09KAMPALA1413_a.html.

9. "SMUG_First_Amended_COMPLAINT.pdf," Center for Constitutional Rights, https://ccrjustice.org/sites/default/files/attach/2014/12/SMUG_First _Amended_COMPLAINT.pdf. A federal judge affirmed that Lively aided and abetted persecution of Ugandan homosexuals, while dismissing the case on a narrow jurisdictional ground.

10. Richard Lusimbo, interview with the author, Kampala, Uganda, June 18, 2019.

11. International Gay and Lesbian Human Rights Commission (IGLHRC), *Off the Map: How HIV/AIDS Programming Is Failing Same-Sex Practicing People in Africa* (New York: IGLHRC, 2007).

12. As a candidate, Barack Obama promised to lift the long-standing bans on federal funding for needle and syringe exchange programs but included language contrary to this in his first budget request to Congress. In 2009, Congress did lift this ban, then reinstated it in legislation signed by Obama in 2012. The ban on funding purchase of syringes and needles didn't preclude other harm-reduction programming, but pendulum swings in policy on interventions with demonstrated public health benefit hurt the HIV response at home and abroad. See Matt Fisher, "A History of the Ban on Federal Funding for Syringe Exchange Programs," *Smart Global Health* (Center for Strategic and International Studies blog), February 7, 2012, www.csis.org/blogs/smart-global-health/history-ban-federal-funding -syringe-exchange-programs, and "New Directions for PEPFAR? Setting the Course of US AIDS Efforts: An Interview with Eric Goosby," *TREAT Asia Report*, amfAR, June 2010, www.amfar.org/articles/around-the-world /treatasia/2010/an-interview-with-ambassador-eric-goosby—new -directions-for-pepfar—setting-the-course-of-u-s—aids-efforts.

13. Makerere University School of Public Health, PEPFAR/Centers for Disease Control and Prevention, and the Ministry of Health, *The Crane Survey Report*, MU-SPH/PEPFAR/MOH, 2010, http://fileserver.idpc.net/library /Crane-Survey-Report-Round-1-Dec10.pdf; President Museveni said, "We have no homosexuals here," in a 1999 speech. IGLHRC, *Off the Map*.

14. Chris Beyrer et al., "The Increase in Global HIV Epidemics in MSM," *AIDS* 27, no. 17 (November 13, 2013). doi: 10.1097/01.aids.0000432449.30239

.fe; Gaston Djomand et al., "HIV Epidemic Among Key Populations in West Africa," *Current Opinion in HIV/AIDS* 9, no. 5 (September 2014). doi: 0.1097/COH.0000000000000090.

15. "Uganda: Homophobe Extremists and Homosexual Scapegoats."

16. Scott Evertz, *How Ideology Trumped Science: Why PEPFAR Has Failed to Meet Its Potential* (Washington, DC: Center for American Progress, 2010), www.americanprogress.org/issues/healthcare/reports/2010/01/13/7214/how -ideology-trumped-science.

17. Lusimbo interview, June 18, 2019.

18. Anthony S. Fauci, "AIDS: Let Science Inform Policy," *Science* 333, no. 6038 (July 1, 2011), 13, https://science.sciencemag.org/content/333/6038/13.

19. "PrEP Can Reduce Risk of HIV Infection Among Heterosexuals," May 13, 2019, Centers for Disease Control and Prevention Newsroom, www.cdc .gov/nchhstp/newsroom/2011/prepheterosexuals.html.

20. Jon Cohen, "New Prevention Data Leads WHO to Delay Guidelines for Couples," *Science*, July 25, 2011, www.sciencemag.org/news/2011/07/new -prevention-data-leads-who-delay-guidelines-couples.

21. Geoff Garnett, phone interview with the author, June 22, 2020.

22. UNAIDS, *A New Investment Framework for the Global HIV Response* (Geneva: UNAIDS, 2011).

23. Timothy B. Hallett et al., "Optimal Uses of Antiretrovirals for Prevention in HIV-1 Serodiscordant Heterosexual Couples in South Africa: A Modelling Study," *PLOS Medicine* 8, no. 11 (November 15, 2011): e1001123. doi: 10.1371/journal.pmed.1001123.

24. Nathan Ford, "HIV Treatment as Prevention: We Urgently Need Policy Guidance," Médecins Sans Frontières Access Campaign, July 21, 2011, https:// msfaccess.org/hiv-treatment-prevention-we-urgently-need-policy-guidance.

25. UNAIDS, *Investing for Results. Results for People. A People-Centred Investment Tool Towards Ending AIDS* (Geneva: UNAIDS, 2012).

26. Roger England, "A Strategic Revolution in HIV and Global Health," *The Lancet* 378, no. 9787 (July 16, 2011): 226. doi: 10.1016/S0140-6736(11)61119-7.

27. Michel Sidibé, "Sustainable Health Care Is a Moral Obligation, Speech at the Pontifical Council for Health Care," UNAIDS, May 28, 2011, www.unaids .org/en/media/unaids/contentassets/documents/speech/2011/20110528 _Sidibe_Vatican_en.pdf.

28. UNAIDS, *A New Investment Framework*.

29. Blandford interview, January 12, 2020.

30. M. Cohen et al., "HIV Treatment as Prevention," 2012.

31. In a December 1, 2011, email sent to USAID administrator Raj Shah and to the Health GAP listserv, veteran AIDS activist and cofounder of the Treatment Action Group Gregg Gonsalves wrote, "But why is [*sic*] Rajiv Shah, the Administrator of USAID, been arguing in the background, plotting

with his former colleagues at Gates Foundation, to derail substantial new investments in ART, even though it is our most powerful tool now for saving lives, preventing new infections? What's going on? Well, if you've been schooled at the Gates Foundation, you've heard countless times from the benefactor that we can't treat our way out of the epidemic, even though the new science says that is exactly what might be possible." Individuals working at the Office of the Global AIDS Coordinator confirm intense resistance from USAID to the proposal to expand the treatment target.

32. Grace Wyler, "Obamas Get Flirty at New York Fundraiser," *Business Insider*, September 20, 2011.

33. Leigh Blake, phone interview with the author, March 10, 2020. Paul Zeitz, Sharonann Lynch, and Matthew Kavanagh all confirmed elements of these events, as do contemporaneous notes provided by Lynch (in the author's possession).

34. Laurie McHugh, phone interview with the author, March 19, 2020.

35. Hillary Clinton, "Remarks on 'Creating an AIDS-Free Generation,'" US Department of State Newsroom, November 11, 2017, https://2009-2017 .state.gov/secretary/20092013clinton/rm/2011/11/176810.htm.

36. David Brown, "Fund Halts New Grants for AIDS, TB and Malaria Treatment in Poor Countries," *Washington Post*, November 23, 2011.

37. Médecins Sans Frontières, "Médecins Sans Frontières Response to Unprecedented Decision to Cancel Funding Round of the Global Fund to Fight AIDS, TB and Malaria, Taken at Board Meeting in Accra, Ghana, November 21–22, 2011," lists.critpath.org, November 22, 2011, https://lists.critpath .org/pipermail/healthgap/2011-November/003176.html.

38. All quotes are from Sharonann Lynch's "running file" of meeting notes, emails, and conversations conducted during this period (in the author's possession).

39. GFATM, "Turning the Page from Emergency to Sustainability: The Final Report of the High-Level Independent Review Panel on the Fiduciary Controls and Oversight Mechanisms of the Global Fund to Fight AIDS, Tuberculosis and Malaria," Global Fund, September 19, 2011, www.theglobalfund.org/me dia/5424/bm25_highlevelpanelindependentreviewpanel_report_en.pdf.

40. Asia Russell, "Funding the Fight to End the AIDS Epidemic," in *AIDS Today: Tell No Lies, Claim No Easy Victories*, ed. Sisonke Msimang (Brighton, UK: International HIV/AIDS Alliance, 2014).

41. Email and notes provided by Sharonann Lynch (in the author's possession).

42. Matthew Kavanagh, interview with the author, December 19, 2019, Washington, DC. Sharonann Lynch was present and had the same recollection; Chris Collins also confirmed hearing about this interaction from Kavanagh at the time.

43. "National AIDS Strategy," Office of National AIDS Policy, White House, https://obamawhitehouse.archives.gov/administration/eop/onap/nhas;

"Remarks by the President on World AIDS Day," White House, December 1, 2013, https://obamawhitehouse.archives.gov/photos-and-video/video/2013/12/02/world-aids-day-2013#transcript.

44. Kellie Moss and Jennifer Kates, "PEPFAR Reauthorization: Side-by-Side of Legislation over Time," Kaiser Family Foundation, January 19, 2019; Peter Troilo, "What's Next for America's Global HIV/AIDS Program?," *Devex*, July 23, 2012, www.devex.com/news/what-s-next-for-america-s-global-hiv -aids-program-78747.

45. PEPFAR, "10th Annual Report to Congress," US Department of State, 2014, www.state.gov/wp-content/uploads/2019/08/PEPFAR-2014-Annual-Report -to-Congress.pdf.

CHAPTER 12: MADAM AMBASSADOR

1. "Remarks at Swearing-in Ceremony for Ambassador-at-Large and Coordinator of the USG Activities to Combat HIV/AIDS Deborah Birx," US Department of State, April 25, 2014, https://2009-2017.state.gov/secretary /remarks/2014/04/225218.htm.

2. Deborah Birx, interview with the author, Washington, DC, March 5, 2018.

3. Sandra Thurman and Cornelius Baker, interview with the author, Washington, DC, January 21, 2020.

4. Deborah Birx and Angeli Achrekar, interview wth the author, New York City, December 5, 2018.

5. Nomo's existence was confirmed in multiple interviews by Goosby-era staffers.

6. John Donnelly, "US Reveals Nearly $1.5 Billion in Unspent AIDS Money," *The World*, April 17, 2012, www.pri.org/stories/2012-04-17/us-reveals-nearly -15-billion-unspent-aids-money.

7. John Donnelly, "A Q&A with US Global AIDS Coordinator Eric Goosby," *The World*, April 18, 2012, www.pri.org/stories/2012-04-18/qa-us-global-aids -coordinator-eric-goosby.

8. Birx interview, March 5, 2018.

9. Deborah Birx and Angeli Achrekar, interview with the author, Washington, DC, July 31, 2019.

10. Sandra Thurman, email to the author, June 20, 2020.

11. Paul Zeitz, interview with the author, Washington, DC, April 15, 2019.

12. Paige Reffe, interview with the author, Washington, DC, January 29, 2020.

13. Paul Zeitz interview, April 15, 2019.

14. Julia Martin, phone interview with the author, August 28, 2020.

15. Eric Goosby, phone interview with the author, September 9, 2020.

16. Birx and Achrekar interview, December 5, 2018.

17. Sandra Thurman and Cornelius Baker, interview with the author, Washington, DC, January 29, 2020.

18. Mike Gehron, phone interview with the author, May 6, 2019.

19. Irum Zaidi, interview with the author, Washington, DC, July 31, 2018.

20. UNAIDS, "Fast Track: Ending the AIDS Epidemic by 2030," UNAIDS, September 25, 2014, www.unaids.org/en/resources/documents/2014/fast_track.

21. UNAIDS, *Fast-Track—Ending the AIDS Epidemic by 2030*. World AIDS Day Report (Geneva: UNAIDS, 2014), www.unaids.org/sites/default/files/media_asset/JC2686_WAD2014report_en.pdf.

22. UNAIDS, "BRICS Health Ministers Adopt the UNAIDS Fast-Track Strategy to End the AIDS Epidemic," UNAIDS, December 10, 2014, www.unaids.org/en/resources/presscentre/featurestories/2014/december/2014 1210_brics.

23. President's Emergency Plan for AIDS Relief, *PEPFAR 3.0: Controlling the Epidemic, Delivering on the Promise of an AIDS-Free Generation* (Washington, DC: Office of the Global AIDS Coordinator, 2014), www.state.gov/wp-content/uploads/2019/08/PEPFAR-3.0-%E2%80%93-Controlling-the-Epidemic-Delivering-on-the-Promise-of-an-AIDS-free-Generation.pdf.

24. Zeitz interview, April 15, 2019.

25. Judith Bruce, phone interview with the author, May 6, 2020.

26. Nina Hasen, phone interview with the author, May 5, 2020.

27. Birx and Achrekar interview, December 5, 2018.

28. Noni Mokati, " 'Blood'-Stained Panties Make a Statement About Victims," *Saturday Star*, February 18, 2013, www.iol.co.za/saturday-star/blood-stained-panties-make-a-statement-about-victims-1472492.

CHAPTER 13: OUR WORK IS FAR FROM DONE

1. "Uganda," Civil Freedom Monitor, International Center for Not-for-Profit Law, accessed on October 15, 2020, www.icnl.org/resources/civic-freedom-monitor/uganda; "Anti Pornography Act, 2014," Uganda Legal Information Institute, https://ulii.org/ug/legislation/act/2015/1-7.

2. "Ugandan President Yoweri Museveni Signs Anti-gay Bill," *BBC News*, February 24, 2014, www.bbc.com/news/world-africa-26320102.

3. The photo essay, titled "We Are Here: LGBTI in Uganda," by D. David Robinson and Sunnivie Brydum won awards for excellence in photojournalism; however, it is no longer posted on the internet. Intrepid searchers can find components of it via the Internet Archive Wayback Machine at archive.org/web.

4. Richard Lusimbo, phone interview with the author, May 6, 2020.

5. Sara Allinder, phone interview with the author, April 8, 2019.

6. "US Imposes Sanctions on Uganda for Anti-gay Law," *BBC News*, June 19, 2014, www.bbc.com/news/world-us-canada-27933051; Andy Kopsa, "Obama's Evangelical Gravy Train," *The Nation*, July 8, 2014. As described in this article, the United States announced additional military aid to

Uganda during the same period in which it imposed sanctions related to the antihomosexuality act.

7. J. Lester Feder, "U.S. Funding Choices Are Challenged in the Wake of Uganda's Anti-gay Law," *BuzzFeed News*, March 6, 2014, www.buzzfeednews.com/article /lesterfeder/us-gave-millions-of-hiv-dollars-to-supporter-of-ugandas-anti.

8. Robert W. Mason, *Agreed-upon Procedures Review of USAID Resources Managed by Inter-religious Council of Uganda Under Cooperative Agreement AID-617-A-10-00002* (Pretoria: USAID Office of the Inspector General, Regional Inspector General, 2013), https://oig.usaid.gov/sites/default/files/2018 -06/4-617-14-001-s.pdf. The review concluded that US government money hadn't gone toward promoting the antihomosexuality bill. It also hadn't located any overtly homophobic content, just a booklet that urged political leaders to "advocate" for the passage of legislation "denouncing all forms of negative cultural practices." The OIG read this as both ambiguous and troubling and recommended that this specific booklet be revised. USAID/Uganda had, in its formal response to the findings, respectfully disagreed. That text appeared in a booklet on the prevention of mother-to-child transmission. It could also refer to genital mutilation, wife inheritance, and child marriage. To remove it would be to invite controversy and erase concerns about these other issues, which did require legislative remediation.

9. Frank Mugisha, "Smoking Out the Gays: How Legislating Against Hatred Has Distracted Ugandans and Reversed Hard-Won Gains in the Fight Against AIDS," in *AIDS Today: Tell No Lies, Claim No Easy Victories*, ed. International HIV/AIDS Alliance (Brighton, UK: International HIV/ AIDS Alliance, 2014), 120.

10. Binyavanga Wainana, "I Am a Homosexual, Mum," *Africa Is a Country*, January 1, 2014, https://africasacountry.com/2014/01/i-am-a-homosexual-mum/. Kevin Mwachiro, "Shaken But Not Stirred: Ugandan LGBTI Activist Richard Lusimbo," *Hivos News*, April 8, 2014, https://east-africa.hivos.org /news/shaken-but-not-stirred-ugandan-lgbti-activist-richard-lusimbo/.

11. Kenneth Mwachiro. "Shaken But Not Stirred: Ugandan LGBTI Activist Richard Lusimbo," *Hivos* blog, April 8, 2014, https://east-africa.hivos.org /news/shaken-but-not-stirred-ugandan-lgbti-activist-richard-lusimbo/.

12. "Uganda Court Annuls Anti-homosexuality Law," *BBC News*, August 1, 2014.

13. "Uganda Pride 2014," Pulitzer Center, November 10, 2014, https://pulitzer center.org/reporting/uganda-pride-2014.

14. PEPFAR's rhetoric on providing HIV prevention and treatment for people who use drugs (PWUD) would change over time—after initially omitting numerical reporting on services to PWUD, the program would begin to tally those services, as well as track ARV delivery to PWUD. From 2008 on, the program did take a more proactive approach, naming harm reduction as a core component of HIV prevention. However, in 2016, these

expenditures amounted to 0.5 percent of the program's overall budget. Even as injecting drug use emerged as a driver of HIV subepidemics in East, Southern, and West Africa, the program would remain cautious and even conservative in its approach to harm reduction. Activists would find more flexibility and opportunities for securing funding for harm-reduction approaches via activism directed at the Global Fund. The global AIDS epidemic will not be brought under control without a comprehensive shift in the legal, health, and human rights context for people who use drugs in every country, a topic that requires more attention than it receives in these pages. For additional context, see Catherine Cook and Charlotte Davies, *The Lost Decade: Neglect for Harm Reduction Funding and the Health Crisis Among People Who Use Drugs* (London: Harm Reduction International, 2018); Joanne Csete et al., "Lives to Save: PEPFAR, HIV, and Injecting Drug Use in Africa," *The Lancet* 373, no. 9680 (June 13, 2009). doi: 10.1016 /S0140-6736(09)61092-8; HIV Guest Writer, "Goosby: PEPFAR Examines Next Steps as Needle Exchange Ban Officially Nixed," *Science Speaks Blog*, December 17, 2009, https://sciencespeaksblog.org/2009/12/17/goosby -pepfar-examines-next-steps-as-needle-exchange-ban-officially-nixed.

15. President's Emergency Plan for AIDS Relief, "PEPFAR Process—How Does It All Relate?," slide presentation, September 8, 2015, https://ng.usem bassy.gov/wp-content/uploads/sites/177/2017/02/2015_09_08-PEPFAR -Annual-Cycle.pdf.

16. Kenneth Mwehonge, interview with the author, Kampala, Uganda, June 20, 2019.

17. Antigone Barton, "State Department Cable to Embassies: Meet with, Document, and Respond to Civil Society When Building Country PEPFAR Plans," *Science Speaks: Global ID News*, June 25, 2013, https://sciencespeaksblog .org/2013/06/25/state-departmentment-cable-to-embassies-meet-with -document-and-respond-to-civil-society-when-building-country-pepfar-plans.

18. Maureen Milanga, phone interview with the author, May 7, 2020.

19. Milanga interview, May 7, 2020.

20. Chamunorwa Mashoko, phone interview with the author, May 3, 2020.

21. Mwehonge interview, June 20, 2019.

22. Sandra Thurman and Cornelius Baker, interview with the author, Washington, DC, January 29, 2020.

23. Felix Mwanza, phone interview with the author, April 28, 2020.

24. In 2003, the South African province of KwaZulu-Natal applied for and was awarded a Global Fund grant over the objections of the then AIDS-denialist-led national government, which challenged the grant on the grounds that the country did not have a CCM.

25. amfAR, *Data Watch: Data Accessibility from Global Funders of HIV, TB and Malaria Programming* (Washington, DC: amfAR, 2019), www.amfar.org

/data-watch-accessibility. As the report notes, "A 2016 review of 50 CCMs by the Global Fund's Office of Inspector General (OIG) found that only 9% of CCMs were fully compliant with eligibility criteria for CCM membership. Eighty-four percent of CCMs surveyed had no clearly defined mechanism for obtaining input from constituencies, and 58% did not share oversight reports with country stakeholders. Among civil society and key population representatives surveyed in these 50 countries, 54% reported that their CCM failed to share pertinent information with constituencies" (citation in the original has been removed).

26. "PEPFAR Watch," Health GAP, https://healthgap.org/resources/pepfar-watch.

27. President's Emergency Plan for AIDS Relief, *PEPFAR 2019 Country Operational Plan Guidance for all PEPFAR Countries* (Washington, DC: Office of the Global AIDS Coordinator, 2019), 358.

28. "Open letter to Ambassador Birx," AVAC, January 13, 2020, www.avac.org /sites/default/files/u3/IndexTestingLetter_Jan2020.pdf.

29. "Ambassador Deborah Birx: 'I Don't Find Anything Impossible,'" *AIDS 2020* (podcast), Center for Strategic and International Studies, February 20, 2020, www.csis.org/node/55560.

30. "FY 2019 PEPFAR Planned Allocations," Memo from S/GAC—Ambassador Deborah L. Birx, MD, to Chargé LaPenn, South Africa, January 16, 2019, www.state.gov/wp-content/uploads/2019/08/South-Africa.pdf.

31. amfAR, *Data Watch*, 11.

32. L. C. Simbayi et al., *South African National HIV Prevalence, Incidence, Behaviour and Communication Survey, 2017* (Cape Town: HSRC Press, 2019); Alain Vandormael et al., "HIV Incidence Declines in a Rural South African Population: A G-Imputation Approach for Inference," *BMC Public Health* 20 (August 6, 2020). doi: 10.1186/s12889-020-09193-4.

33. M. Kate Grabowski et al., "HIV Prevention Efforts and Incidence of HIV in Uganda," *New England Journal of Medicine* 377, no. 22 (November 30, 2017): 2154–2166. doi: 10.1056/NEJMoa1702150.

34. Adam Akullian et al., "The Effect of 90-90-90 on HIV-1 Incidence and Mortality in ESwatini: A Mathematical Modelling Study," *The Lancet* 7, no. 5 (February 13, 2020), www.thelancet.com/journals/lanhiv/article/PIIS2352 -3018(19)30436-9/fulltext.

35. Sara M. Allinder, *South Africa's Future at the Brink: Emergency in the World's Largest HIV Epidemic* (Washington, DC: CSIS Global Health Policy Center, Center for Strategic and International Studies, 2020), 15.

36. J. P. Lawrence, "Claim: Denied: Wounded in Iraq, Ugandans Fight for Compensation from America," *The Intercept*, February 22, 2016.

37. I visited Tororo in May 2018 and June 2019. Information about the shift in data use comes from an interview with Dr. Rebecca Amongi, Tororo, Uganda, June 19, 2019.

38. "Ambassador Deborah Birx: 'I Don't Find Anything Impossible.'"
39. Mike Igoe, "PEPFAR Chief Wants 70 Percent 'Indigenous' Funding in 30 Months," *Devex*, July 16, 2018.
40. David Serwadda, interview with the author, Kampala, Uganda, June 24, 2019.
41. US Department of State, *Audit of the Department of State's Coordination and Oversight of the US President's Emergency Plan for AIDS Relief* (Washington, DC: OIG, February 2020).
42. Joshua Musinguzi, interview with the author, Kampala, Uganda, June 24, 2019.
43. David Okumo, interview with the author, Tororo, Uganda, May 25, 2018.
44. "Star Report: Malawi Compact," Millennium Challenge Corporation, April 2020, www.mcc.gov/resources/story/section-mwi-star-report-executive-summary.
45. Sanyu Mojola, *Love, Money and HIV: Becoming a Modern Woman in the Age of AIDS* (Oakland: University of California Press, 2014), 178.
46. In the 2020 report cited below, a government team surveying four PEPFAR country programs found that "across the four missions, PEPFAR country teams consistently expressed the belief that their input was not considered during the COP development process, especially regarding the attainability of performance targets and changes to the OGAC-developed preparation tools" (p. 10). In response to this report, the Office of the Global AIDS Coordinator said that it changed the target-setting process in order to give country teams more flexibility and control. US Department of State, *Audit of the Department of State's Coordination and Oversight*.
47. Deborah Malac, interview with the author, Kampala, June 20, 2019.
48. Matthew Kavanagh, interview with the author, Washington, DC, March 7, 2018.
49. Lillian Mworeko, phone interview with the author, April 30, 2020.
50. Katy Talento, interview with the author, Washington, DC, October 15, 2019.
51. Katy Talento, "Here's How to Prepare if the Coronavirus Comes to a Quarantine," *The Federalist*, March 2, 2020.
52. Shepherd and Anita Smith, interview with the author, Sterling, Virgina, May 16, 2019. The Smiths had known Birx since her days working at the Walter Reed Army Institute for Research when she'd briefly served as an advisor for their group, ASAP, and on at least one occasion wrapped Christmas presents with them for their charitable mission. This association would emerge in the context of an internal investigation of Birx's then supervisor, Dr. Robert Redfield, an ASAP board member, prompted in part by allegations that he'd shared confidential information on a vaccine candidate with the Smiths. Redfield would ultimately be cleared of wrongdoing but sanctioned for an improper relationship with the Smiths. The investigation did

not result in any findings of impropriety for Birx, the public records of which would remain the primary source for descriptions of her as part of the "Christian Right." An extensive array of primary sources, including letters of concern and testimony, can be found in the University of Michigan's Jon Cohen AIDS Research Collection online archive (https://quod.lib .umich.edu/c/cohenaids).

53. Michael Gerson, "Trump Team's Compassionate Act Will Keep Up the Momentum on AIDS Prevention," *Washington Post*, January 20, 2017.

54. Helen Cooper, "Trump Team's Queries About Africa Point to Skepticism About Aid," *New York Times*, January 13, 2017.

55. "U.S. Global AIDS Coordinator Birx Addresses Potential Impacts of Mexico City Policy, Budget Cuts on PEPFAR Operations, Highlights Importance of Data," Kaiser Family Foundation, March 14, 2017, www.kff .org/news-summary/u-s-global-aids-coordinator-birx-downplays-potential -impacts-of-mexico-city-policy-budget-cuts-on-pepfar-operations -highlights-importance-of-data.

56. "Remarks by Vice President Pence at World AIDS Day Event," White House, December 1, 2018, www.whitehouse.gov/briefings-statements/remarks-vice -president-pence-world-aids-day-event.

57. "H.R.6651–115th Congress (2017–2018): PEPFAR Extension Act of 2018," Congress.gov, www.congress.gov/bill/115th-congress/house-bill/6651.

58. Megan Twohey, "Mike Pence's Response to H.I.V. Outbreak: Prayer, Then a Change of Heart," *New York Times*, August 7, 2016; Associated Press, "Pence's Handling of 2015 HIV Outbreak Gets New Scrutiny," *NBC News*, February 28, 2020, www.nbcnews.com/politics/white-house/pence-s-hand ling-2015-hiv-outbreak-gets-new-scrutiny-n1144786.

59. International AIDS Society, "New Evidence Shows Far-Reaching Impact of Expanded US 'Global Gag Rule,'" media alert, AIDS 2018, July 27, 2018, http://www.aids2018.org/Media-Centre/The-latest/Press-releases/Article ID/194/New-evidence-shows-far-reaching-impact-of-expanded-US-%E 2%80%9Cglobal-gag-rule%E2%80%9D; amfAR, *The Effect of the Expanded Mexico City Policy on HIV/AIDS Programming: Evidence from the PEPFAR Implementing Partners Survey* (Washington, DC: amfAR, 2019), www.amfar .org/uploadedFiles/_amfarorg/Articles/On_The_Hill/2019/IB-1-31-19a.pdf.

60. Paul Zeitz, interview with the author, Washington, DC, April 15, 2019.

61. "DREAMS Partnership," PEPFAR, 2019, www.state.gov/pepfar-dreams -partnership/#:~:text=Data%20released%20on%20World%20AIDS,by% 20greater%20than%2040%20percent. "Making DREAMS a Reality: Supporting Determined, Resilient, Empowered, AIDS-Free, Mentored and Safe Girls," CDC Division of Global HIV & TB, 2018, www.cdc.gov /globalhivtb/who-we-are/resources/keyareafactsheets/Making-DREAMS -a-Reality.pdf.

As of 2020, PEPFAR's reports on incidence reduction in DREAMS districts had not been validated as a direct causal impact of the program's work. In-depth evaluations designed to deliver a more direct assessment of impact were ongoing and are described here: Isolde Birdthistle et al., "Evaluating the Impact of the DREAMS Partnership to Reduce HIV Incidence Among Adolescent Girls and Young Women in Four Settings: A Study Protocol," *BMC Public Health* 18, no. 912 (July 2018). doi: 10.1186/s12889-018-5789-7.

62. PEPFAR, "Key Populations Investment Fund Fact Sheet," US Department of State, 2020, www.state.gov/wp-content/uploads/2020/07/PEPFAR_Key -Populations-Investment-Fund_Fact-Sheet_2020.pdf; Kate Sosin, "Trump Has Gutted LGBTQ+ Rights: Could a Biden Presidency Undo the Damage?" *USA Today*, October 10, 2020.

63. Yvette Raphael, phone interview with the author, October 13, 2020.

CHAPTER 14: THE BEGINNING

1. UNICEF, *Averting a Lost COVID Generation: A Six-Point Plan to Respond, Recover and Reimagine a Post-pandemic World for Every Child* (New York: UNICEF, November 2020), www.unicef.org/media/86881/file/Averting-a-lost -covid-generation-world-childrens-day-data-and-advocacy-brief-2020.pdf.

2. UNFPA, with contributions from Avenir Health, Johns Hopkins University (USA), and Victoria University (Australia), "Impact of the COVID-19 Pandemic on Family Planning and Ending Gender-Based Violence, Female Mutilation, and Child Marriage," Interim Technical Note, UNFPA, April 27, 2020, www.unfpa.org/sites/default/files/resource-pdf/COVID-19_impact_brief _for_UNFPA_24_April_2020_1.pdf.

3. This figure was reported at a media briefing by Dr. Tedros Adhanom Ghebreyesus, WHO director-general, and tweeted the same day by the World Health Organization. @WHO, "A survey of responses from 103 countries," Twitter, August 3, 2020, 1:27 p.m., https://twitter.com/who/status/1290232 744274870273?lang=en.

4. Jasmine Aly et al., "Contraception Access During the COVID-19 Pandemic," *Contraception and Reproductive Medicine* 5, no 17 (October 8, 2020). doi: 10.1186/s40834-020-00114-9.

5. See, for example, Adrian Dunlop et al., "Challenges in Maintaining Treatment Services for People Who Use Drugs During the COVID-19 Pandemic," *Harm Reduction Journal* 17, no. 26 (May 6, 2020). doi: 10.1186 /s12954-020-00370-7; Haifeng Jiang et al., "Challenges of Methadone Maintenance Treatment During the COVID-19 Epidemic in China: Policy and Service Recommendations," *European Neuropsychopharmacology* 35 (June 2020). doi: 10.1016/j.euroneuro.2020.03.018.

6. "COVID-19 Response Mechanism," Global Fund, www.theglobalfund
.org/en/covid-19/response-mechanism.

7. Office of the Global AIDS Coordinator, "PEPFAR Technical Guidance in Context of COVID-19 Pandemic," US Department of State, October 7, 2020, www.state.gov/wp-content/uploads/2020/10/10.07.2020-PEPFAR-Technical-Guidance-During-COVID.pdf (launched in April 2020, the PEPFAR guidance was updated on a regular basis).

8. Dr. Tiffany G. Harris, "Resilience of HIV Activities During COVID-19 Pandemic at Health Facilities in Africa," presented at Virtual Conference on Retroviruses and Opportunistic Infections, March 2021, *Late-Breaker Abstract* 186.

9. PEPFAR's data for select program indicators are presented and regularly updated on "PEPFAR Panorama Spotlight" (https://data.pepfar.gov).

10. Winnie Byanyima, phone interview with the author, March 18, 2020.

11. UNAIDS, *Prevailing Against Pandemics by Putting People at the Centre: World AIDS Day Report 2020* (Geneva: UNAIDS, 2020).

12. "Covid-19 Situation Report #32," Global Fund, November 2020, www
.theglobalfund.org/media/10304/covid19_2020-11-11-situation_report
_en.pdf?u=637408006351070000.

13. Ewen Callaway, "The Unequal Scramble for Coronavirus Vaccines—by the Numbers," *Nature News Explainer*, August 24, 2020, www.nature.com/articles
/d41586-020-02450-x.

14. Aruna Kashyap and Margaret Wurth, "Waiving Intellectual Property Rules Key to Beating Covid-19," Human Rights Watch, November 16, 2020, www.hrw.org/news/2020/11/16/waiving-intellectual-property-rules-key-beating-covid-19#.

15. Paige Reffe, interview with the author, Washington, DC, January 29, 2020.

16. Tim Murphy, "Has Deborah Birx Crossed the Line?," *TheBodyPro*, March 30, 2020, www.thebodypro.com/article/deborah-birx-coronavirus-task-force-crossed-the-line.

17. Sarah Schlesinger, phone interview with the author, December 2, 2020.

18. Gregg Gonsalves (@gregggonsalves), "So apparently #DeborahBirx...," Twitter, March 27, 2020, 2:35 p.m., https://twitter.com/gregggonsalves/status
/1243516937788940298.

19. Charles Piller, "The Inside Story of How Trump's COVID-19 Coordinator Undermined the World's Top Health Agency," *Science*, October 14, 2020, https://www.sciencemag.org/news/2020/10/inside-story-how-trumps-covid-19-coordinator-undermined-cdc.

20. Elise Reuter, "HHS Renews $10.2M TeleTracking Contract for COVID-19 Data Collection," *MedCity News*, October 5, 2020, https://medcitynews
.com/2020/10/hhs-renews-10-2m-teletracking-contract-for-covid-19-data
-collection.

21. Alexis C. Madrigal, "America's Most Reliable Pandemic Data Are Now at Risk," *Atlantic*, January 18, 2021.

22. James Bandler et al., "Inside the Fall of the CDC," *ProPublica*, October 15, 2020, www.propublica.org/article/inside-the-fall-of-the-cdc.

23. Jonathan Mermin, interview with the author, Atlanta, Georgia, June 6, 2020.

24. PEPFAR, "PEPFAR Uganda Country Operational Plan (COP) 2019: Strategic Direction Summary," US Department of State, April 12, 2019, www .state.gov/wp-content/uploads/2019/09/Uganda_COP19-Strategic -Directional-Summary_public.pdf.

25. Stanford University, "Statement Regarding Scott Atlas," *Stanford University News*, November 16, 2020, https://news.stanford.edu/2020/11/16/statement -regarding-scott-atlas/.

26. Kate Bennett and Elizabeth Cohen, "Birx Cedes White House Turf to Atlas While Hitting the Road to Spread Her Public Health Gospel," *CNN*, October 29, 2020, www.cnn.com/2020/10/29/politics/deborah-birx-task-force -scott-atlas/index.html.

27. Adam Cancryn, "'It's Complicated': Biden Team Weighs Whether to Retain Deborah Birx," *Politico*, November 18, 2020, www.politico.com/news /2020/11/18/biden-coronavirus-team-deborah-birx-437923.

28. David M. Morens and Anthony S. Fauci, "Emerging Pandemic Diseases: How We Got to COVID-19," *Cell* 182, no. 5 (September 3, 2020): 1077–1092. doi.org/10.1016/j.cell.2020.08.021.

29. Kenneth Bernard, phone interview with the author, October 30, 2020.

30. Bill Frist, email to the author, November 23, 2020.

31. Peter Sands, "COVID-19 Must Transform the Definition of Global Health Security," *The Global Fund* (blog), November 19, 2020, www.theglobalfund .org/en/blog/2020-11-19-covid-19-must-transform-the-definition-of-global -health-security.

32. Richard Jolly and Deepayan Basu Ray, *The Human Security Framework and National Human Development Reports* (Geneva: UNDP, 2006).

33. See, for example, the challenges to implementing a "human security" approach to public health in this article: Kenneth W. Bernard, "Health and National Security: A Contemporary Collision of Cultures," *Biosecurity and Bioterrorism: Biodefense Strategy, Practice and Science* 11, no. 2 (November 2, 2013). doi: 10.1089/bsp.2013.8522.

34. Cissy, interview with the author, Brooklyn, New York, March 6, 2020.

INDEX

INDEX

INDEX

Helms Amendment, 116
Hemphill, Essex, 37–38
Heywood, Mark, 35, 108
Hirnschall, Gottfried, 309
HIV diagnoses, 11, 301, 362; Cissy experience
  around, 76, 77, 108, 352; Fauci on
  survivability and, 9–10; for Katana, 68–69;
  for Mworeko, 78, 108; PEPFAR impact for
  adolescent girls/young women, 390; Raphael
  response to, 38–39; stigma and persecution
  around, 4–5, 347, 348–349, 352–353
HIV origins, 18–19
HIV Plus, 8, 10–13, 17, 31, 32, 140, 201
HIV Prevention Trials Network (HPTN),
  299–303, 307–313, 328
HIV/AIDS activism, 10–11, 14–16, 21, 24,
  67, 302. *See also specific individuals and
  organizations*; discipline and expertise with,
  303–304; frustrations with power brokers,
  310–311; human security and, 410; inside-
  outside game in, 26, 328; lessons from, 4,
  404–405, 407–408; "90-90-90" targets and,
  362–363; around treatment as prevention,
  302–304, 309–310, 312
HIV/AIDS in Africa. *See also* President's
  Emergency Plan for AIDS Relief; *specific
  countries and topics*: AIDS in US contrasted
  with, 70; Bush, G. W., 2003 PEPFAR
  speech on fighting, 1–6, 53, 108–113, 300,
  379; coercive sex for young women in,
  128; environmental degradation relation
  to, 375–376; gender gap in, 124; housing
  activism and, 39–40; 9/11 and US aid for, 85;
  South African government denialism with,
  33, 34, 39, 40, 42, 100, 157; US and global
  initial negligence in fight against, 3, 5–6
HIV/AIDS in US: Black Americans and rates
  of, 11, 228–229; *HIV Plus* coverage of, 8–9;
  HIV/AIDS in Africa contrasted with, 70;
  Obama, B., successes with, 320–321
Hogan, Carlton, 14
Holmes, Charles, 262, 276, 301, 316
Home-Based AIDS Care (HBAC) Project,
  175, 179, 184–185, 281–282; about, 99,
  171–172, 193–194; client stories, 194,
  198–199, 411–412; Mugeni on future of, 194,
  197, 204–205, 410, 413
Homeland Security Council, 56, 247
Hoover, John, 273
House International Relations Committee,
  96, 115, 126, 130, 245
Housing Works, 8, 10, 39–40, 142, 155

HPTN. *See* HIV Prevention Trials Network
HR1298. *See* President's Emergency Plan for
  AIDS Relief and HR1298
Hughes, Langston, 170–171
human security, 409–410
Hyde, Henry, 50, 95–96, 97, 114–115, 120, 242

IDI. *See* Infectious Disease Institute
IMF. *See* International Monetary Fund
Infectious Disease Institute (IDI), 269–270,
  280–281, 332
Institute of Medicine (IOM), 231–233
Inter-American Development Bank, 89, 90
International AIDS Conference: 1996 in
  Vancouver, 9–10, 21; 1998 in Geneva, 21;
  2000 in Durban, South Africa, 31, 34–36,
  40–45, 47–48, 50–51, 67, 100; 2002 in
  Barcelona, 99–102; 2010 in Vienna, 287;
  2012 in Washington, DC, 321
International AIDS Vaccine Initiative, 44, 67
International Conference on AIDS and
  Sexually Transmitted Infections in Africa,
  Côte d'Ivoire, 267
International Conference on Financing for
  Development in Monterrey, Mexico, 90, 92
International Monetary Fund (IMF), 48–49,
  59–60, 73
investment framework, 311–314, 317–318, 319,
  322, 376
IOM. *See* Institute of Medicine
Iraq War, 5, 147, 161; Ugandans serving in,
  364; US global image impacted by, 254;
  US preparation for and start of, 1–2, 106,
  110–111, 129, 153

Jacobson, Jodi, 243–244, 246, 262
James, John, 13–14, 20
JCRC. *See* Joint Clinical Research Center
Jefferson, Thomas, 1
Johnson, Nkosi, 41–42
Joint Clinical Research Center (JCRC),
  44, 82, 104; ACE assistance to, 279–280,
  287; clinic, staff, and patients at, 68–69,
  179–183, 205–216, 277–279, 281, 294–299,
  363–364, 366, 373, 382; funding sources,
  178–182, 214, 279, 281; Mugyenyi
  leadership of, 44–46, 68, 173, 178–180,
  183, 281; orphan and vulnerable children
  care at, 179, 211–216, 294–299; outreach
  coordinator position and experience at,
  277–279, 295–298, 366, 382
Jubilee 2000, 49, 58

INDEX

INDEX

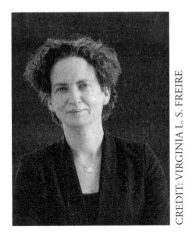

CREDIT: VIRGINIA L. S. FREIRE

EMILY BASS has spent more than twenty years writing about and working on HIV/AIDS in America and East and Southern Africa. Her writing has appeared in numerous books and publications including the *Washington Post, The Lancet, Esquire*, and *n+1*, and she has received notable mention in *Best American Essays*. She has served as an external expert for the World Health Organization and is the recipient of a Fulbright journalism fellowship and a Martin Duberman Visiting Research Fellowship from the New York Public Library. She lives in Brooklyn with her family.